Atlas of Endoscopic Perforator Vein Surgery

Springer

London
Berlin
Heidelberg
New York
Barcelona
Budapest
Hong Kong
Milan
Paris
Santa Clara
Singapore
Tokyo

ATLAS OF
Endoscopic Perforator Vein Surgery

Edited by

Peter Gloviczki, MD, FACS

Professor of Surgery
Mayo Medical School
Vice-Chair, Division of Vascular Surgery
Mayo Clinic and Foundation
Rochester Minnesota
USA

John J. Bergan, MD, FACS, FRCS (Hon.) Eng.

Professor of Surgery
Loma Linda University Medical Center
Loma Linda, California

Clinical Professor of Surgey
University of Southern California, San Diego
San Diego, California

Clinical Professor of Surgery
Uniformed Services University of the Health Sciences
Bethesda, Maryland

Professor of Surgery Emeritus
Northwestern University Medical School
Chicago, Illinois

Scripps Memorial Hospital
La Jolla, California
USA

With 236 Figures

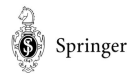 Springer

Peter Gloviczki, MD
Division of Vascular Surgery, Mayo Clinic & Mayo Foundation,
200 First Street SW, Rochester, Minnesota, MN 55905, USA

John J. Bergan, MD
North Coast Surgeons, 9850 Genesee Avenue, Suite 800,
La Jolla, California, CA 92037, USA

The illustrations reproduced on the cover are (from top to bottom): color Dopplers of a large incompetent perforator vein demonstrate reversed flow with distal augmentation; division of a medial calf perforator vein with endoscopic scissors; Olympus endoscope for division of perforator veins; ascending venogram of a patient with nonhealing venous ulcer demonstrates incompetence of medial and lateral calf perforator veins.

ISBN 3–540–76171–3 Springer-Verlag Berlin Heidelberg New York

British Library Cataloguing in Publication Data
Atlas of endoscopic perforator vein surgery
  1.Endoscopic surgery 2.Veins – Surgery
  I.Gloviczki, Peter II.Bergan, John J.
  617.1'14'059
  ISBN 3540761713

Library of Congress Cataloging-in-Publication Data
Atlas of endoscopic perforator vein surgery / Peter Gloviczki and John
  J. Bergan (eds). – 1st ed.
     p.   cm.
    Includes bibliographical references and index.
    ISBN 3–540–76171–3 (hardback   : alk. paper)
    1. Venous insufficiency—Endoscopic surgery—Atlases. 2. Venous
insufficiency—Pathophysiology—Atlases. I. Gloviczki, Peter.
II. Bergan, John J., 1927–
    [DNLM: 1. Varicose Ulcer—surgery—atlases. 2. Varicose Ulcer—
physiopathology—atlases. 3. Venous Insufficiency—surgery—
atlases.   4. Venous Insufficiency—physiopathology—atlases.
5. Surgery, Endoscopic—methods—atlases. WG 17 A88435 1997]
  RD560.A897 1997
  617.4'14059—dc21
  DNLM/DLC   97-16185
  for Library of Congress   CIP

Typeset by EXPO Holdings, Kuala Lumpur, Malaysia
Printed and bound at SNP Printing Pte Ltd., Singapore
28/3830-543210 Printed on acid-free paper

DEDICATION

*To Marta for her remarkable patience and understanding,
to Peter Jr. and Julia for their inspiration and love,
to Zoltan and Eva, who made it all possible*

and

*to EMB and RB in California
who provided good humored back up support.*

Acknowledgement

Both of us owe much to the colleagues mentioned in the preface. Their cooperation in managing to submit intelligent and timely contributions suggests that interest in the venous system is increasing and that patients in the future will profit from physician interactions and exchange of information.

Putting this volume together has depended greatly on the support of our technical staff, particularly Marcia Simonson in Rochester, Minnesota and Monica Vickers in California. The burden of putting together the manuscripts has fallen on their shoulders. However, bringing order to the entire project has been the responsibility of Susan Parmentier who displayed an unobtrusive dedication to the project while always reacting to the demands of the editors with unfailing good humor.

We are also grateful for the research efforts of Jae-Sung Cho, M.D. who compiled several of the biographies, and a very special thanks to Professor Jurgen Weber for his biography of Professor Dr. May.

From the Mayo Clinic, it is most appropriate to acknowledge here the assistance of an enthusiastic and innovative operating team, that included Terry Sweno, Cynthia Reed, Nancy Tscharner and Brenda Mathews, who helped to develop the endoscopic technique with gas insufflation. A special thanks goes to the members of the Division of Vascular Surgery at Mayo, Kenneth Cherry, John Hallett and Thomas Bower for their support of this project and for referring patients for the endoscopic procedure. Finally, in this era of managed care and decreasing reimbursement, we should be grateful to Department Chairs like Peter Pairolero who has the vision and conviction to support promising new procedures with appropriate allocation of funds.

We have particularly enjoyed working with the Springer-Verlag team based in England. Nick Mowat recognized the worth of the project and spurred us on with e-mail messages. Christopher Greenwell, Brian Dowling and Roger Dobbing provided invaluable organizational assistance and advice. Without their backing, our efforts to complete this Atlas would not have been successful.

Preface

Readers of this volume already know that chronic venous insufficiency is one of the most prevalent of medical conditions. Of the 100 000 patients with some form of venous disease who are admitted annually to non-federal United States hospitals, almost 20 000 are hospitalized for chronic venous insufficiency. The number of ambulatory patients is much higher. In the United States an estimated 14.6 million work-days are lost annually due to venous disease. Yet until the 1990's, information on the pathophysiology and treatment of chronic venous insufficiency could be classified as surgical dogma rather than surgical science. Knowledge of pathophysiology and treatment was handed down, for the most part, from non-randomized studies with concurrent or historic controls. Worse yet, most were case series with no controls.

After the mid 1980's and with the advent of Duplex scanning, accurate knowledge of pathophysiology of chronic venous insufficiency began to emerge. Effectiveness of different treatment modalities has also been evaluated more objectively in scientifically designed studies and a few small, randomized trials have been published.

Today in an era of evidence-based medicine, guidelines for management can only be derived from prospective, randomized, Level I multicenter studies. That type of information on the effectiveness of specific medical or surgical therapies of chronic venous disease is currently unavailable. The purpose of this atlas is not to claim the superiority of a minimally invasive operation over other procedures to treat venous ulcers and other complications of chronic venous insufficiency. Rather, the objective of the editors is to present the latest information available on evaluation and management of chronic venous disease at a time when there has been increased interest in the study of venous physiology and documentation of new forms of venous treatment.

Surgery has changed in recent years. Minimally invasive technology has emerged along with general availability of endoscopic instruments. Some of these instruments have been introduced for use in perforator vein surgery and resurrection of a modified, minimally invasive operation for interruption of incompetent perforators has occurred. Valuable data on early safety and efficacy by the NASEPS (North American Subfascial Endoscopic Perforator Surgery) Registry brought physicians with interest in venous disease together to share information on a promising surgical technique.

This volume is designed to assemble a summary of developing knowledge focusing on endoscopic vein surgery between the covers of an illustrated atlas so that interested practitioners can more effectively treat this widely prevalent condition.

The classic, open technique of perforator vein interruption was described five decades ago by Robert R. Linton. The first chapter on historic perspectives guides us through these five decades, depicting the continuously changing surgical techniques leading ultimately to the development of endoscopic vein surgery. At the beginning of a volume on surgical technique it is logical to insert a description of anatomy. In this instance, special dissections with the subfascial perforator vein operation in mind are described by Dr. Géza Mózes and his colleagues with illustrations by David Factor.

It is logical to describe the epidemiology of the condition being treated. Although recent epidemiologic studies emanating from North America have not been available, Peter Lawrence of the University of Utah Health and Sciences Center compiled data on the prevalence of this condition in Europe and added important, new information from the United States using the comprehensive database of the National Hospital Discharge Summary. Although modern knowledge regarding the pathophysiology of chronic venous insufficiency has been scattered in journal articles, it is combined in this book so as to place the operation of perforator vein interruption on a firm scientific basis.

Science, to paraphrase Lord Kelvin, begins with measuring and classification. Classification of venous insufficiency was accomplished by a group of prominent venous scientists headed by experts at the Straub Clinic and Hospital in Hawaii, and early experienced with this classification has been achieved. This subject is described in detail by Robert Kistner. User of this classification in describing the results of perforator vein surgery will go far towards organizing information rapidly for prompt dissemination.

Clinically, patients with severe chronic venous insufficiency must be evaluated before surgery, and here Robert Hobson and colleagues describe their methods of evaluation. The Mayo Clinic group describes in detail preoperative evaluation using Duplex scanning. They also discuss the role and indications for phlebography.

Ultimately, surgical intervention is the most effective therapy for chronic venous insufficiency. Such therapy includes correction of superficial venous reflux which is dealt with a full chapter in this volume.

New operations, as mentioned before, have their origin in older techniques. In this instance, Linton's operation and it's modification are detailed here by Ralph DePalma. There is a vast array of technical armamentaria which is useful in performing perforator vein surgery. Alan Lumsden describes some of the available and most commonly used instrumentation.

Techniques of endoscopic perforator vein interruption vary between use of laparoscopic instrumentation with gas insufflation to enlarge the subfascial space and the use of a single scope without gas insufflation. Chapters by Peter Gloviczki and John Bergan detail technique and results of both methods. A third technique is mentioned for potential future use.

Thomas Fogarty, always a surgical innovator, has created a device for enlarging the subfascial plane. He and his colleagues, describe its use. Credit goes to Thomas O'Donnell for introducing laparoscopic instrumentation in endoscopic vein surgery in the United States. The experience, including the use of ultrasonic coagulation, of O'Donnell and colleagues at New England Medical Centre is detailed in a well-illustrated chapter. Ultimately, new techniques must be compared to old standards. Comparison of the new endoscopic technique with the open Linton operation has been accomplished by Cees Wittens and colleagues in Amsterdam. Wittens describes the comparison in this book.

A sizable proportion of patients having subfascial perforator vein surgery will be in the highest risk category for deep venous thrombosis and pulmonary embolism. Therefore, it is appropriate to describe new methods of thromboembolism prophylaxis in this book. Dependable, level I evidence is available now on the effectiveness of unfractionated and low-molecular-weight heparin as discussed by Russell Hall and colleagues.

Compression therapy has been generally accepted as effective physical treatment of patients with chronic venous insufficiency. It is employed before and after surgical treatment as well. Colleagues at Oregon Health Sciences University have long advocated conservative care of patients with venous ulcers and their experience is detailed in an enlightened chapter in this volume. The medical management of ulcers at the Mayo Clinic and experience with the use of new techniques, such as intermittent pneumatic compression treatment is presented by Thom Rooke. This is supplemented by an illustrated presentation of plastic surgical procedures on local management of chronic leg ulcers by Craig Johnson.

A unique way of collecting information from a large experience was achieved by formation and implementation of the North American Registry of Subfascial Endoscopic Perforator Surgery. Its first report was given to the Society for Vascular Surgery in 1996, and experience gleaned from the registry is described in the last chapter in this volume.

Thus, the editors have succeeded in their objective of producing a book which contains virtually all the available information relevant to endoscopic perforator vein surgery. We sincerely hope that this atlas will be of help in treating patients with severe, disabling and painful chronic venous insufficiency.

Peter Gloviczki, M.D.   John J. Bergan, M.D.

Contents

Section 4 Supportive Therapy

Section 5 North American Subfascial Endoscopic Perforator Surgery (NASEPS) Registry

Profiles

Contributors

Robert C. Allen, MD
Endovascular Associate
Vascular Surgery Division
Stanford University Medical Center
Stanford, California, USA

Clifford T. Araki, MD
Clinical Assistant Professor, Department of
Health Technologies
University of Medicine and Dentistry of
New Jersey
Technical Director, Vascular Laboratory
University Hospital
Newark, New Jersey, USA

Jeffrey L. Ballard, MD
Associate Professor of Surgery
Loma Linda University Medical School
Loma Linda, California, USA

John J. Bergan, MD, FACS, FRCS (Hon) Eng.
Professor of Surgery
Loma Linda University Medical Center
Loma Linda, California
Clinical Professor of Surgery
University of Southern California, San Diego
San Diego, California
Clinical Professor of Surgery
Uniformed Services University of the Health
Sciences, Bethesda, Maryland
Professor of Surgery Emeritus
Northwestern University Medical School
Chicago, Illinois
Scripps Memorial Hospital
La Jolla, California, USA

Robert A. Cambria, MD
Assistant Professor of Surgery
Medical College of Wisconsin
Milwaukee, Wisconsin, USA

Linda G. Canton, RN, BSN
Division of Vascular Surgery
Mayo Clinic and Foundation
Rochester, Minnesota, USA

Steven W. Carmichael, PhD, DSc
Professor and Chair of Anatomy
Mayo Medical School
Department of Anatomy
Mayo Clinic and Foundation
Rochester, Minnesota, USA

Jae-Sung Cho, MD
Fellow, Division of Vascular Surgery
Mayo Clinic and Foundation
Rochester, Minnesota, USA

Ralph G. DePalma, MD, FACS
Professor of Surgery, Associate Dean
Vice Chair, Department of Surgery
University of Nevada School of Medicine
Reno, Nevada, USA

Bo Eklof, MD, PhD
Clinical Professor of Surgery
University of Hawaii
Vascular Surgeon
Straub Clinic and Hospital
Honalulu, Hawaii, USA

Cindy Felty, MSN, RN, C-ANP
Adult Nurse Practitioner, Director, Vascular
Ulcer/Wound Healing Center
Mayo Clinic and Foundation
Rochester, Minnesota, USA

Thomas J. Fogarty, MD, FACS
Professor of Surgery
Vascular Surgery Division
Stanford University Medical Center
Stanford, California

Christine E. Gazak, MA
Research Associate, Health Research Center
University of Utah Health Sciences Center
Salt Lake City, Utah, USA

Peter Gloviczki, MD, FACS
Professor of Surgery
Mayo Medical School
Vice-Chair, Division of Vascular Surgery
Mayo Clinic and Foundation
Rochester, Minnesota, USA

Robert W. Hobson II, MD
Professor of Surgery & Physiology
Chief, Section of Vascular Surgery
University of Medicine & Dentistry of New Jersey/New
Jersey Medical School
Newark, New Jersey, USA

Russell D. Hull, MD
Professor, Department of Medicine
University of Calgary
Foothills Hospital
Calgary, Alberta, Canada

Mark D. Iafrati, MD
Instructor in Surgery
Tufts University School of Medicine
Vascular Surgery Fellow
New England Medical Center
Boston, Massachusetts, USA

Craig H. Johnson, MD
Assistant Professor
Mayo Medical School
Consultant
Division of Plastic Surgery, Department of Surgery
Division of Hand Surgery, Department of Orthopedic
Surgery
Mayo Clinic and Foundation
Rochester, Minnesota, USA

Robert L. Kistner, MD
Clinical Professor of Surgery
University of Hawaii
Department of Surgery
Straub Clinic and Hospital
Honolulu, Hawaii, USA

Anna Kádár, MD
Professor of Pathology, Associate Dean
Semmelweis University of Medicine
2nd Central Electron Microscope Lab
2nd Department of Pathology
Budapest, Hungry

Mark J. Kulbaski, MD
Fellow, Division of Vascular Surgery
Emory University School of Medicine
Atlanta, Georgia, USA

Peter F. Lawrence, MD
Professor of Surgery
Chief of Vascular Surgery
University of Utah Health Sciences Center
Salt Lake City, Utah, USA

Bradley D. Lewis, MD
Assistant Professor of Radiology
Mayo Medical School
Senior Associate Consultant
Diagnostic Radiology
Mayo Clinic and Foundation
Rochester, Minnesota, USA

John R. Lindsey, RDMS, RVT
Instructor in Radiology
Mayo Medical School
Supervisor, Vascular Ultrasound
Mayo Clinic and Foundation
Rochester, Minnesota, USA

Alan B. Lumsden, MD, CHB
Associate Professor of Surgery
Emory University of School of Medicine
Associate Head General Vascular Surgery
Emory University Hospital
Atlanta, Georgia, USA

Michael A. McKusick, MD
Assistant Professor in Radiology
Mayo Medical School
Consultant in Diagnostic Radiology
Mayo Clinic and Foundation
Rochester, Minnesota, USA

Sunil S. Menawat, MD
Fellow, Mayo Medical School
Mayo Clinic and Foundation
Rochester, Minnesota, USA

Gregory L. Moneta, MD
Associate Professor, Division of Vascular Surgery
Oregon Health Sciences University
Portland, Oregon, USA

Géza Mózes, MD
Research Fellow,
Division of Vascular Surgery
Mayo Clinic and Foundation
Rochester, Minnesota, USA

Resident
2nd Department of Pathology
Semmelweis University of Medicine
Budapest, Hungary

Mark R. Nehler, MD
Fellow, Division of Vascular Surgery
Oregon Health Sciences University
Portland, Oregon, USA

Alexander D. Nicoloff, MD
Resident, Division of Vascular Surgery
Oregon Health Sciences University
Portland, Oregon, USA

Thomas F. O'Donnell Jr MD
Andrews Professor of Surgery and Chairman,
Department of Surgery
Tufts University School of Medicine
Surgeon-in-chief
New England Medical Center
Boston, Massachusetts, USA

Graham F. Pineo, MD
Professor, Departments of Medicine and Oncology
University of Calgary
Calgary General Hospital
Calgary, Alberta, Canada

John J. Porter, MD
Professor of Surgery and Head of Division of Vascular
Surgery
Oregon Health Sciences University
Portland, Oregon, USA

Robert Y. Rhee, MD
Assistant Professor of Surgery
Division of Vascular Surgery
Presbyterian University Hospital
Pittsburgh, Pennsylvania, USA

Thom W. Rooke, MD
Associate Professor of Surgery
Mayo Medical School
Director, Gonda Vascular Center
Mayo Clinic and Foundation
Rochester, Minnesota, USA

Atsushi Seyama, MD
Postdoctoral Research Fellow, Section of Vascular
Surgery
University of Medicine & Dentisty of New Jersey
New Jersey Medical School
1st Department of Surgery, Yamaguchi University
School of Medicine
Yamaguchi, Japan

Stephen Sparks, MD
Assistant Clinical Professor
University of California, San Diego
San Diego, California, USA

Roy L. Tawes, MD, FACS
Chief of Surgery
Mills/Peninsula Hospital
San Mateo/Burlingame, California, USA

Jurgen Weber, MD
Professor of Radiology
Institute for Diagnostic and Interventional Radiology
DRK and Froimauer Hospital Rissen
Hamburg, Germany

L. Albert Wetter, MD, FACS
Faculty Proctor
University of California, San Francisco
San Francisco, California
Mills/Peninsula Hospital
San Mateo/ Burlingame, California, USA

Cees H. A. Wittens, MD, PhD
Vascular Surgeon
Sint Fransiscus Gasthuis
Rotterdam, The Netherlands

Fundamental Considerations

Profile

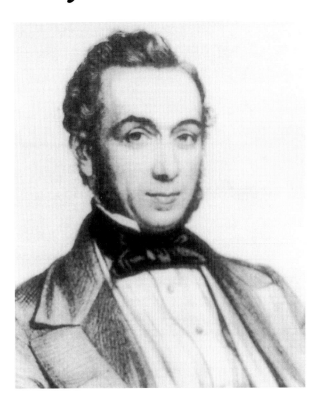

John Gay
1812–1885

It was John Gay, a London physician, who made the first scientific investigations of venous insufficiency. He noted that varicosities could exist without ulceration, a fact which is amply confirmed today. He has been much quoted as saying, "ulceration is not a direct consequence of varicosity but of other conditions of the venous system." His observations preceded by 150 years the theories of genesis of leg ulcer which explain those differences today.

His Lettsomian lectures were delivered in 1867 and summarized his thinking at the time. His drawings, published in his monograph *Varicose disease of the lower extremities* (Lettsomian Lecture, London, Churchill 1866) were hand drawn by him from autopsy dissections. These not only show the posterior arch vein but also the perforating veins and, in the case of a 56-year-old woman who died of erysipelas of the leg, the detailed drawing shows perforating veins with enclosed thrombus. In another dissection, Gay shows a superficial vein connecting to the posterior tibial vein in immediate proximity to a leg ulcer. He wrote, "there is one rule which is applicable to all leg ulcers – namely, that rest is an essential part of their treatment – with the foot elevated above the pelvis." He advised intervention in the case of venous ulceration saying "the radical cure of these ulcers contemplates their permanent cicaturization. The principle of treatment involves the destruction of any veins which pass from the margin of the diseased skin tissue and especially from the ulcer itself." He added, "the blood will flow freely from the veins which will thus be divided but this can be very readily controlled by elevating the leg, plugging, and a temporary application of a firm bandage."

In an observation that preceded experience with the open Linton procedure, Gay said, "whatever the condition of the diseased skin tissue, … a wound made (in it) … it not infrequently happens that the ulcer heals first in consequence of some … sloughing on the surface of the artificial wounds."

In addition to his work on perforating veins of the calf and ankle, Gay also described thrombus formation and post-thrombotic recanalization and was the first to describe compression of the left common iliac vein beneath the right common iliac artery. Further, he called attention to the subfascial course of the proximal lesser saphenous vein.

John J. Bergan and Jeffrey L. Ballard

After man had an ulcer … for a long time, the veins lying above it which were varicose, were excised. Immediately, the ulcer healed. Yet the incision … did not get well.

Claudius Galen, AD 130 to 200

Evolution of medical thought through the ages can be traced through the descriptions of treatment of leg ulcers. Hippocrates (460 to 377 BC), in a much quoted phrase, wrote "in the case of an ulcer, it is not expedient to stand." He was a keen observer; for example, he noted that varicose veins did not occur before puberty and that they occurred in riders of horses whose feet were always hanging down. Galen, who knew the writings of Hippocrates, tore out varicose veins with a blunt hook and applied wine to leg ulcers. He was opposed to frequent dressing changes and therefore diminished epidermal damage. Unfortunately, Galen followed in the footsteps of Hippocrates with his strong interest in diet. When looked at through the magnifying glass of time, one sees that their diets actually produced vitamin deficiencies. They found fault with most vegetables, and fruits were considered even worse. Galen believed seriously in starving, purging, and bleeding the patient. He once wrote that he could not understand how anyone could be so thickheaded as not to understand that leg ulcers called for bleeding the patient.[1]

Jean Fernal (1506–1588) observed that a varix might come from a blow or from a contusion. This has been amply confirmed in modern times. He also preceded today's knowledge of coach-class thrombosis as he wrote that the varix might come from hard work and much travelling. On the other hand, in 1555, Marianus Sanctus alternated truth with fiction, saying that the varices might come from childbearing and "standing too much before kings." The theory of humors prevailed at that time, and Thomas Vicary (1495–1561) noted that "their legges

… when they are offended or wounded, are very perilous, because unto them runneth a great quantity of humors." The humoral theory held it would be risky to cure leg ulcer even though ancient physicians worked strenuously to heal the ulcer. Humors were thought to be outside of the main venous channels and deleterious humors were thought to be safe unless pressed back by bandaging. If this were done, it might lead to "madness or other disasters." Even as late as 1768, Heister in Germany considered the leg ulcer to be a drain for humors which, if not expelled, would cause serious illness.[2] Today, as an explanation for that, the final stages of healing of venous ulcer may be accompanied by invasive infection, erythema, increased warmth, and tenderness which command prescription of antibiotics.

Among those who felt that ulcer healing was deleterious to the general health of the patient was Ambrose Paré (Fig. 1.1). This is curious considering that he gained great fame by healing the leg ulcer of his captor, Lord Vandeville. His advice, given 400 years ago, holds true today, "(in bandaging) roule the leg beginning at the foot and finishing at the knee, not forgetting a little bolster upon the varicose veins."[3]

Wiseman (1676) apparently understood that valvular incompetence was caused by dilation of a vein and may have been the first to consider that leg ulcers might be the direct result of a circulatory defect. He used the term "varicose ulcer." Acting on his observations, he introduced the method of compressing the leg by a laced-up stocking usually made of soft leather such as dog skin. His prescient observation that nonelastic compression was effective in leg ulcer healing was adopted widely and was used on the European

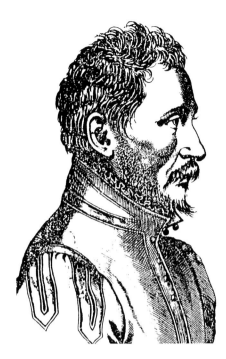

Fig. 1.1. Ambrose Paré, seen here at age 45, was the leading surgeon of the Renaissance. His expression, "I dressed the wound, God healed it" applies to the management of venous ulcers today.

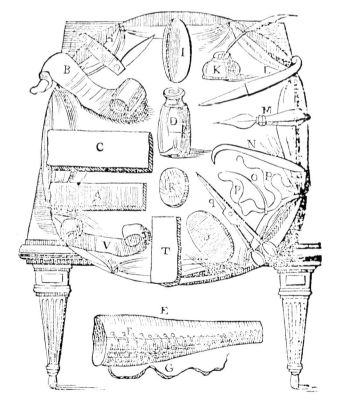

Fig. 1.2. This illustration shows a collection of instruments used in treating venous ulceration in the mid-seventeenth century. Notice the lace-up stocking of soft leather which gave effective, non-stretch compression therapy to be adjusted by the lacings.

continent for more than 100 years. Petit (1790) preferred Wiseman's technique because the degree of compression could be varied by the lacing, thus anticipating today's use of Velcro closures on non-elastic compression for treatment of leg ulcer (Fig. 1.2).

In retrospect, it can be seen that a considerable step forward was achieved by John Gay (1812–1885).[4] He published an outstanding investigation on the etiology of leg ulcers in 1868. This work is credited as being the first painstaking scientific investigation of leg ulcers in England. Gay pointed out that severe, long-standing varicosities might exist without producing ulceration and, in fact, this was the rule rather than the exception. Today we understand that additional conditions, such as leukocyte trapping and activation, must come into play before the skin will become heavily pigmented and induration develop. Gay can be quoted as saying, "ulceration is not a direct consequence of varicosity, but of other conditions of the venous system with which varicosity is not infrequently a complication, but without which neither one of the allied skin afflictions (induration and hyperpigmentation) is met with." Gay went further and described the deep veins in the leg after venous thrombosis, providing an accurate anatomical description of ankle perforating veins (Fig. 1.3). He introduced the term "venous ulcer."

In the early years of the seventeenth century, William Harvey travelled to the University of Padua where Fabricius of Aquapendente (1533–1620) was teaching surgical anatomy in an anatomical amphitheatre which he built at his own expense. Fabricius had made many contributions to comparative and human anatomy as well as to embryology, physiology, and medicine and, therefore, attracted students such as Harvey to Padua. It is acknowledged that despite the many contributions of Fabricius, the most important was his study of the venous valves, and there is no doubt that William Harvey's discovery and explanation of the circulation grew directly out of the observations of Fabricius (Fig. 1.4A). Therefore, there is no doubt that the study by Fabricius and Harvey of the veins and their valves was the very beginning of all modern cardiovascular medicine and surgery. Harvey correctly reasoned that because valves opened toward the heart and functioned to prevent flow away from the heart, the arteries must carry blood in one direction, and that is away from the heart (Fig. 1.4B).

Dodd and Cockett[5] hold that there were few advances from the time of Gay until the present

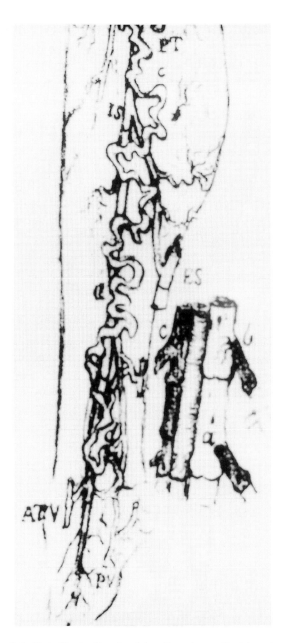

Fig. 1.3. This illustration by John Gay shows that he clearly understood the relationship of perforating veins to varicose veins and further shows the relationship of venous thrombosis to leg ulcer. The thrombi can be seen in perforating veins emanating from the posterior tibial vein. This dissection was made at autopsy on a 56-year-old woman who died of erysipelas of the affected left leg.

century when John Homans presented his study of the pathology of thrombosis of the deep veins of the leg in 1917.[6] Homans' influence over the years was profound. His observations on re-canalization with destruction of valves were strikingly similar to those of Gay. With emphasis on venous thrombosis as a precursor to venous leg ulcer, Dodd and Cockett present

the figures of 30% to 87% of patients giving a definite history of previous thrombosis as they entered into treatment for venous leg ulcer.[5] They acknowledged that the criteria as to what constitutes a history of deep venous thrombosis might vary widely and that various clinics were different one from another.

Today, we might look at the reverse and conclude that in approximately 40% to 60% of patients, deep venous thrombosis has not been the cause of the chronic venous insufficiency. This has been confirmed by many reports of duplex scanning in limbs with severe chronic venous insufficiency.

The text by Dodd and Cockett, first published in the mid-1950s, had a profound influence on the training of English surgeons. In their illustration of ankle veins, they pointed out that "the effect of incompetence or destruction of the valves in one or more of the direct ankle perforating veins will be to transmit the high exercise venous pressure within the lower third of the calf during contraction of the soleus, directly to the mesh of fine subcutaneous venules in the gaiter area. This will lead to their gradual dilation, including the small subcuticular venules." They followed saying, "this is the essential and basic pathology of venous ulcers and induration of the ankle."

Dodd and Cockett were acquainted with the physiologic studies performed by Wells, Youmans and Miller.[7] These workers measured intramuscular pressure by placing a needle in the muscles of the leg. They found that in the lower third of the soleus muscle, the rise of pressure on contraction was 90 mmHg. Dodd and Cockett added that if there is an incompetent ankle perforating vein and incompetence of the greater saphenous vein, the addition of these two sources of increased venous pressure would take place in the medial aspect of the ankle. They carried their observations further to say that the same forces would be acting on the lateral aspect of the ankle if there were incompetence of the lateral ankle perforating veins in association with short saphenous venous incompetence.

During the early 1950s at St Thomas's Hospital,[8] ankle perforator exploration was done on 135 limbs with indurative lesions and ankle ulcers. This group of cases did not have incompetent greater saphenous system superficial veins. Incompetent ankle perforating veins were found and proven to be incompetent by the Turner Warwick test. Turner Warwick had described this at operation. When a normal perforating vein was cut across during surgery, the end which

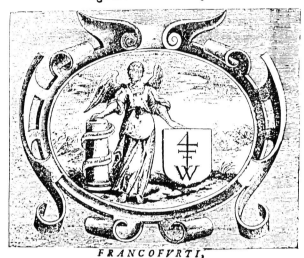

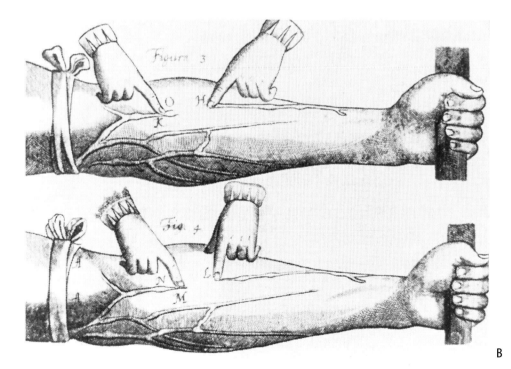

disappeared through the hole in the deep fascia would not bleed because its valve, if competent, was held shut by the venous pressure within the calf. If a probe was gently inserted in the lumen of that perforator vein and the valve held aside, bleeding would immediately occur. If an incompetent perforating vein was cut across, the result was quite different. Profuse steady bleeding occurred outwards from the deep vein. If the calf was suddenly squeezed, a jet of blood was ejected with surprising force. English surgeons learned that this was a practical demonstration of what happens in normal circumstances when the calf pump is put into action.

The findings of the modern St Thomas's study were that either the middle or upper internal ankle perforating vein was most likely to be incompetent but it was unusual for both to be found to be incompetent and in the same leg. It was found that these varied inversely in size. When the upper vein was large, the middle vein was small. Furthermore, the lower ankle perforating vein located just below and posterior to the medial malleolus was hardly ever found to be incompetent.

Fig. 1.4.A. This illustration is the title page from William Harvey's 1628 masterpiece which describes his theory of circulation. His thinking derived from the teachings of Fabricius whose own work beautifully illustrated the structure and function of venous valves. **B.** Harvey's illustration of the function of venous valves was elegant in its simplicity and utterly convincing. Thus, study of the function of the venous system cast light on the physiology of the arterial system as well.

In Boston, Linton advocated perforator vein interruption but also focused on deep venous ligation in an attempt to decrease lower leg venous hypertension. Linton gave credit to Buxton and Coller of Michigan[9] as the first to report interruption of the femoral vein as a method of treating post-thrombotic ulcerations. Further, Linton gave credit to Homans who had insisted for a number of years that the canalized post-thrombotic femoral vein was a useless structure and should be interrupted.

Although deep venous interruption has been abandoned today, some lessons were actually learned from that experience. Linton and Hardy advocated interruption of the superficial femoral vein with the complete removal of the long saphenous vein and the short saphenous vein, and they said that "from the experience gained by the study of these cases … it is believed that the varicose saphenous veins rarely, if ever, constitute collateral channels necessary for the return of blood from the extremity."[10] Linton also emphasized the chronic destruction of the lymphatic system of the lower extremity in cases of advanced chronic venous insufficiency. He found that chronic lymphedema was present in 100% of the extremities in which he performed operations. Confessing that it was one of the least well understood pathological conditions, he rationalized that it resulted from lymphatic obstruction due to scarring and fibrosis of the perivascular tissues. The lymphatic destruction was secondary to the inflammatory process affecting the superficial and deep veins. Further, he said, "it would appear that it (lymphedema) alone is not the sole cause because chronic ulcerations are rarely seen in the presence of elephantiasis of the lower extremity without venous pathology."[10]

Linton's operation was carried out only after healing of the ulceration or excision and grafting.[11] The objectives of his operation as stated by him were: (1) to remove all of the enlarged superficial veins, especially in the lower leg, namely the long and short saphenous veins and their tributaries; (2) to sever the communications between the deep and superficial systems of veins by dividing and ligating the communicating veins (perforating veins), especially those on the inner and posterior sides of the lower leg; (3) to interrupt the canalized and valveless venous system in the thigh in order to prevent reflux of blood through it from the larger proximal venous reservoirs; and (4) to attempt restoration of the lymphatic drainage from the superficial tissues in the skin into those of the deeper muscular structures by resecting the deep fascia of the lower leg.

The incision for performing the superficial to deep disconnection was made from just distal to the level of the tibial tubercle. It extended distally 2 cm posterior to the inner edge of the tibia. It proceeded halfway between the medial malleolus and the inner tuberosity of the os calcis where it curved forward to extend just beyond the medial malleolus. This incision was carried through the deep fascia along its entire length. The posterior tibial perforating veins were located directly under the incision where, in Linton's words, "one or several large, incompetent communicating veins will be found." Further, he emphasized that some very large veins may be encountered coming out along the posterior edge of the tibia (paratibial perforators) in the upper and middle thirds of the leg. These latter veins might be tightly bound to the periosteum of the tibia.

Linton's work was presented to the American Surgical Association meeting in Los Angeles in 1953, and among the discussants was Dr Harris B. Shumaker, Jr of Indianapolis. He rose to question the advisability of ligation of the superficial femoral vein. Dr Linton welcomed that question and admitted that "I don't know just what interrupting the deep venous circulation does. I am sure that the interruption in itself is not sufficient."

Frank Cockett remarks of this time in the history of venous surgery as follows, "the high point of my (venous) career was undoubtedly my visit to Bob Linton in 1953." At that time, Cockett had completed a series of dissections on fresh cadaver legs, including the injection of arteries and veins. He had identified the importance of ankle perforating veins in 1951 and had developed a new operation to correct the perforator outflow at that time. The dissections and study of the injected limbs had identified the ankle perforating veins and when Cockett arrived in Boston, he found that Linton had arrived at similar conclusions to his own but his operation in Boston was based on brilliant clinical observation and deduction only. The scientific dissections of Cockett, therefore, supported the deductions of Linton and gave strong scientific background to the Linton perforator interruption (Linton flap) operation.

In 1955, D. A. Felder proposed a modification of Linton's medial incision, placing his own in the posterior aspect of the calf (Fig. 1.5). This has been referred to as the stocking-seam incision.[12] Although

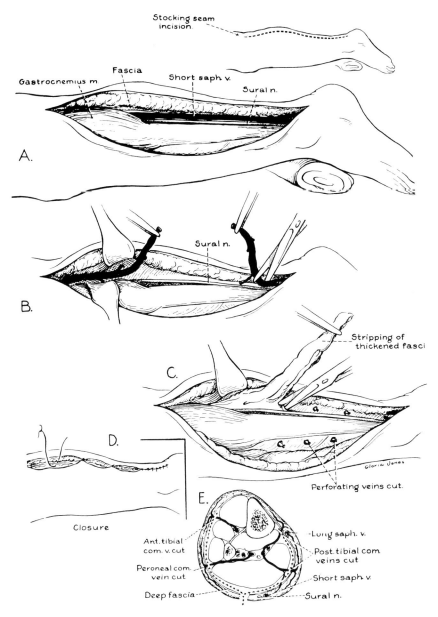

Fig. 1.5. These drawings illustrate the old operation of subfascial interruption of perforating veins through a stocking seam incision. In A the longitudinal incision made from the popliteal fossa to the ankle level was made in the midline and deepened through the deep fascia. Thus, the short saphenous vein and sural nerve were exposed. The short saphenous vein was excised completely as shown in B and subfascially, the medial, lateral, and anterior groups of perforators were identified, ligated, and cut. As shown in C if the fascia was markedly thickened, a wide strip was excised at the same time as dictated by Linton, and subcutaneous and cutaneous stitches closed the stocking seam incision (D) which was then placed under a compression dressing. The cross-section illustration seen in E shows the perforating and superficial veins and their relationships to the anterior, peroneal and posterior tibial veins.

this incision was designed to decrease wound complications, in fact it did not. In 1960, Felder reported 60 operations in 52 patients. There were four instances of postoperative infection. In two of these, there was complete separation of the wound edges. Twelve of the extremities in addition developed sloughs of the wound edge in the lower third of the operative site,

usually in the medial skin flap. Felder and Bernstein confessed that "the high incidence of sloughs of the wound edges has been disconcerting."[13]

By 1967, a group from Argentina reported a large experience with the subfascial perforating vein operation.[14] In 207 operations to interrupt perforating veins, 73 were performed by the technique proposed by Linton with skin necrosis occurring in 34 cases. Fifty-seven were done by the modification described by Felder, and in 24 of these there was skin necrosis, either at the site where trophic changes persisted or elsewhere.

DePalma, operating in Cleveland, recognized the wound healing complications of the Linton procedure and its modifications. Therefore, in 1966, he began a modified approach to the problem. Rather than creation of longitudinal flaps for ligation of communicating veins, a series of parallel bipedicle skin flaps were created in natural skin lines of the extremity. Perforating veins from the crest of the tibia to the Achilles tendon were ligated. Concomitant skin grafting was done if necessary, and stripping of the incompetent long and short saphenous veins was accomplished at the same operation.[15] He reported this technique at the Annual Meeting of the Society for Vascular Surgery in Chicago in 1974. Thirty-eight operations were performed on 31 patients. No major wound infection occurred, necrosis of skin flaps was absent, and the skin line incisions favored primary healing of the flaps.

In the past, perforator vein interruption has seldom been carried out without concomitant correction of superficial reflux. Usually this is done by excision of refluxing saphenous veins and superficial varicosities. Until recently, such an approach was entirely empiric. However, duplex scanning has uncovered the rationale for such superficial reflux correction. Superficial reflux may be the only abnormality uncovered by diagnostic testing. This is almost always true in simple varicose veins and telangiectasias. It is also a surprising fact that in advanced chronic venous stasis, superficial reflux may be the only abnormality present. Obviously, correction of such pathophysiology will go a long way towards permanent relief of chronic venous dysfunction and its cutaneous effects. Using duplex technology, Menzoian[16] found that in 95 extremities with recurrent venous ulceration, 16.8% had only superficial incompetence and another 19% showed superficial incompetence combined with perforator incompetence. Similarly, the Middlesex group, in a study of 118 limbs, found that "in just over half of the patients with venous ulceration, the disease was confined to the superficial venous system."[17]

Historically, most of the treatment of severe chronic venous insufficiency was focused on ablation of superficial reflux and elimination of perfora-

tor incompetence. An opposite approach has been explored by some surgeons. This is the direct surgical reconstruction of refluxing venous segments.[18–21] Long-term results of valveplasty are available. Personal and recorded experience suggests that excellent results defined as return to full activity without elastic support is to be expected in about one-third of patients. An additional 25% of patients will be able to return to full activity but will have to continue to wear external elastic support.

Kistner was the first to describe direct valveplasty in 1975, and by 1993 was able to report that the results were maintained long-term in 70% of patients. He summarized available reports from the literature in which follow-up was longer than 2 years. He noted that good results were obtained in from 70% to 90% of limbs subjected to valveplasty.[22] As in those cases the saphenous veins were either ligated or removed by nearly all surgeons performing the valveplasty, the good results cannot be attributed to the valve repair alone. Deep venous incompetence may correct itself as the superficial reflux is treated.[23] The role of perforator veins in reports of valve repair is still not clear as there has been much variability in management of perforator veins when valveplasty was being done. Most surgeons interrupt the perforating veins selectively. Some reserve valveplasty for failures of perforator interruption.

Direct venous reconstructive surgery should be performed only in patients with intractable, severe and incapacitating venous stasis. Superficial venous incompetence and perforator incompetence should be searched for and corrected prior to embarking on the course which leads to deep venous reconstruction.

Kistner was able to evaluate the results of other types of reflux correction including valve transplantation and valve transposition. He summarized the results as good in 75% in valve transplantations. However, the number of cases ranged only from 12 to 48 interventions. The results of valve transposition have not been as good. Only a small number have been done with good results being obtained in 17% to 78% of cases, but mostly in the 50% range. Kistner thoughtfully evaluated the present status of valve repair in 1993 saying, "it appears that patients who have repair of all the venous reflux abnormalities in the extremity have an improved long-term result when compared with those who only have repair of some of the reflux deficits. It appears preferable to treat the saphenous, perforator, and the deep veins in patients in whom all the systems are significantly abnormal at the time of the initial venous evaluation."

Therefore, at this time the historical precedents for perforator vein interruption have been established. Experience with perforator vein interruption is much larger than the published reports would indicate but even these reveal general success of the operation (Table 1.1). The effect of the operation on ulcer healing cannot be established either from the publications or from personal experience in the era in which complete ulcer healing prior to surgical intervention was advocated. However, prevention of ulcer recurrence is established by the reports except in those limbs in which severe deep venous reflux remains uncorrected.[42] It is in these limbs in which the surgical challenge remains to be answered.

Table 1.1.   The results of perforator vein interruption, arranged according to recurrences

Author	Number of limbs	% recurrence	Follow-up (yr)
Wilkinson[24]	134	2	<9
Field[25]	52	2	6
Felder[26]	28	3.6	1–2
Blumenberg[27]	25	4	0–6
Healey[28]	18	5.6	0–5
DePalma[29]	68	6	12
Lim[30]	29	10	>6
Silver[31]	31	10	1–15
Cikrit[32]	32	12	1–15
Szostek[33]	105	14	10
Hansson[34]	59	19	>5
Cranley[35]	175	30	10
Negus[36]	109	31 (15% minor)	3–4
Hyde[37]	83	33	1–19
Bowen[38]	71	34	15
Linton[39]	49	47	5
Johnson[40]	47	51	>5
Burnand[41]	41	55	2–6

References

1. Majno G (1975) The healing hand. Harvard University Press, Cambridge, p 419
2. Bergan JJ (1991) Historical highlights in treating venous insufficiency. In: Venous disorders. Bergan JJ, Yao JST (eds) WB Saunders Co, Philadelphia, pp 6–7
3. Malgaigne JF (1840) Oeuvres completes dé Ambroise Paré, *Paris*. J-B Baillière, p 269
4. Gay J (1868) Varicose disease of the lower extremities and its allied disorders: Skin discoloration, induration, and ulcer. London, Churchill
5. Dodd H, Cockett FB (1956) The pathology and surgery of the veins of the lower limb. E&S Livingstone, Ltd, Edinburgh and London, p 344
6. Homans J (1917) The etiology and treatment of varicose ulcers of the leg. Surg Gynecol Obstet 24:300
7. Wells, Youmans and Miller (1938) J Clin Invest 17:489
8. Dodd H, Cockett FB (1956) The pathology and surgery of the veins of the lower limb. E&S Livingstone, Ltd, Edinburgh and London, p 357
9. Buxton RW, Coller FA (1945) Surgical treatment of long-standing deep phlebitis of the leg. Surgery 18:663–672
10. Linton RR, Hardy IB (1948) Postthrombotic syndrome of the lower extremity: Treatment by interruption of the superficial femoral vein and ligation and stripping of the long and short saphenous veins. Surgery 24:452–468
11. Linton RR (1953) The postthrombotic ulceration of the lower extremity: Its etiology and surgical treatment. Ann Surg 138:415–432
12. Felder DA, Murphy TA (1955) The evaluation of a method of phlebography of the lower extremities. Surgery 37:198–205
13. Felder DA, Bernstein EF (1960) A reevaluation of the posterior subfascial approach for the ligation of the communicating veins in the leg. Surgery 47:349–352
14. Quiros RS, Kitainik E, Swiatlo MR, Breyter E (1967) Cutaneous complications of the subaponeurotic surgery of the communicating venous system. J Cardiovasc Surg 8:206–208
15. DePalma RG (1974) Surgical therapy for venous stasis. Surgery 76:910–916
16. Hanrahan LM, Araki CT, Rodriguez AA, et al. (1991) Distribution of valvular incompetence in patients with venous stasis ulceration. J Vasc Surg 13:805–812
17. Shami SK, Sarin S, Cheatle TR, et al. (1993) Venous ulcers and the superficial venous system. J Vasc Surg 17:487–490.
18. Hallberg D (1972) A method for repairing incompetent valves in deep veins. Acta Chir Scand 138:143–145
19. Ferris EB, Kistner RL (1982) Femoral vein reconstruction in the management of chronic venous insufficiency. Arch Surg 117:1571–1577
20. Johnson D, Queral LA, Flinn WR, Yao JST, Bergan JJ (1981) Late objective assessment of venous valve surgery. Arch Surg 116:1461–1466
21. Taheri SA, Lazar L, Elias SM, Marchand P (1982) Vein valve transplant. Surgery 91:28–33
22. Kistner RL (1993) Late results of venous valve repair. In: Yao JST, Pearce W (eds) Long-term results in vascular surgery. Appleton-Lange, Norwalk, chapter 39
23. Walsh JC, Bergan JJ, Beeman S, Comer TP (1994) Femoral venous reflux is abolished by superficial venous ablation. Ann Vasc Surg 8:566–570
24. Wilkinson GE, Maclaren IF (1986) Long-term review of procedures for venous perforator insufficiency. Surg Gynecol Obstet 163:117–120
25. Field P, Van Boxel P (1971) The role of the Linton flap procedure in the management of stasis dermatitis and ulceration in the lower limb. Surgery 70:920–926
26. Felder DA, Murphy TO, Ring DM (1995) A posterior subfascial approach to the communicating veins of the leg. Surg Gynecol Obstet 100:730–734
27. Blumenberg RM, Gelfand ML (1978) The posterior stocking seam approach to radical subfascial clipping of perforating veins. Am J Surg 136:202–205
28. Healey PJ, Healey EH, Wong R, et al. (1979) Surgical management of the chronic venous ulcer. The Rob procedure. Am J Surg 137:556–559

29. DePalma RG (1979) Surgical therapy of venous stasis: Results of a modified Linton operation. Am J Surg 137:810–813

30. Lim RC, Blaisdell FW, Zubrin J, et al. (1970) Subfascial ligation of perforating veins in recurrent stasis ulceration. Am J Surg 119:246–249

31. Silver D, Gleysteen JJ, Rhodes GR, et al. (1971) Surgical treatment of the refractory postphlebitic ulcer. Arch Surg 103:554–560

32. Cikrit D, Nichols K, Silver D (1988) Surgical management of refractory venous stasis ulceration. J Vasc Surg 7:474–478

33. Szostek M, Skorski M, Zajac S, et al. (1988) Recurrences after surgical treatment of patients with postthrombotic syndrome of the lower extremities. Eur J Vasc Surg 2:191–192

34. Hansson LO (1964) Venous ulcers of the lower limb: A followup study five years after surgical treatment. Acta Chir Scand 128:269–277

35. Cranley JJ (1975) Chronic venous insufficiency in vascular surgery. In: Peripheral venous diseases. New York, Harper & Row Publishers, Inc., vol 2, p 293

36. Negus D, Friedgood A (1980) The effective management of venous ulceration. Br J Surg 70:623–627

37. Hyde GL, Litton TC, Hull DA (1981) Long-term results of subfascial vein ligation for venous stasis disease. Surg Gynecol Obstet 153:683–686

38. Bowen FH (1975) Subfascial ligation (Linton operation) of the perforating leg veins to treat postthrombophlebitic syndrome. Am Surg 41:148–151

39. Linton RR (1938) The communicating veins of the lower leg and the operative technique for their ligation. Ann Surg 107:582–593

40. Johnson WC, O'Hara ET, Corey C, Widrich WC, Nabseth DC (1985) Venous stasis ulceration. Arch 120:797–800

41. Burnand K, O'Donnell T, Thomas ML, et al. (1976) Relation between postphlebitic changes in the deep veins and results of surgical treatment of venous ulcers. Lancet 1:936–938

42. Bradbury AW, Ruckley CV (1993) Foot volumetry can predict recurrent ulceration after subfascial ligation of perforators and saphenous ligation. J Vasc Surg 18:789–795

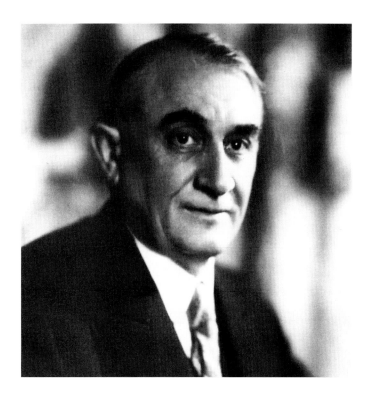

Charles Horace Mayo
1865–1939

Known as Dr Charlie, the younger of the two Mayo brothers Dr Charles H. Mayo was a lovable man. Gifted with the common touch in human contacts he comforted and relieved the fears and disturbed emotions of those around him by employing his knowledge of human psychology and his charming personality. He embodied every noble and admirable quality in a physician: patience, great modesty, ingenuity and humor.

Born in Rochester, Minnesota, to a physician father, William Worrall Mayo, Dr Charlie was reared in medicine. Along with his older brother, William James, he assisted his father's medical and surgical practice from boyhood. He received his medical degree at the Chicago Medical College, later the Northwestern University Medical School, in 1888 and returned to Rochester to join his father and, with his brother, gradually took over the father's practice.

Master at the craft of surgery, Dr. Charlie originated many operations, and excelled in surgery of the chest and of the thyroid gland. He contributed to venous surgery by developing an extraluminal vein stripper and described results of saphenous vein excision and stripping in a large number of patients. His work led to the formation of a unique Section of Peripheral Vein Surgery at the Mayo Clinic, devoted entirely treatment of venous disorders.

The monumental contribution of Charles Mayo with his brother was the establishment of the Mayo Clinic, the first integrated practice focusing on all the skills of a group to treat patients with multiple medical problems. When the patient load reached beyond their capacity, they rapidly expanded recruitment of a collection of capable and highly-trained physicians. With a belief that no man has any right to great wealth when others are living in poverty, the Mayo brothers established the Mayo Foundation for Medical Education and Research in 1915.

It has been said that the honor and recognition of merit awarded to the Mayo brothers has never been matched in extent anywhere in modern era. Virtually every honor in medicine was bestowed upon Charles H. Mayo and he held the presidency of many major medical and surgical societies. A host of universities and societies conferred honorary degrees and memberships on him.

The legacy of Dr. Charles H. Mayo is cherished throughout the world where the Mayo name immortalized.

Surgical Anatomy of Perforating Veins

2

Géza Mózes, Peter Gloviczki, Anna Kádár and Stephen W. Carmichael

A thorough knowledge of topographical anatomy is essential for learning new surgical procedures. Operations on the venous system of the legs require understanding the anatomy of the main groups of veins, their location and relationship to adjacent structures within the different compartments of the leg. Veins in few regions of the human body have more variability than in the lower limbs, and few areas in the body have a more complex topographical anatomy than the subfascial leg compartments.

Venous drainage of the leg is maintained by two systems, the superficial and the deep. Unidirectional flow in both is secured by valves. Perforating veins, most of which also contain valves, connect the two venous systems. In perforating veins, except some of those in the foot, blood normally flows from the superficial to the deep venous system.[1,2]

Superficial Veins of the Leg

Superficial veins of the sole form a venous network, that is connected by numerous small veins to deep plantar and superficial dorsal veins of the foot.[2] On the dorsum of the foot, digital veins form the dorsal metatarsal veins that empty into the dorsal venous arch (Fig. 2.1). The medial end of this arch continues in the greater, the lateral end in the lesser saphenous vein. The greater saphenous vein accompanied by the saphenous nerve ascends anterior to the medial malleolus, crosses the tibia and ascends medial to the knee (Fig. 2.2).[3] In the thigh it ascends anteri-

orly, enters the fossa ovalis below the inguinal ligament and empties into the femoral vein.[4] Just before it ends, the greater saphenous vein receives one or two large tributaries from the thigh, the lateral and medial accessory saphenous veins and several smaller ones from the inguinal and pudendal regions.[5] The posterior arch vein, or Leonardo's vein (presumably first depicted on Leonardo da Vinci's drawings) drains a fine network around the medial malleolus, ascends on the posteromedial aspect of the leg and joins the greater saphenous vein distal to

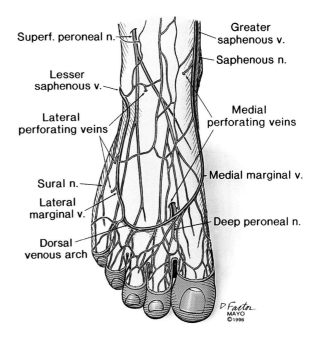

Fig. 2.1. Anatomy of the superficial and perforating veins of the foot.

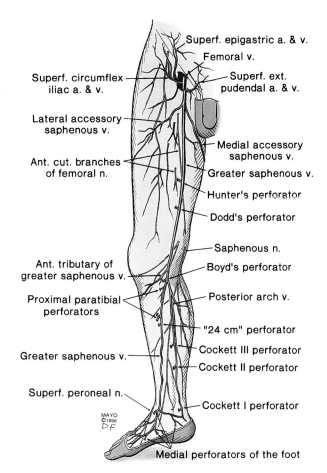

Fig. 2.2. Anatomy of medial superficial and perforating veins of the leg.

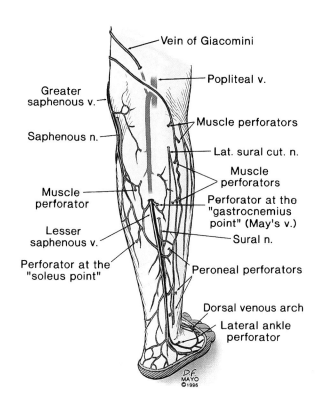

Fig. 2.3. Anatomy of posterior superficial and perforating veins of the leg.

the knee (Fig. 2.2).[6] Major medial perforating veins connect the posterior arch vein with the posterior tibial veins. An anterior vein also ascends from the dorsum of the foot and joins the greater saphenous vein at the knee.[7]

The lesser saphenous vein ascends on the postero-lateral aspect of the leg, close to the sural nerve, and usually joins the popliteal vein in the proximal popliteal fossa (Fig. 2.3).[8] The vein of Giacomini, a communicating vein in the posterior thigh, may connect the lesser to the greater saphenous vein.[9] There can be other, smaller, direct connections (communicating veins) between the lesser and greater saphenous veins.

Deep Veins of the Leg

Deep veins accompany the arteries and their branches (Fig. 2.4). In the foot plantar digital veins unite into four plantar metatarsal veins, that form the deep plantar venous arch. This continues into the medial and lateral plantar veins, that empty into the posterior tibial veins behind the medial malleolus. The main deep veins on the dorsum of the foot are the dorsalis pedis veins, which form the paired anterior tibial veins at the ankle.[10]

In the calf the paired posterior tibial veins, accompanying the posterior tibial artery, run between the edges of the flexor digitorum longus and tibialis posterior muscles, under the fascia of the deep posterior compartment. They penetrate the soleus close to its origin and continue to the popliteal vein following union with the paired peroneal and the anterior tibial veins.[10] The soleus muscle has several large venous sinuses, that are drained by the soleal veins into the posterior tibial and peroneal veins. In the lower third of the leg they

The popliteal vein ascends to an aperture in the adductor magnus and continues into the femoral vein, that changes its name at the inguinal ligament to become the external iliac vein. It is important to remember that the segment of the femoral vein between the adductor canal and the profunda femoris vein is also called superficial femoral vein although this segment is part of the deep venous system. The profunda femoris and the greater saphenous veins are main tributaries to the femoral vein.[2,10]

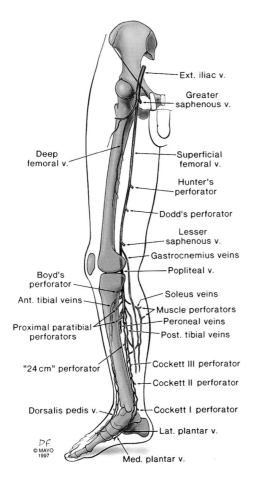

Fig. 2.4. Anatomy of the deep veins of the leg.

frequently join direct perforating veins before they enter the deep veins.[7] Bilateral gastrocnemius veins usually drain directly into the popliteal vein, distal to the confluence of the lesser saphenous vein with the popliteal vein.[11]

Perforating Veins

Perforating veins connect the superficial to the deep venous system.[12] The term "communicating vein" is reserved for venous tributaries that connect veins within the same system, i.e. veins of the superficial or those of the deep system.[13,14] *Direct* perforating veins connect superficial to deep axial veins, whereas *indirect* perforators connect superficial veins to veins of leg muscles.[15] Direct perforating veins showed a relatively constant location in most anatomic studies (Table 2.1), whereas the more frequent indirect perforators are irregularly distributed.[2] There are four groups of perforating veins in the leg: those of the foot, of the medial and lateral calf, and of the thigh.

In the foot, perforating veins either have no valves or have valves directing blood from the deep to the

Table 2.1. Studies on the location of direct medial perforating veins of the leg

Author (Year)	Number of Legs		Location of medial perforating veins[a]		
	Anatomic dissections	Surgical findings	Cockett II	Cockett III	Proximal paratibial perforating veins (PVs)
Linton (1938)[12]	10	50	Distal third of the leg	Middle third of the leg	Proximal third of the leg
Sherman (1949)[26]	92	901	13.5 cm	18.5 cm	24 cm, 30 cm, 35 cm, 40 cm
Cockett (1953)[19]	21	201	13–14 cm	16–17 cm	At the knee
O'Donnell (1977)[21]	–	39	Half of the incompetent PVs are between 10–15 cm[b] (15–20 cm[a])		Few incompetent PVs
Fischer (1992)[22]	–	194	Random distribution of incompetent PVs		
Mozes (1996)[17]	40	–	7–9 cm[b] (12–14 cm[a])	10–12 cm[b] (15–17 cm[a])	18–22 cm[b], 23–27 cm[b], 28–32 cm (23–27 cm[a]), (28–32 cm[a]), (33–37 cm)

[a] Distances measured from the sole.
[b] Distances measured from the lower tip of the medial malleolus

superficial system. Direct perforators connect the superficial veins, such as the dorsal venous arch, the greater and lesser saphenous veins to the dorsalis pedis veins or to the medial and lateral plantar veins (Fig. 2.1).[16]

The most important leg perforators are located in the medial calf (Figs 2.2 and 2.4). The number of these perforators in our anatomic study, that included dissections of 40 normal limbs in 24 cadavers, averaged 13.8 (range: 7–22).[17] However, only 25% of all medial perforators measured >2 mm in size. This confirms our clinical experience, that division of 2 to 4 incompetent medial perforators in the leg is usually satisfactory to treat perforator incompetence.[18]

The same anatomic study also revealed that of 552 medial perforating veins that were identified in 40 limbs, 287 (52%) were direct perforators (Fig. 2.5), connecting the superficial with the deep systems, 228 (41%) were indirect muscle perforators (Fig. 2.6), and the anatomy of 37 perforators (7%) could not be determined.[17]

In the distal half of the medial side of the leg, there are four important groups of direct perforating veins. The lowest, the retromalleolar group (Cockett I) is located just behind the medial malleolus (Fig. 2.2).[19-22] The Cockett II and III perforators are usually at 7–9 cm and 10–12 cm proximal from the medial malleolus, in a distance within 2–4 cm from the medial edge of the tibia (Figs. 2.2, 2.4 and 2.5).[17] These perforating veins connect the posterior arch vein or other tributaries of the greater saphenous vein with the posterior tibial veins. The fourth group is that of the paratibial perforating veins, locating usually within 1 cm of the medial edge of the tibia. In our anatomic studies it consisted of three independent clusters of perforators (Figs 2.2 and 2.5). The lowest group, located at 18–22 cm from the medial malleolus, was described as the "24 cm perforators" because of their usual distance from the sole.[13] Two other groups are located at 23–27 and 28–32 cm from the medial malleolus.[17] Less than half of these perforators make direct connections between the greater saphenous and the posterior tibial veins; the majority of them connect the tributaries of the greater saphenous vein to the deep veins. There is an additional group of perforators (Boyd perforator) located distal to the knee, at 35 cm

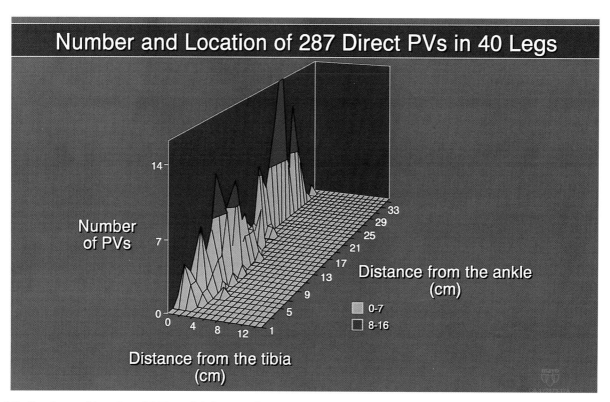

Fig. 2.5. Number and location of 287 medial direct perforating veins in 40 legs. The distance of the perforators from the medial malleolus was corrected for differences in leg length.

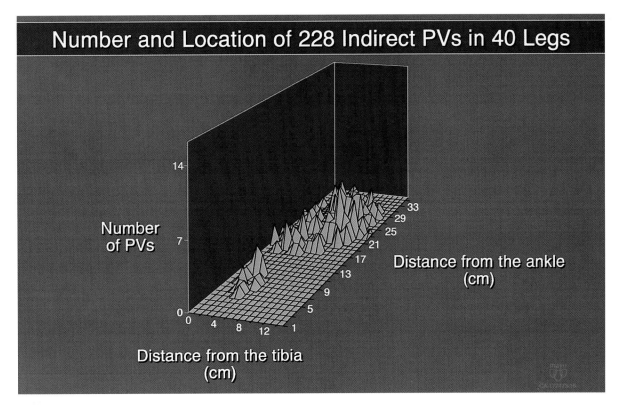

Fig. 2.6. Number and location of 288 indirect muscle perforating veins in the medial side of 40 legs. The distance of the perforators from the medial malleolus was corrected for differences in leg length.

from the medial malleolus, 1–2 cm medial to the medial edge of the tibia (Fig. 2.2).[23,24] The Boyd perforator connects the main trunk or a tributary of the greater saphenous vein and the posterior tibial, the tibioperonal or popliteal veins. Indirect muscle perforators, as mentioned, are randomly distributed, although most are located in the proximal half of the calf (Fig. 2.3 and 2.6).

On the posterolateral side of the calf proximal indirect perforating veins take their origin from the tributaries of the lesser saphenous vein (Fig. 2.3). These perforators make connections either with muscular venous sinuses or with veins draining the gastrocnemius and soleal muscles into the deep veins.[2,25] The location of the greatest muscular perforators in this area are referred as the gastrocnemius and soleus points (Fig. 2.3).[13] More distally in the posterolateral region direct perforating veins (peroneal perforators) connect the tributaries of the lesser saphenous to the peroneal vein (Bassi's perforator at 5–7 cm and the "12 cm perforator" at 12–14 cm from the lateral ankle).[2,13] On the anterolateral side of the calf direct perforators connect the anterior tributaries of the greater saphenous to the paired anterior tibial veins.[25]

Perforating veins of the thigh are less numerous than those of the calf, but clinically they can be equally or even more important (Fig. 2.2 and 2.4). Two major groups at the medial aspect of the thigh are the Dodd's perforators and the Hunterian perforators, connecting directly the greater saphenous vein with the proximal popliteal or distal superficial femoral vein.[7,13,26]

Surgical Anatomy for Subfascial Endoscopic Surgery

During endoscopic procedures the endoscope is inserted into the superficial posterior compartment (Figs 2.7 and 2.8A–D) through the deep fascia (also called the lamina superficialis of the deep fascia). While 63% of the medial perforators (including most indirect medial muscle perforators) are accessible from this compartment, anatomic dissections of normal legs revealed that 68% of the Cockett II, 16% of the Cockett III and 75% of the proximal paratibial

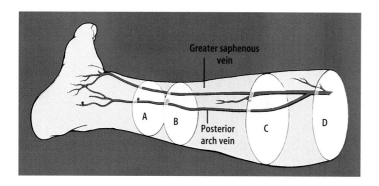

Fig. 2.7. Superficial and perforating veins in the medial side of the leg (cross-sections at levels A through D are shown in Fig. 8).

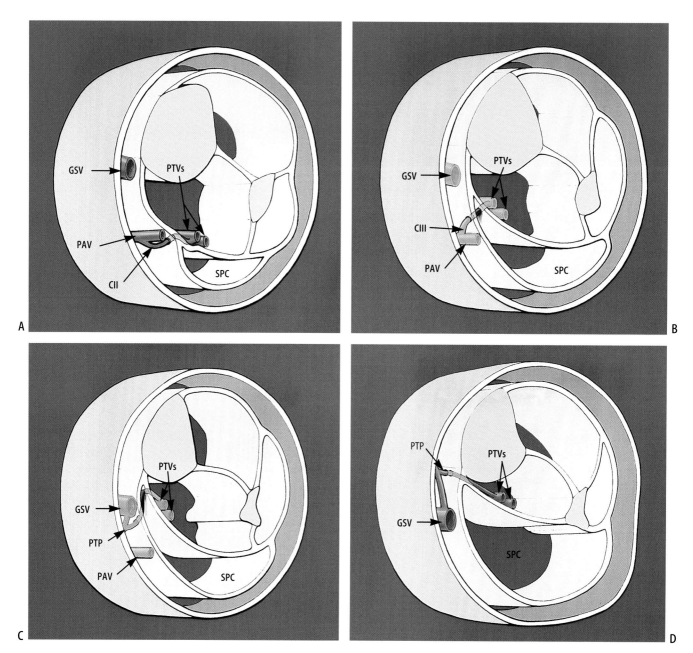

Fig. 2.8. A–D. Compartments and medial veins of the leg. Cross-sections at the level of Cockett II (**A**), Cockett III (**B**), "24 cm" (**C**) and more proximal paratibial (**D**) perforating veins. GSV: Greater Saphenous Vein, PAV: Posterior Arch Vein, PTVs: Posterior Tibial Veins, SPC: Superficial Posterior Compartment, CII: Cockett II, CIII: Cockett III, PTP: Paratibial Perforator.

Table 2.2. Occurrence and accessibility of direct medial perforating veins in 40 legs. (Distances measured from the lower tip of the medial malleolus.)

	Cockett II	Cockett III		Proximal paratibial perforating veins	
	(7–9 cm)	(10–12 cm)	(18–22 cm)	(23–27 cm)	(28–32 cm)
Occurrence	75%	75%	53%	93%	68%
Perforating veins not accessible from the superficial posterior compartment	68%	16%	57%	83%	85%

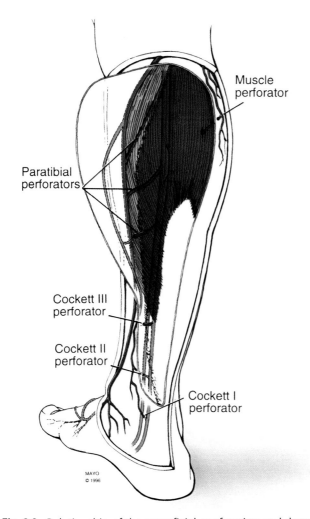

Fig. 2.9. Relationship of the superficial, perforating and deep veins to the fascia of the superficial posterior compartment. Note Cockett III and the lowest proximal paratibial perforator ("24 cm perforator") are readily accessible from the subfascial space.

perforators were not readily accessible (Figs 2.7, 2.8 A–D, 2.9 and Table 2.2).[17] The Cockett II and III perforators were located either in the deep posterior compartment or they were within a duplication of the deep fascia (intermuscular septum) between the superficial and deep posterior compartments (Figs 2.8A and 2.10 A,B). To gain access to these perforators the fascia of the deep posterior compartments frequently has to be incised (paratibial fasciotomy) (Figs 2.11 A–C and 2.12).[17,18] If they are located within the intermuscular septum, this has to be incised to dissect and divide perforating veins. Access to the Cockett I perforator is rarely possible through the endoscope because of the retromalleolar position of this perforating vein (Fig. 2.8). Proximal paratibial perforators can be hidden from endoscopic view by the insertion of the soleus muscle on the tibia or they may be located between the periosteum of the tibia and the deep fascia of the superficial posterior compartment (Figs 2.8D and 2.12).[17] To access these paratibial perforators the detachment of the soleus from the tibia by proximal paratibial fasciotomy may be necessary (Fig. 2.13 A–C).

Incision of the fascia of the deep posterior compartment in the distal third of the leg just distal to the belly of the soleus muscle may reveal the deep neurovascular structures, the paired posterior tibial veins, the posterior tibial artery and the tibial nerve. Injury to these structures during dissection and clipping of the perforators should be carefully avoided.

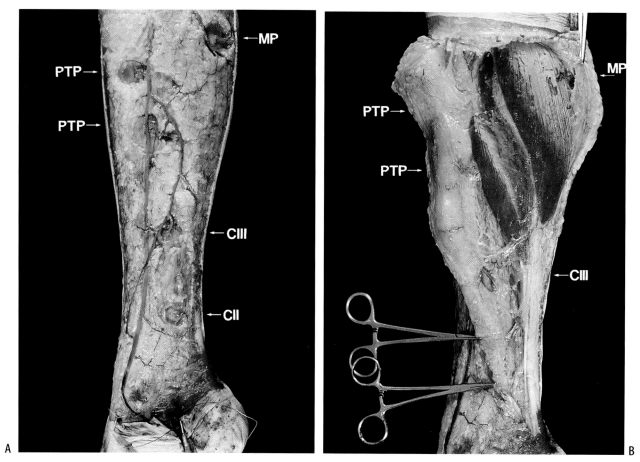

Fig. 2.10

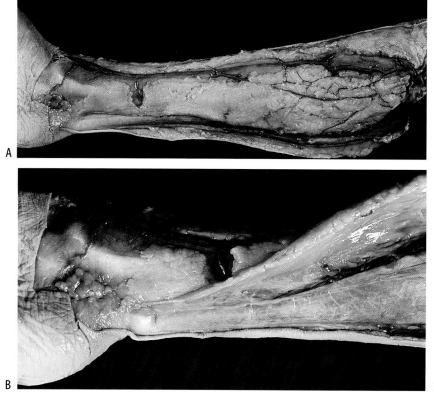

Fig. 2.11

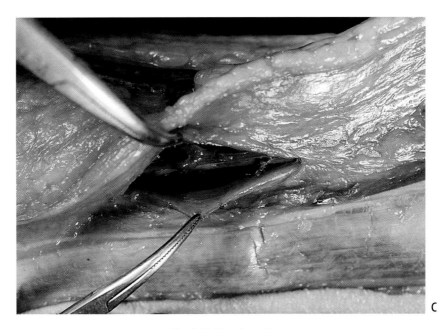

C

Fig. 2.11 *(Continued)*

◀ **Fig. 2.10A, B.** Corrosion cast of the leg veins. **A** Skin and portion of subcutaneous fat were removed. MP: muscle perforator, PTP: paratibial perforator, CII: Cockett II, CIII: Cockett III. **B** Fascia has been incised and rolled anteriorly to expose superficial posterior compartment. Note that the only lower paratibial perforator and Cockett III perforators are now accessible in the superficial posterior compartment.

◀ **Fig. 2.11A–C** Venous corrosion cast of the leg. **A** Note Cockett II perforator draining the greater saphenous vein. **B** Fascia has been rolled to expose superficial posterior compartment. **C** Note that the Cockett II perforator is hidden by the fascia between the superficial and deep posterior compartments and an incision is needed to uncover it.

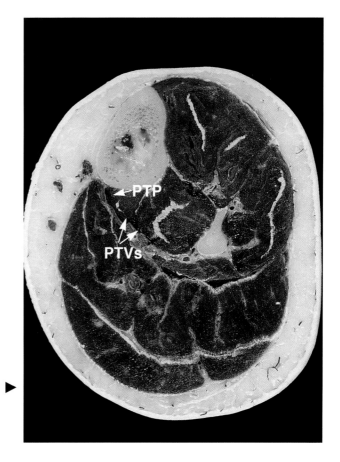

Fig. 2.12 Cross-section of the upper third of the leg. Note a ▶ paratibial perforating vein passing between the periosteum of the tibia and the fascia of the superficial posterior compartment. PTP: paratibial perforator, PTVs: posterior tibial veins. Veins were filled with blue latex.

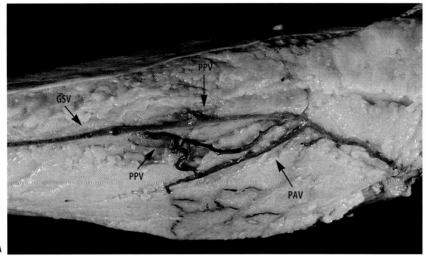

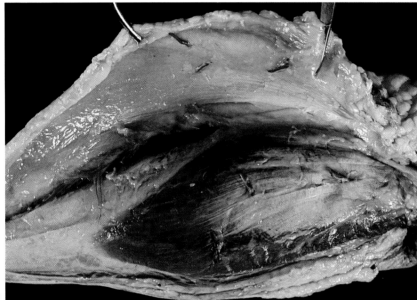

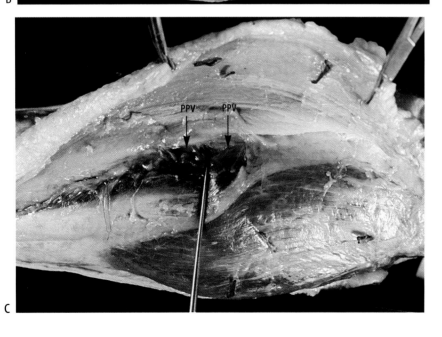

Fig. 2.13A–D. Venous corrosion cast of the leg. **A** Note two paratibial perforators draining the main trunk and a primary tributary of the greater saphenous vein. **B** Fascia has been rolled to expose superficial posterior compartment and dissected muscle perforators. **C** Note the lack of view on paratibial perforators. Soleus has to be detached to uncover these paratibial perforators. **D** Magnified view of paratibial perforators. PPV = paratibial perforating veins; GSV = greater saphenous vein; PAV = posterior arch vein.

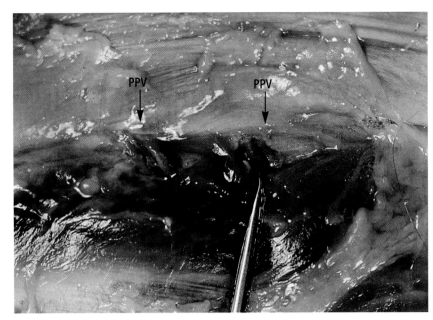

Fig. 2.13 *(Continued)*   **D**

References

1. Gay J (1868) John Churchill and Sons, On varicose disease of the lower extremities. London
2. Hollinshead WH (ed) (1969) Anatomy for surgeons: The back and limbs, Volume 3. Harper & Row Publishers, New York, pp 617–631, 754–758, 803–807
3. Garnjobst W (1964) Injuries to the saphenous nerve following operation for varicose veins. Surg Gynec Obst. 119:359–361
4. Gardner E, Gray DJ, O'Rahilly R (1986) Anatomy – A regional study of human structure, 5th edn: Vessels and lymphatic drainage of the lower limb. WB Saunders, Philadelphia, pp 190–196
5. Daseler EH, Anson BJ, Reimann AF, Beaton LE (1946) The saphenous venous tributaries and related structures in relation to the technique of high ligation: Based chiefly upon a study of 550 anatomical dissection. Surg. Gynec. Obst. 82:53–63
6. Negus D (1995) The blood vessels of lower limb: applied anatomy. In: Negus D, ed. Leg ulcers: A practical approach to management. 2nd edn Butterworth-Heinemann, London, pp 14–29
7. Dodd H, Cockett FB (1956) Surgical anatomy of the veins of the lower limb. In: Dodd H, Cockett FB (eds). The pathology and surgery of the veins of the lower limb. E & S Livingstone, London; pp 28–64
8. Kosinski C (1926) Observations on the superficial venous system of the lower extremity. J Anat 60:131–142
9. Bergan JJ (1996) Surgical Management of primary and recurrent varicose veins In: Gloviczki P, Yao ST (eds) Handbook of venous disorders. Chapman and Hall, London, pp 394–415
10. Williams PL, Warwick R, Dyson M, Bannister LH (eds) (1989) Gray's anatomy. Churchill Livingstone, New York, pp 812–814
11. Tibbs DJ (1992) Varicose veins and related disorders. Butterworth-Heinemann, Oxford, pp 204–232
12. Linton RR (1938). The communicating veins of the lower leg and the operative technic for their ligation. Ann Surg 107:582–593
13. May R (1981) Nomenclature of the surgically most important connecting veins. In: May R, Partsch H, Staubesand J (eds) Perforating veins. Urban & Schwarzenberg, Baltimore, pp 13–18
14. May R, Nissl R (1973) Phlebography of the lower limb (In German). 2nd edition Thieme, Stuttgart
15. Le Dentu A (1867) Anatomic research and physiologic considerations of the venous circulation of the foot and leg (In French). Thèse Agrégat, Paris: 1867
16. Kuster G, Lofgren EP, Hollinshead WH (1968) Anatomy of the veins of the foot. Surg Gynec Obst. 127:817–823
17. Mozes G, Gloviczki P, Menawat SS, Fisher DR, Carmichael SW, Kadar A (1996) Surgical anatomy for endoscopic subfascial division of perforating veins. J Vasc Surg 24:800–808
18. Gloviczki P, Cambria RA, Rhee RY, Canton LG, McKusick MA (1996) Surgical techniques and preliminary results of endoscopic subfascial division of perforating veins. J Vasc Surg 23:517–523
19. Cockett FB, Jones DEE (1953) The ankle blow-out syndrome: A new approach to the varicose ulcer problem. Lancet 1:17–23
20. Cockett FB (1956) The pathology and treatment of venous ulcers of the leg. Br J Surg 44:260–278
21. O'Donnell TF, Burnand KG, Clemenson G, Thomas ML, Browse NL (1977) Doppler examination vs clinical and phlebographic detection of the location of incompetent perforating veins. Arch Surg 112:31–35
22. Fischer R, Fullemann HJ, Alder W (1992) About a phlebological dogma of the localization of the Cockett perforators (In French). Phlébologie 45:207–212
23. Boyd AM (1948) Discussion on primary treatment of varicose veins. Proc Royal Soc Med 41:633–639

24. Stolic E (1981) Terminology, division and systematic anatomy of the communicating veins of the lower limb. In: May R, Partsch H, Staubesand J (eds). Perforating veins. Urban & Schwarzenberg, Baltimore, pp 19–34

25. Sherman RS (1944) Varicose veins: anatomic findings and an operative procedure based upon them. Ann Surg 120:772–784

26. Sherman RS (1949) Varicose veins: Further findings based on anatomic and surgical dissections. Ann Surg 130:218–232

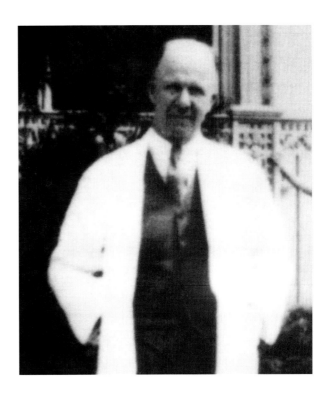

John Homans
1877–1954

John Homans was the fourth Boston physician of that name, and throughout his lifetime as a general surgeon, he continued to add laurels to it. He was among the first American surgeons to develop investigative and clinical interest in vascular surgery, and his particular concerns were the venous and lymphatic systems. His background, his manners, his speech, and his dress were Bostonian in every way. He brought to his bedside teaching, patient care, and surgery, his singularly personal and original observations.

Homans was not only a fifth-generation Boston physician, but he was a gentleman of supreme intelligence. He graduated from Harvard with honors and from medical school first in his class. Subsequently, the Moseley Professor of Surgery, Maurice Richardson, sent Homans to Baltimore for training. When Harvey Cushing became Chief of Surgery at Harvard, he chose as one of his two principal assistants, John Homans. While at Harvard, he developed a truly great *Textbook of Surgery* which was first published in 1931 and continued subsequently. In commenting on that book, Harvey Cushing said, "just as *Osler's Medicine* was the best existent book on surgery, so was the Homans' *Textbook of Surgery* a book which a physician could not be without."

In his 1939 monograph, *Circulatory Disorders of the Extremities*, Homans made a strong case for the fact that a correct diagnosis in vascular diseases could be made solely from a good history and physical examination. Among his contributions was the classification of varicose veins as primary if the deep veins were normal and secondary if the deep veins showed evidence of post-thrombotic damage. It was he who suggested that leg ulcers were caused by post-thrombotic deep vein damage and that venous stasis was the ultimate cause of venous ulceration. Homans strongly influenced Linton and many generations of surgeons who trained at the Massachusetts General Hospital. The highest award given by the Society of Vascular Surgery carries his name.

Epidemiology of Chronic Venous Insufficiency

3

Peter F. Lawrence and Christine E. Gazak

Chronic venous disease in the lower limbs is one of the most common diseases affecting adults in the industrialized world. It has been estimated that 40% of the US population has some form of venous disease, and that 4.6 million work-days are missed due to illnesses related to venous diseases.[1] However, the significance of venous disease (excepting venous thrombosis and pulmonary embolism) is not appreciated by a majority of physicians and health care workers since it is rarely limb- or life-threatening.

Epidemiologic studies can provide information on the spectrum and frequency of venous disease in the population and help physicians better understand the scope and incidence of the disease. Such information not only contributes toward an understanding of the mechanisms that cause the clinical sequelae of venous disease; it also assists in the development of screening and treatment strategies. To better understand the impact of venous disease on productivity in the form of lost work-days, medical costs, and its cost on society in general, we must understand the prevalence and incidence of venous disease in the general population and be able to identify subgroups who have or who are likely to develop venous disease. Prevalence of venous disease (e.g., a cross-sectional measurement of the number of cases in a population from one point in time) has been calculated extensively in Europe and Israel. To date, unfortunately, there have been few studies that have focused on the incidence of venous disease in the US. Consequently, most information about the epidemiology of venous disease comes from Europe,[2] where population demographics such as occupation, environment, and lifestyle differ in

many ways from the United States. While the first major study of venous disease took place in the US National Health Survey of 1935–36,[3] no recent study into the prevalence of venous disease in the US has been conducted. The incidence of venous disease, or its occurrence in a population longitudinally through time, has yet to be thoroughly explored in the Western world. Studies on rates of increase in venous disease in specific populations have been measured in New Guinea and other areas of the world[4] that, in recent years, have rapidly become westernized and subject to changes in health status.

There are several reasons for the paucity of data on venous disease, the first due to the nature of the disease itself. Although, venous disease has a high frequency in the US, there is debate as to whether or not a diagnosis of a non-morbid venous complaint is simply a normal variation in the population at large, much like a diagnosis of fibrocystic disease in a female patient. In addition, screening strategies for venous disease (i.e., ultrasound) can be costly and impractical for an entire population. Other, lower-cost screening tools, such as the physical examination, are often neglected by the physician who perceives venous disease as an insignificant problem or a "vanity complaint."

Another difficulty in calculating venous disease rates lies in difficulties in definitions of scope. There is a broad spectrum of venous complaints, ranging from minor cosmetic blemishes to chronic venous ulcers and deep vein thrombosis, all of which are often grouped in the same category of diseases. To provide a precise evaluation of venous disease, it is important to clearly delineate between types of venous complaints. Definitions of the types of venous disease and veins follow at the end of this section.

Finally, the pathogenesis of many venous complaints has only recently been elucidated. Because this information has not been widely understood, many physicians take a nihilistic approach in diagnosis and are unaware that treatment options exist for most types of venous complaints.

Definitions of Veins

Estimates of the prevalence of varicose veins depend on the definition of varicose veins – since dilated veins ranging from telangiectasias to huge varicosities may fall in the general category of varicose veins. The population under study must be defined as well, since risk factors such as age, sex, and number of pregnancies may change the incidence of varicose veins.

Varicose vein refers to any dilated, tortuous, elongated vein, irrespective of size.

Telangiectasias or *hyphen-webs* ("spider-veins") refer to intradermal varicose veins which are small and rarely symptomatic. Because of their relatively benign nature, the epidemiology of telangiectasias may or may not be included in papers describing the epidemiology of venous disease. Since telangiectasias are very common, studies that include these veins in their epidemiologic analysis will report a much higher incidence and prevalence of varicose veins than those that do not.

Trunk veins are the greater or lesser saphenous veins, or their named tributaries.

Reticular veins are subcutaneous veins that enter tributaries of trunk veins.

Prevalence of Venous Disease

Due to the variety of definitions of varicose veins and the numerous methods used in assessing venous disease, it is difficult to determine exact prevalence. One study conducted in a West London community[5] used self-report questionnaires to find the incidence

and distribution of venous disease for that community. A random sample of 2103 patients selected from three general practice sites were asked to complete a questionnaire on venous disease, including any previous self-report or physician diagnosis and usage of support hose. Of the 1338 returned questionnaires, 31% reported having some form of venous disease. Twenty-five percent reported having varicose veins, 5% noted a history of phlebitis, 4% had a current or prior leg ulcer, 4% percent reported venous thrombosis and 1% reported a pulmonary embolism.

A study based in Finland sought to assess the reliability of self-reporting of varicose veins.[6] A random sample of 166 patients who previously reported having varicose veins using a self-report questionnaire were examined by a surgeon to determine what variables in the questionnaire predicted misclassification; that is, the self-reported variables which were unreliable in correlating a given condition to a diagnosis of varicose veins. The researchers found that the only statistically significant variable associated with mis-classification was a positive reporting of family history of varicose veins, i.e., those patients who reported a family history of varicose veins were more likely to assume they had varicose veins when they did not. Other self-reported variables such as height, weight, occupational status and age did not appear to be subject to mis-classification.

Risk Factors for Varicose Veins

There are definite risk factors for varicose veins. Although there is disagreement about the significance of some of these factors, a strong argument can be made that a combination of several risk factors can be a strong predictor of varicose veins. Stvrtinová *et al.*[7] found several variables positively associated with a diagnosis of varicose veins. In a survey of 696 Czechoslovakian women employed at a large department store, 421 were diagnosed with varicose veins. Women who were older, had at least one pregnancy, who stood at work or who were obese had a statistically higher prevalence of trunk varices than their thinner, younger seated-worker counterparts. While mitigating factors such as differences in diet, economic status and genetic history must be taken into account, variables such as age

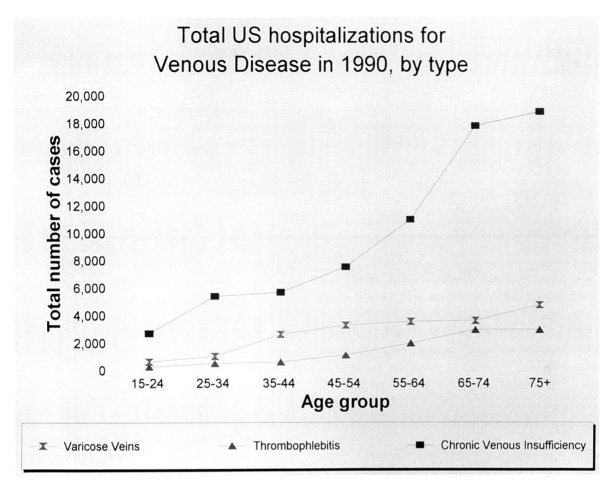

Fig. 3.1. Total US hospitalizations for varicose veins, thrombophlebitis and chronic venous insufficiency distributed in age-specific groups.

and weight are considered significant predictors of varicose veins in other studies.[2] Below are the risk factors reported in a number of studies. They are listed in decreasing importance.

Age. There is an increase in prevalence of varicose veins with age. In virtually all studies, varicose veins increase in both men and women with age, independent of other risk factors. The link between an increase in age and an increase in varicose veins is unknown, but probably reflects an inherited weakness in the vein wall or valve cusp, which, as it is subjected to lifestyle-related physical stress, eventually weakens until valve incompetence and varicose veins occur (Fig. 3.1).

Sex. The majority of epidemiologic studies indicate that women have more varicose veins than men of comparable age. This difference can range from a 1 to 1 to a 10 to 1 ratio, but most studies find that women have a three- to four-fold greater risk for

varicose veins than men. While there is a chance that women may be more likely to notice varicose veins and self-report them, independent examinations have verified a higher incidence of varicose veins in women. There are many potential explanations for this difference, but pregnancy appears to be the most frequent and important stress that leads to a greater prevalence of varicose veins in women.

Geography. Some epidemiological studies have shown a greater incidence of varicose veins in some countries than in others. A study that compared English and Egyptian cotton-mill workers found a greater incidence of varicose veins in the English population.[8] Another survey conducted in Jerusalem found that migrant men born in North Africa had significantly lower rates of varicose veins than their immigrant counterparts who were born in Europe, America and Israel.[9] These studies have been interpreted to show a genetic or hereditary etiology for varicose veins; an individual with a genetic predisposition will develop varicose veins more frequently when exposed to physical stresses such as pregnancy, obesity, etc.

Occupation. Studies correlating occupation and risk for varicose veins have reported conflicting results. The previously mentioned Czech study found a correlation between prolonged standing and an increased risk for varicose veins. Another study that looked at chair sitting, with its resultant stasis and increase in venous pressure in the calf veins found that in New Guinea, where women sat cross-legged on the ground and men sat on low stools or logs with their legs dangling, it was men who were diagnosed with varicose veins.

Parity. Women with multiple pregnancies may be at an increased risk for varicose veins, but the etiology is unclear. Pregnancy-related varicose veins may be due to an increased blood volume and venous pressure, or to hormonal factors. In addition, once varicose veins have developed, they tend to increase in size with pregnancy. Stvrtinova[7] found a positive correlation between pregnancy and varicose veins. Other studies have found no evidence of a link between pregnancy and varicose veins. It would seem that, until evidence proves otherwise, pregnancy exacerbates the risk factor for varicose veins only in combination with other risk factors such as occupation.

Diet. There is fair evidence that the Western diet, with its refined foods and reduced fiber content results in constipation, which, in turn, results in increased intra-abdominal pressures and straining during a bowel movement. Cleave[10] suggests that the increase in bowel pressure causes compression of the iliac veins, which over the years, results in the development of varicose veins. Another theory by Burkitt[11] suggests that raised intra-abdominal pressure from straining during constipation (Valsalva maneuver) is transmitted to the veins of the legs and eventually leads to dilation and valvular incompetence of the veins.

Other Factors. Many other factors have been suggested as causes for varicose veins including obesity, heredity, heavy lifting and hematologic factors. Each of these proposed etiologic factors has less evidence supporting it than the previously mentioned factors. Until further research provides substantiation for them, these links can only be suggested as likely causes, and not directly linked to an increased likelihood of varicose veins.

Venous Thrombosis and Post-thrombotic Syndrome

Acute deep venous thrombosis (DVT) has been reported to occur in 1.6/1,000 persons in the general population – although there are subgroups of patients undergoing hip or knee prosthetic replacement who have a higher incidence of DVT. There has been considerable debate, though, about the relationship between deep venous thrombosis and the development of chronic venous ulcers. What proportion of patients with DVT develop chronic venous insufficiency, and can a patient without prior DVT develop chronic venous insufficiency?

Prevalence of Chronic Venous Insufficiency

As mentioned previously, a self administered questionnaire to a West London community[5] identified 6% of patients who had a prior episode of DVT, 6% who had been treated with anticoagulation, and 4% who had a prior or current leg ulcer, although the etiology of the leg ulcer was not determined by this questionnaire.

Relationship of Valve Incompetence to Prior Venous Thrombosis

Markel *et al.*[12] studied patients with DVT longitudinally over time to determine the location and timing of valvular incompetence. They found that 6% of patients with "normal" legs have deep valve incompetence in spite of no prior DVT. These patients have now been recognized to have primary valve incompetence, which is frequently congenital, and can lead to the same sequelae as the post-thrombotic leg. When DVT occurs, valve incompetence develops over time as the thrombosed segments recanalize. At the time of DVT 17% of deep valves are incompetent, while at 12 months 69% are incompetent. They also showed that valves in prior thrombosed segments are the ones that develop incompetence. (Fig. 3.2 A–D)

Relationship of Valve Incompetence to Venous Insufficiency and Venous Ulcers

Patients with chronic ulcers in the lower extremities often have chronic venous insufficiency as the cause. A Swedish epidemiologic study investigated the frequency and etiology of limb ulcers. Eight hundred and twenty seven ulcers were found in 270,800 people in a rural and urban Swedish population, for a prevalence of 0.16% with a male/female ratio of 1:1.9. Fifty four percent of ulcers were due to venous disease; 60% had deep venous insufficiency and 40% had superficial or perforator vein incompetence.

The prevalence of venous ulcers increases with age, as it does in non-venous ulcers (Fig. 3.3). The median age of first venous ulcers was 59 (vs 73 for non-venous ulcers). Fifty four percent of patients had a venous ulcer for more than 1 year, while only 8% had a venous ulcer less than 3 months. Recurrence of venous ulcers is common (72%), particularly when there is deep venous involvement. The location of venous ulcers is usually in the "gaiter" zone (95%), while non-venous ulcers occur most commonly in the foot. Interestingly, only 37% of patients with venous ulcers had a history of DVT; consequently, many venous ulcers are either associated with primary valvular incompetence, incompetent superficial veins, or some may have had unrecognized DVT.

Venous Disease in Hospitalized Patients

Venous disease is a frequent cause for admission to the hospital, and is identified in many more patients admitted for other causes while they are in the hospital. What has not been recently mapped out in a US population is the variation in admissions by such factors as gender, race, region, and type of condition.

The National Hospital Discharge Summary is a comprehensive database that includes all care delivered at non-federal short-stay hospitals, including out-patient surgical procedures. Since data are available from samples of all patients who require hospital treatment of venous disease, this data set can provide information on the most severe forms of venous disease; i.e., those that require hospitalization. Consequently, we have reviewed the 1990 admissions of all patients in the US who sought care (in-patient or out-patient) in a hospital setting, to determine the frequency of venous disease.

In 1990, 99,903 patients were admitted to hospitals with a primary diagnosis of venous disease. Table 3.1 shows the distribution of diagnostic categories. Over 270,000 US. patients had venous disease identified as a secondary or other diagnosis. This is 49% of the more than one-half million total vascular surgery arterial procedures performed on US patients each year. Roughly as many patients are admitted to hospitals for a primary diagnosis of venous disease as are admitted for angioaccess procedures (98,000 cases in 1992; source, NHDS). In general categories, 67,098 patients were admitted for thrombophlebitis (presumably for anti-coagulation), 8647 for varicose veins (presumably requiring surgery), and 9631 for chronic venous insufficiency (presumably for limb care and/or surgery).

There are marked regional variations in the diagnosis of venous disease in hospitalized patients (Fig. 3.4) which may represent differences in population characteristics, admitting practices, billing techniques, or lifestyle. Since each region has a different population distribution by age, an expected frequency of venous admissions can be compared to the actual number of admissions in each region. Patterns of admission in the East and Mid-West areas of the country indicate that they either have more venous disease in those regions, or that they admit more patients to the hospital than their counterparts in the South and West.

The prevalence of venous disease in hospitalized patients increases with age (Fig. 3.1), which is consistent with other epidemiologic studies in non-hospitalized patients reporting a venous complaint. Studies have shown that some races are less likely to report venous disease. This variation may represent

Superficial femoral vein

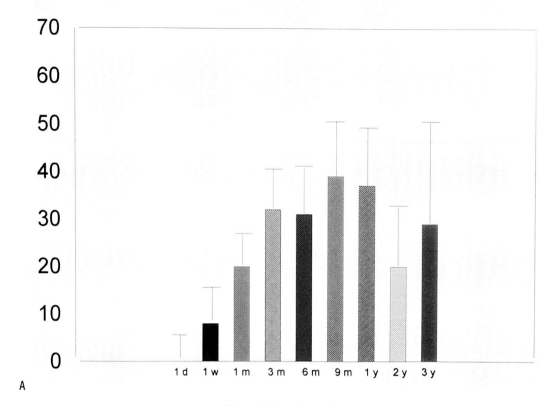

A

Popliteal vein

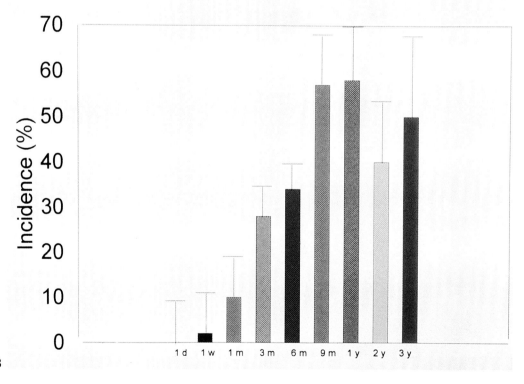

B

Fig. 3.2A, B, C, D. Incidence of reflux in four different deep veins after DVT. Follow-up visits were recorded 1 day, 1 week, 1 months, 3 months, 6 months, 9 months, 1 year, 2 years and 3 years after surgery. Standard errors for each time interval are shown.

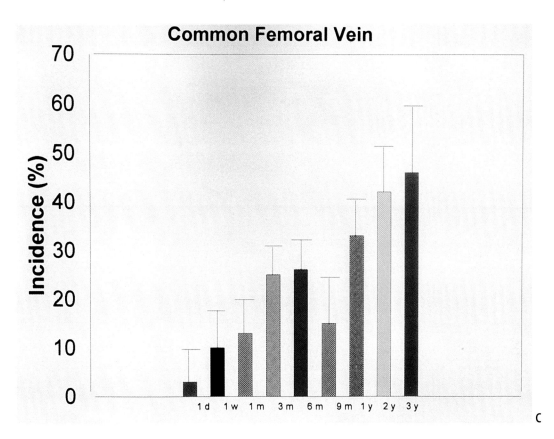

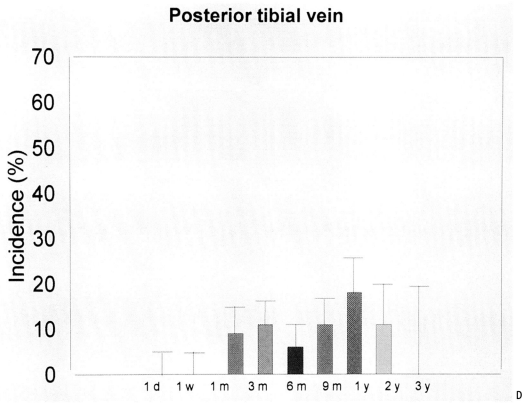

Fig. 3.2 (*Continued*)

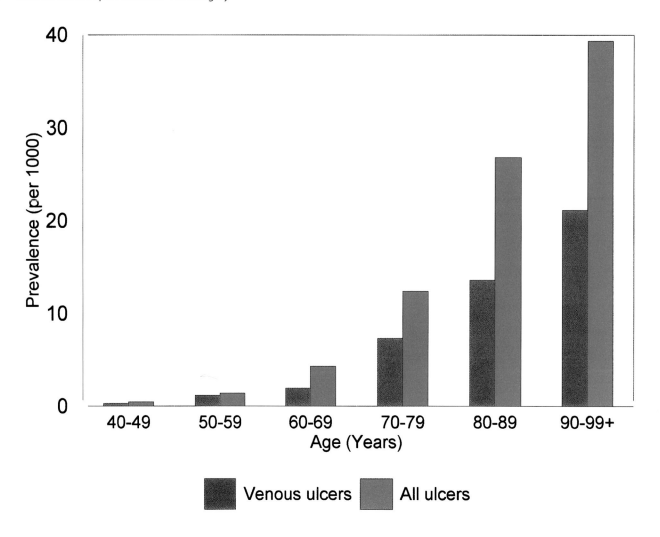

Fig. 3.3. Distribution of patients with venous ulcers as compared to all patients with non-venous ulcers in an age-specific Swedish population.

differences in genetic susceptibility, lifestyle, occupation, or admission patterns. With the exception of its Native American population, US data from 1990 shows no statistically significant difference between reportings of venous disease by race and population distribution by race. (Fig. 3.5).

The spectrum of venous disease ranges from acute, life-threatening problems such as venous thrombosis to less severe problems like reticular varicose veins (Table 3.1 shows different ICD codes for venous disease).

Procedures on the venous system were performed in 59,901 patients or two-thirds of hospitalized patients reporting with a primary diagnosis of a venous complaint. Many of these procedures, such as those for varicose complaints, were performed on

an ambulatory basis, but are included in this data set since the procedure was hospital-based. Among cases with a primary diagnosis of thrombophlebitis 51.1% had one or more procedures performed.

Seventy eight point three percent of cases with a primary diagnosis of varicose vein, with or without ulcer, had 1 or more procedures performed and 64% of cases with a primary diagnosis of a chronic venous insufficiency had 1 or more procedures performed.

Morbidity and complications related to venous disease were common but mortality rare when the venous problem was the indication for admission (Fig. 3.6).

In-hospital morbidity and mortality as related to surgical procedures was directly linked to the mag-

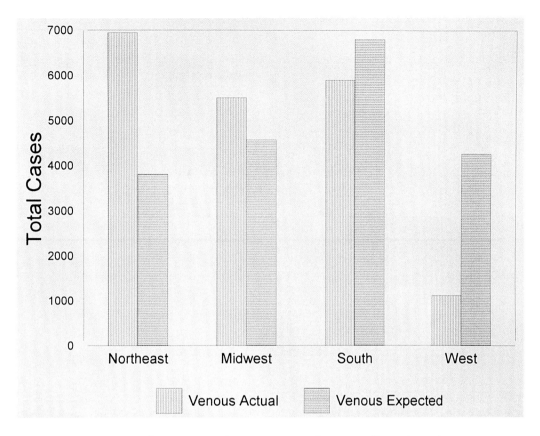

Fig. 3.4. Difference in US admitting practices for venous disease by region.

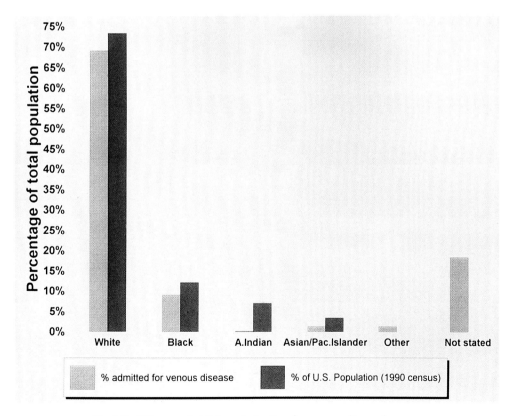

Fig. 3.5. Difference in US hospitalization for venous disease by race.

Table 3.1.   Venous complaints that have specific ICD-9 codes and may require hospitalization

Iliac vein thrombophlebitis (DVT)
Superficial thrombophlebitis of the Lower Extremities
Deep vein thrombophlebitis (DVT)
Upper extremity DVT
Unspecified phlebitis (Superficial or Deep)
Portal vein thrombosis
Budd-Chiari syndrome
Thrombophlebitis migrans
Thrombophlebitis of vena cava
Thrombophlebitis of other specified veins
Varicose vein of the leg (with ulcer)
Varicose vein of the leg (with inflammation)
Varicose vein of the leg (with both)
Varicose vein with inflammation and ulcer not mentioned
Compression of the vein (stenosis)
Venous insufficiency (unspecified)

nitude of the procedure, the age of the patient and the length of stay. Longer length of stay rates were positively correlated to higher mortality rates. Length of stay for all venous complaints varied. When only one procedure code was used and the primary diagnosis was venous disease, the hospital length of stay ranged from less than 1 day to 8 days, depending on the severity of the complaint. Typically, varicose complaints, with or without ulcer, required a length of stay of 1 day or less, chronic venous insufficiency required a stay of 4 days or less while thrombophlebitis required stays of up to 7 days, presumably for anticoagulation.

Conclusion

Venous disease is predominately found in industrialized societies. Varicose veins occur in 25% of the population. Risk factors such as age, pregnancy, and genetic predisposition have been shown to increase the likelihood of varicose veins.

Deep vein thrombosis occurs in 4%–6% of the population over their lifetime. The effect of DVT is mostly valvular damage, which occurs in 2/3 of patients 1 year after the episode. In addition, 6% of "normal" people have an incompetent deep valve, which may lead to the same sequelae of chronic

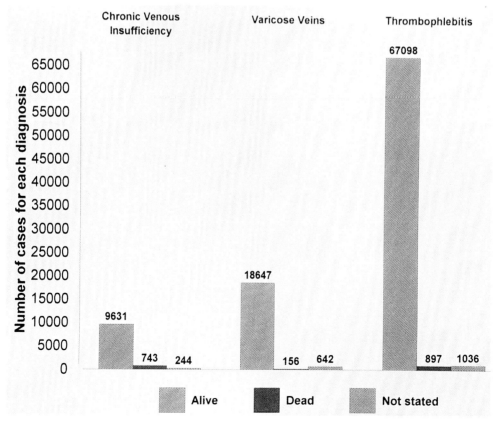

Fig. 3.6. Discharge status of in-patient cases for chronic venous insufficiency, varicose veins, and thrombophlebitis by status: alive, dead, unknown.

venous insufficiency, limb swelling, pigmentation, lipodermatosclerosis and limb ulceration. Limb ulcers have a prevalence of 0.16%, and 55% are due to venous disease, mainly chronic deep venous insufficiency. Venous ulcers increase in frequency with age, require more than 1 year to heal in most patients, and recur in 70%. The most severe forms of venous disease require hospitalization. As many patients require annual hospitalization for venous disease as for angio access and aortic procedures. The length of hospital stay is dependent on the type of venous complaint. Typically, varicose veins with venous ulcers require 1–2 days in the hospital, while DVT requires 4–5 days for anticoagulation. In spite of the high frequency of hospitalization for all venous complaints, the identified in-patient mortality is low.

Both physicians and patients must be made aware that there are methods of treatment for venous disease that should be promoted early in the course of the disease so as to reduce the cost and trauma associated with its progression.

References

1. Stanley JC, Barnes RW; Ernst CB (1996) Vascular surgery in the United States: Workforce issues. J Vasc Surg 23:172–181
2. Callam MJ (1994) Epidemiology of varicose veins. Br J Surg 81:167–173
3. US Department of Health, Education and Welfare (1938) National Health Survey 1935–1936. Preliminary Reports. The magnitude of the chronic disease problem in the United States. Washington DC
4. Stanhope JM (1975) Varicose veins in a population of lowland New Guinea. Int J Epidemiol 4:221–225
5. Franks PJ, Wright DI, Moffatt CJ (1992) Prevalence of venous disease: A community study in West London. Eur J Surg 158:143–147
6. Laurikka J (1995) Misclassification in a questionnaire survey of varicose veins. J Clin Epidemiol 48:1175–1178
7. Stvrtinová V, Kolesár J (1991) Prevalence of varicose veins of the lower limbs in the women working at a department store. Int Angiol 10:2–5
8. Mekky S, Schilling RS, Walford J (1969) Varicose veins in women cotton workers: An epidemiological study in England and Egypt. Br Med J 2:591–595
9. Abramson JH, Hopp C, Epstein LM (1981) The epidemiology of varicose veins – a survey of western Jerusalem. J Epidemiol Comm Hlth. 35:213–217
10. Cleave TL (1959) Varicose veins – nature's error or mans? Lancet ii:172–175
11. Burkitt DP (1972) Varicose veins, deep vein thrombosis, and hemorrhoids: epidemiology and suggested aetiology. Br Med J 2:556–561
12. Markel A, Manzo RA, Bergelin RO and Strandness Jr DE. Valvular reflux after deep vein thrombosis: incidence and time of occurrence. J Vasc Surg 1992; 15(2):377–82; discussion 383–4

Profile

4

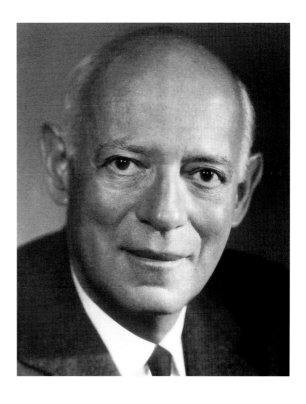

Geza DeTakats
1892–1985

Born into a distinguished medical family in Hungary, Geza DeTakats carried a courtly manner, great wisdom, marvelous humor, and a deferential attitude into his daily living and scientific investigations. Although he knew of vascular trauma and the effect of wounds through personal experience in the Balkan campaigns of the second decade of this century, his long-standing interest was blood coagulation and venous disorders.

In the 1930s, he established the Vascular Clinic at Northwestern University in Chicago. The clinic flourished and later expanded in the Department of Surgery of the University of Illinois. This led to the establishment of one of the first cardiovascular surgical services in the country at the St Luke's Hospital in Chicago. It is a credit to DeTakats' vision and foresight that a cardiovascular research unit was attached to this service.

Although DeTakats participated in many of the technical advances of the early days of modern vas-

cular surgery, including the establishment of a blood vessel bank in Chicago, it was his broader view of the entire cardiovascular scene that stimulated many of his pupils. Commenting on the technical advances of the 1960s, he said, "I have been borne up by the conviction that it is in the very areas where technical advances are most frequent that there is greatest need for a statement of fundamental principles." Commenting on the need for technical skill in cardiovascular surgery he said, "But boldness and manual dexterity in the human cannot be substituted for sound judgment and sound judgment can only be acquired by knowing the natural course of the disease."

DeTakats met his beloved wife, Carol, while on a fellowship at the Mayo Clinic in Rochester, Minnesota. It was from there that he established his practice and his investigations in Chicago. His broad interests included the effect of sympathectomy on vascular tone, the effects of heparin and the varying response of individual patients to that agent, venous thromboembolic disease and its prevention and treatment, as well as the neurovascular lesions of the extremities, including acrocyanosis, erythromelalgia, and the vasoneuropathies. His textbook, entitled *Vascular Surgery*, was published by WB Saunders in 1959 and was the first such textbook to appear in North America.

DeTakats rose to local leadership in medicine and surgery and was acknowledged as a national leader in the earliest days of vascular surgery. Locally, he was President of the Chicago Heart Association and the Chicago Surgical Society. Nationally, he became President of the Society for Vascular Surgery in 1952 and at one time was the Society's oldest surviving member.

In a tribute to Rudolph Matas, DeTakats summarized what others thought was a cogent summary of his own influences in vascular surgery. He said, "The history of surgery can be written in various ways. It is possible merely to record the development of ideas, impersonally, dispassionately, without reference to the lives of men who created them. It seems obvious, however, that the impetus which certain dominant figures have given to progress is only effective if their ideas and activities rapidly permeate contemporary thought and if these ideas then readily serve as building stones for the work of successive generations."

Pathophysiology of Chronic Venous Insufficiency

John J. Bergan and Jeffrey L. Ballard

Disorders of arteries, veins, and lymphatics are loosely termed peripheral vascular disease. Yet the connotation of that phrase is arterial occlusive disease. The functions of arteries, veins, and lymphatics are as different, one from another, as the disorders which afflict them. Arterial disease is dominated by occlusions and dilations. Lymphatic disorders are characterized by fluid accumulation. Venous disorders have a much wider spectrum of dysfunction, ranging from a distasteful appearance, inculcated by beliefs and mores, to frank epidermal loss, rampant infection, disability and amputation.

Only in recent years, when the study of venous dysfunction turned away from the lessons learned in analyzing arterial disorders, has progress been made in understanding. The arterial system, with its unicycle pump and pipe system, is relatively easy to understand. The venous system, with its multiplicity of pumps, tanks, and monodirectional valves, is much more complex. Its collecting system is not just a pipe system but a network. And any strand in the net may be taken away or duplicated without producing dysfunction. Its conduit system can be shown to overflow with its contents progressing away from the heart only to re-enter the deep system and overload deep reservoirs and pipes. Furthermore, the severe changes of chronic venous dysfunction are produced by phenomena almost totally unrelated to dysfunction of arteries and lymphatics. Yet from this background of confusing and often contradictory ideas comes a unifying concept which links all forms of venous dysfunction and explains the differences between simple varicose veins and the stigmata of severe chronic venous insufficiency.

Stasis Ulcers are not Stasis Ulcers

As late as 1995, a chronic venous leg ulcer was defined as a "discontinuity of epidermis, persisting for four weeks or more, occurring as a result of venous hypertension and calf muscle pump insufficiency."[1] Yet by the time this was written and agreed to by a distinguished panel of investigators, much more was known. Many past theories were discarded and new theories were clarified sufficiently that interventional treatments could be codified. Fortunately, the definition given does not mention stasis, yet venous ulcerations have been termed stasis ulcers for the better part of the twentieth century. The concept of stasis suggested stagnant blood lying within tortuous, non-functioning, dilated channels close to the skin. The hypothesis was that tissue anoxia caused cell death. Blalock showed that the oxygen content of blood in patients with varicose veins was higher, not lower, than oxygen content of normal veins.[2] Others confirmed those findings and recent studies have shown a faster circulation time in limbs with varicosities and stigmata of chronic venous insufficiency than normals.[3,4]

Postphlebitic is not Postphlebitic

Another discarded term used in the past to describe venous ulceration was post-thrombotic ulcer. This

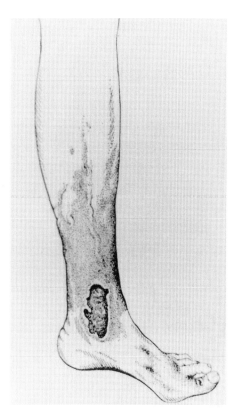

Fig. 4.1. This drawing, taken from the most recent descendant of Homans' *Textbook of Surgery (Warren's Surgery,* WB Saunders Co., Philadelphia, 1963) was labeled "postphlebitic syndrome." It shows the evidences of chronic edema, dilated superficial veins, hyperpigmentation, and ulceration.

was also generalized to name the entire extremity as being postphlebitic (Fig. 4.1). This was also referred to as the post-thrombotic syndrome. Such terminology was dominant in the 1950s when Anning reported a series of 715 leg ulcer patients in which a venous disorder was responsible for the cutaneous ulceration in more than 86%. It was thought that the ulcers were post-thrombotic in greater than 79% of limbs. Anning described true varicose ulceration in only 7%.[5] In light of present-day duplex findings, this could not be true.

Venous Hypertension: The Calf Pump

Old terms die slowly, and the term "postphlebitic" is still in use on both sides of the Atlantic.[6-9] Just as the terms postphlebitic state and venous stasis die slowly,

so does the concept that venous hypertension is the sole cause of severe venous insufficiency.[10] It derives from the past when studies of venous pressure were virtually the only objective means of assessing venous insufficiency. Those studies did show that at rest in the erect position, the superficial and deep venous systems had approximately the same hydrostatic pressure, defined as weight of a column of blood between the point of measurement and the right atrium. During calf muscle contraction, a transient pressure rise would occur in the deep veins which would propel the blood cephalad. The mechanism by which this occurred was called the calf muscle pump. It was known that valves in perforating veins closed during such muscle contraction and this prevented the transmission of high pressure to the superficial system. After calf pump contraction and ejection of a large percentage of the blood, the deep venous pressure was known to fall abruptly to a very low level during muscular relaxation. This allowed the valves in the perforating veins to open and blood from the superficial system to rush into the deep system. This caused superficial venous pressure to drop to approximately 30% of static pressure. Calf muscle dysfunction was thought to occur when either ejection was incomplete or residual volume was maintained at a high level after calf contraction. It was said as late as 1993 that "studies … clearly show that calf pump failure leads to venous ulceration."[11]

Current studies using both ambulatory venous pressure and duplex examination have attempted by statistical methods to show that there is a linear relationship between ambulatory venous pressure and severity of venous dysfunction.[10] Unfortunately, this is not exactly true. In a recent report, a statistically significant difference between normal limbs and limbs with pigmentation and eczema was seen. But, in fact, there were no differences between the latter limbs and those with lipodermatosclerosis nor between those limbs with lipodermatosclerosis and those with ulceration. It is to the authors' credit that they confirmed that tourniquet testing to separate superficial from deep venous dysfunction was inconstant and unreliable. As they say, "there was no greater reduction in ambulatory venous pressure with the application of a tourniquet in the patients with superficial reflux, compared either with those who had deep venous reflux or those who had no reflux." The authors suggested using ambulatory venous pressure (AVP) measurement as a reference standard but even they recognized that pressure measurement was a global assessment and did not give specific information about individual venous segments. Van Bemmelen has said, "The correlation of a high AVP with ulceration is evident but the contribution of the superficial and deep systems to an increased AVP is unclear."[12] Fascination with venous pressure as an index of venous dysfunction has been carried even to continuous pressure measurements.[13] However, such studies have added little to the fundamental knowledge of venous ulceration.

Today, the best explanation of how venous hypertension may be linked to the severe changes of chronic venous insufficiency is found in the studies of Raju and Fredericks.[14] They have suggested that, "velocity of reflux (water hammer effect) may be important". (Fig. 4.2). They studied the relationship between ambulatory venous pressure and Valsalva-induced foot venous pressure. They showed that 20%–25% of patients with venous ulceration had ambulatory venous pressures that were considered to be normal. The Valsalva-induced venous pressure was an improvement in showing a relationship of

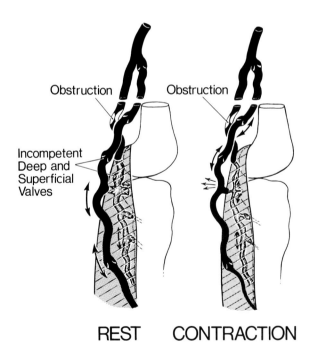

REST   CONTRACTION

Fig. 4.2. These diagrams show the situation found in the true post-thrombotic state in which there is a proximal obstruction, complete or partial, in association with incompetent superficial and deep valves. At rest, pressures in the superficial veins are not elevated but during muscular contraction, the water-hammer effect of muscle systole is observed. Pressures exerted on the skin by the failed check valve of the perforator vein can be enormous, even three to four times the pressure exerted by a compressive stocking.

pressures to ulceration. When both parameters of ambulatory venous pressure and Valsalva-induced venous pressure were considered, the ensuing index provided an excellent correlation with venous ulceration and other evidences of severe venous dysfunction. The concept of the water hammer effect has proven to be an excellent explanation for the initiation of changes as described below. It was referred to in the past as an ankle venous blowout by Negus.[15]

Changes in the Microcirculation

It is surgeons who care for venous ulcerations for the most part, and it is surgeons who think mechanistically. Thus, calf pump function deficiency and ulceration have been linked. However, the mechanisms by which ulcerations occur are not explained. On stepping back and viewing the scene, it is difficult to see how an inefficient calf pump can cause tissue necrosis on the medial aspect of the leg. Recently, while modern arterial vascular surgery was preparing for the twenty-first century, the study of venous pathophysiology was mired in the dogma of the first half of this century. The common explanations for necrotic ulcers on the medial aspect of the leg were venous stasis,[16] venous hypertension,[17] and tissue ischemia secondary to microscopic arteriovenous fistulae.[18] Investigation of venous pathophysiology developed slowly after 1970. Phlebography showed that deep venous channels were destroyed by thrombosis. It showed narrow, irregular, valveless channels or tortuous, dilated collateral veins with incompetent valves. Venous hypertension was correlated with these changes by measurement of pressure in foot veins during exercise. It could be seen that the normal flow of blood from superficial to deep and then to proximal was reversed, leaving the superficial veins distended by high pressure.[19]

An explanation which linked venous hypertension to cause of venous ulceration was reported and still leaves its mark today. This was proposed by Browse and Burnand from St Thomas's Hospital in London. Browse tells the story, "The late Ian Whimster reminded me of an observation he had made in the 1950s of a pronounced increase in number of capillary loops visible in a cross-section of skin adjacent to a venous ulcer.[20] At the same time, I had been impressed by the similarity of the clinical appearance of the tissues of the lower medial third of the leg in patients likely to develop venous ulcers to those of venous thrombosis and acute cellulitis, although neither were occurring. The pioneering work of George Fearnley[21] had shown that there was a level of fibrinolytic activity in normal blood which might play a part in any disease which included the deposition of fibrin." Ultimately, and after much study,[22,23] the fibrin cuff theory was formulated. In Browse's explanation, a vicious cycle was described in which poor systemic fibrinolytic activity led to deep venous thrombosis which led to disordered calf pump function, hyperpermeable capillaries, and excess interstitial fluid fibrin which was not removed because of poor fibrinolysis and exhaustion of fibrinolytic activator stores. This, in turn, led to further thrombosis. The spinoff from this vicious cycle was tissue death from poor oxygenation – the venous ulcer.[24]

The fibrin cuff theory was succinctly described by Kevin Burnand in a leading article in the British Journal of Surgery in 1990.[25] Subsequently, letters to the editor called attention to the fact that the fibrin cuff was not likely to block the passage of oxygen and other nutrients to the skin. Professor C.C. Michel of the Department of Physiology and Biophysics of St Mary's Hospital said, "while not impossible, it seems most unlikely that pericapillary fibrin can reduce the diffusion of oxygen to such critical levels." His conclusion was, "at present, it seems that there is no evidence for the existence of a pericapillary diffusion barrier in tissues associated with venous ulceration and no evidence that the fibrin concentration in pericapillary cuffs can be high enough to seriously impair the diffusion of oxygen."[26]

Simultaneously, other objections were raised. The Middlesex Hospital group[27] observed that Mr Burnand paid little attention to perforating veins, perpetuated the "unlikely suggestion that pericapillary fibrin cuffs are primary in pathogenesis of venous ulcers," and dismissed white blood cell trapping observations too lightly (Fig. 4.3). In support of their argument that the fibrin cuff theory was inadequate and white blood cell trapping and activation was of greater importance, Coleridge Smith and Scurr pointed out that the profibrinolytic, anabolic steroid, Stanozolol, was unable to improve the management of venous ulceration and did not influence healing.[28] They reviewed the observation that white blood cell trapping could be demonstrated in normal lower extremities by raising the venous pressure on sitting with the lower limbs dependent.[29] Additionally, investigations at the Middlesex showed that white blood cell trapping could be induced in the upper extremity by applying a cuff to the arm and inflating it to 80 mmHg for a period of 15 min.[27] Further, they emphasized that biopsies of liposclerotic skin in the supramalleolar area of patients with and without liposclerotic changes showed the number of white cells visible per unit area were 8–40 times as numerous in liposclerotic skin than in normal-appearing skin.[28]

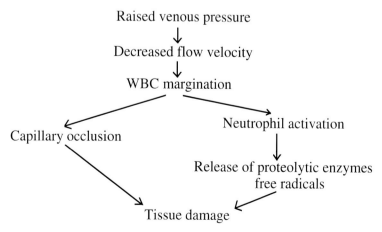

Fig. 4.3. The white cell trapping hypothesis is illustrated in this diagram. The importance of raised ambulatory venous pressure is stressed as is leukocyte activation and release of proteolytic enzymes and free radicals, thus causing tissue damage. (Courtesy Philip Coleridge Smith, Middlesex Hospital Vascular Laboratory.)

Effects of Leukocyte Trapping

A summary of the support for the white blood cell trapping theory was published in a leading article in the *British Journal of Surgery* in 1994 by Coleridge Smith.[29] Citing the use of electron microscopy and immunohistochemical techniques, he stated that, "the perivascular cuff of skin capillaries is much more complex than previously suspected." Fibrin was indeed present but only along with a number of other elements such as collagen Type IV, laminin, fibronectin, tenascin, macrophages and some T-lymphocytes. Further, the endothelium of capillaries in the area was seen to be very prolific and expressed intracellular and endothelium-leukocyte adhesion molecules as well as an upregulation of Factor VIII-related antigen. In addition, the cytokine interleukin 1 and tumor necrosis factor α were reported. These studies confirmed the obvious – that is, that lipodermatosclerosis is a chronic inflammatory process. While not mentioning the role of perforating veins, Coleridge Smith stated that, "in individuals with calf muscle pump failure, venous hypertension will occur whenever the patient stands, presumably leading to neutrophil activation."

Immunohistological methods have investigated the white blood cells surrounding capillaries in regions of venous hypertension (Fig. 4.4). These have shown that the cells are mainly macrophages and T-lymphocytes. Although the metabolism of the

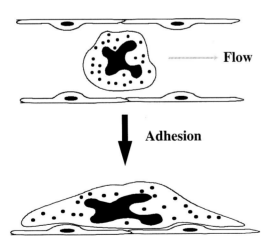

Fig. 4.4. In the white cell trapping hypothesis, selectins cause the leukocyte to begin to roll along the endothelium of the post capillary venule and eventually, the cell adheres to the endothelium. (Courtesy Philip Coleridge Smith, Middlesex Hospital Vascular Laboratory.)

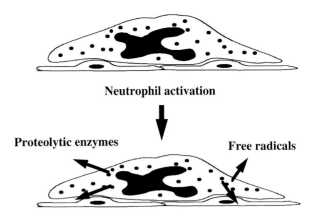

Fig. 4.5. Molecules that promote leukocyte adhesion are the free types of adhesion molecules. The selectins initiate cell rolling but integrins and immunoglobulins effect firm binding of cell to the endothelial surface. Also, intercellular adhesion molecules and vascular cell adhesion molecules also produce firm cell adhesion. The activated leukocyte releases proteolytic enzymes and free radicals. (Courtesy Philip Coleridge Smith, Middlesex Hospital Vascular Laboratory.)

leukocytes within the circulation is difficult to assess, in fact, plasma levels of enzymes from within neutrophils can be measured. Using these techniques, it has been shown that patients with venous disorders have greater neutrophil activation than age- and sex-matched controls (Fig. 4.5).

Experimental venous hypertension produces neutrophil degranulation, and it is possible that increased venous hypertension can result in the neutrophil degranulation which, in turn, may cause local endothelial injury. Minor damage could be easily repaired in normal subjects but in those limbs with an impaired venous system characterized by severe venous hypertension, the damage may be impossible to reverse. Since endothelium in skin with liposclerotic change exhibits increased adhesion molecule expression (ICAM and ELAM) and increased Factor VIII-related antigen production a significant inflammatory response would be produced which would result in lipodermatosclerosis. These factors favor adhesion of increased numbers of leukocytes, thus explaining the observation of increased leukocyte trapping with increased severity of venous disorders.

It is hypothesized that massive activation of large numbers of macrophages present in lipodermatosclerotic skin results in severe destruction of tissues by free radical attack. Other triggering events such as minor trauma might contribute. While the explanation is partly speculative at the present time, it still is a useful explanation when designing strategies of treatment for the individual patient.[30,31]

It is curious that some investigators most interested in the study of severe chronic venous insufficiency remain silent on the role of perforating veins in reporting their studies. For example, in a comprehensive review of the microvascular changes in chronic venous insufficiency, investigators reported that, "skin capillaries in areas of lipodermatosclerosis are dilated, elongated, and tortuous."[32] Observations of elongated, dilated, tortuous vessels apply to telangiectasias, varicosities and all veins in the region of incompetent perforating veins. Similarly, in a comprehensive review of the role of the leukocyte in pathogenesis of vascular disease, the Edinburgh group summarized histologic changes observed in lipodermatosclerotic skin and in skin adjacent to venous ulcerations.[33] They also

observed that the dermal capillaries were tortuous and elongated and so presented an increased surface area of endothelium to circulating blood (Fig. 4.6A, B). They did not link the abnormalities to perforating veins.

As mentioned previously, calf muscle pump failure has been related by many to venous ulceration. Yet there has been little explanation of the exact mechanism of such calf muscle pump failure. There is little evidence that it is the muscle itself or muscular innervation. Instead, as shown in the St Mary's laboratory, there is a relationship between ulceration and increasing values of reflux and decreasing values of venous ejection. In those limbs with minimal axial reflux (saphenous reflux), a poor ejection fraction was directly related to venous ulceration. Conversely, a good ejection fraction significantly reduced the incidence of ulceration in

Fig. 4.6.A. This phlebogram shows the region of the medial malleolus and the vessels associated with the inframalleolar and retromalleolar perforating veins. Note the elongation and tortuosity of the vessels in this area. **B** In this photograph, the maximum concentration of hyperpigmentation and early atrophie blanche is in the region of the inframalleolar perforating vein where the elongation and tortuosity of vessels allows a greater surface area for leukocyte adherence and activation.

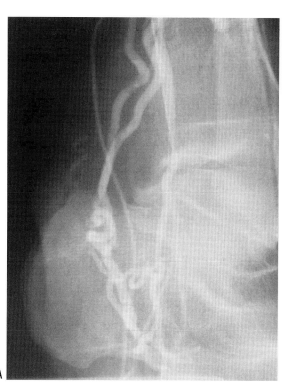

A

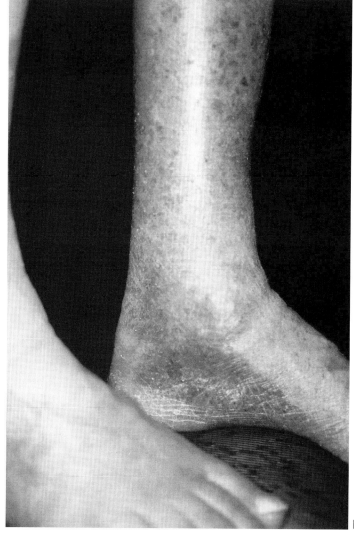

B

limbs with marked reflux.[34] Those studies were done using an air plethysmograph with an air chamber that included the whole leg. Therefore, the reports are silent on the role of perforating veins which fail to eject blood in a proximal direction while instead fill the superficial venous system and increase venous volume.

Difficulty in assessing the presence of perforating veins and their direction of flow has in the past hampered investigations designed to study perforating veins. However, more recent work has begun to show the relationship of perforating veins and venous ulceration. For example, a reflux study in Melbourne under Myers showed that a comparison of limbs with uncomplicated varicose veins to those with lipodermatosclerosis or past ulceration could be very revealing and had therapeutic implications. For example, isolated deep reflux was found in only 2% of uncomplicated varicose veins, only 7% in limbs with lipodermatosclerosis, and 8% in limbs with past ulceration.[35] Presumably, those limbs with isolated deep reflux would be those in which direct surgical therapy would be most difficult. This pathophysiology might require valve transplantation or perhaps valveplasty. In contrast, superficial reflux alone was found in 55% of limbs with uncomplicated varicose veins. Limbs with lipodermatosclerosis had superficial reflux only in 39% and the same was true for limbs with past ulcerations which showed only superficial reflux in 38%. Limbs with ulcerations more frequently showed superficial reflux, lesser saphenous reflux and deep reflux in the posterior tibial veins. In this study, of telling importance was the fact that outward flow was seen in medial calf perforating veins in 57% of complicated varicose veins, 67% of limbs with lipodermatosclerosis, and 66% of limbs with healed ulceration. Such outward flow in perforating veins occurred more frequently in limbs with complications. Isolated flow in perforating veins without any other abnormality was found in 10% of varicose veins, 10% of limbs with lipodermatosclerosis and 2% of limbs with ulceration.[35] Clearly, correction of superficial reflux and perforator outward flow could have a profoundly beneficial effect.

In a study performed almost simultaneously, the Middlesex group also examined limbs with venous ulceration. They found that isolated deep venous reflux was present in only 15% of limbs while in 53% of such limbs, isolated superficial venous reflux was present. The remaining limbs had combinations of deep and superficial reflux. While pointing out that, "large calf perforating veins permitting outward flow are commonly associated with venous disease," they admitted that, "we do not systematically map or treat these vessels."[36]

Perforating Veins and Leukocyte Sequestration

The same group did perform a separate study on the role of medial calf perforating veins in initiation or promotion of venous disorders. The direction of blood flow in the medial calf perforating veins was assessed during compression of the foot and calf by a cuff that inflated to 60 mmHg. Blood flow was assessed during deflation of the cuff. These studies showed that blood flow within medial calf perforating veins could be both inward and outward even in limbs with no evidence of venous disease. Fifteen percent of normal limbs showed flow outward in perforating veins but the most telling finding was the fact that "a significant number of perforating veins demonstrated outward flow, particularly in those limbs with deep venous insufficiency with or without superficial venous insufficiency."[37] This observation was made after compression of the calf proximal to the perforating vein. During the relaxation phase after proximal compression, many perforating veins demonstrated reverse flow from deep to superficial. While describing the difficulties of assessing perforator vein anatomy, these authors concluded that, "large, dilated perforating veins were seen and it is our experience that they were commonly, though not always, associated with lipodermatosclerosis and previous ulceration." (Fig. 4.7).

In light of the concept of white blood cell trapping and activation, it is not surprising that normal limbs might have perforating veins with outward flow. These might not suffer from white cell trapping. Conversely, large, dilated perforating veins would be associated with cutaneous changes and even ulceration if leukocyte sequestration and activation were present. As these authors have said, that phenomenon (of inward and outward flow) appears to extend across the entire spectrum of venous disease but is more common in those limbs with deep venous insufficiency.

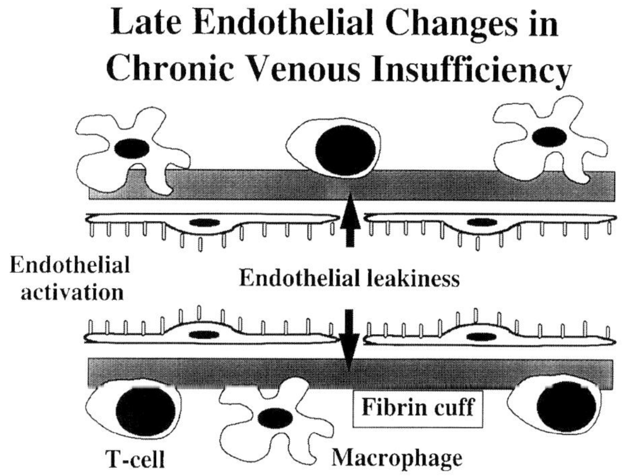

Late Endothelial Changes in Chronic Venous Insufficiency

Fig. 4.7. After leukocyte adhesion and activation takes place, there are endothelial leukocyte interactions which allow penetration of leukocytes into tissue and endothelial leakiness which allows the passage of fluid, plasma, and plasma proteins into the interstitial tissue where secondary changes occur. (Courtesy Philip Coleridge Smith, Middlesex Hospital Vascular Laboratory.)

One aid in assessing perforating veins in the future would be the observation of these investigators that, "after distal compression, flow during the relaxation phase does not occur in the perforating veins of limbs without objective evidence of venous disease. Flow during the relaxation phase was present in 33% to 44% of perforating veins in those limbs where there was evidence of venous disease in the superficial or deep venous system. Demonstration of flow within a medial calf perforating vein during the relaxation phase therefore cannot be considered to be normal and is associated with venous disease."[37]

Assuming that superficial reflux and deep reflux produce distal venous hypertension and that perforating vein incompetence transmits both static and dynamic exercise pressure to the skin, it is not surprising that in some limbs, lipodermatosclerosis and ulceration occur and in others, skin changes are absent. The differentiating factor between these extremes could be white blood cell trapping and activation. Limbs with normal skin would have an absence or decrease in trapping and activation while those with the most profound changes would have maximal tissue destruction by the toxic factors liberated by activated leukocytes.

With that concept in mind, one can take a therapeutic view of studies such as those at Newcastle.[38] There, a total of 300 limbs in 153 patients were examined by duplex ultrasonography. Focus was on the presence of venous reflux in superficial veins, deep veins, and medial perforating veins, both above and below the knee. In the 98 limbs with skin changes of hyperpigmentation, lipodermatosclerosis, atrophie blanche, and ulceration, only 2% had no evidence of venous reflux. These may have had undetected perforator dysfunction. In contrast, 39% had deep venous reflux and 57% had superficial venous incompetence. Two percent of this group had isolated medial perforating vein reflux. More important was the fact that of 25 limbs with ulceration, 13 had superficial reflux and 12 had deep venous reflux. In the 202 limbs, which included 20 normal controls, there were no skin changes. Of these, 22.3% had no venous reflux, and 8.4% had deep vein incompetence while 65.3% had superficial incompetence and 4% isolated medial calf perforating vein incompetence.

The differentiating factor, leukocyte trapping and activation, between those limbs with intact skin and those with advanced skin changes was not assessed and could not be assessed by this study. The implications are clear, however. A very large number of patients with advanced skin changes could profit by removal of the superficial reflux. If this were done, 52% of the limbs with ulceration and 57% of those with skin changes would be improved. Further, treatable superficial reflux combined with perforator vein incompetence was present in 77% of ulcerated limbs. The inescapable conclusion of this observation is that ablation of superficial reflux and interruption of perforator veins could be of benefit in those limbs with the most advanced skin changes.

Across the Atlantic, similar findings were found in Boston where McMullin[39] demonstrated that two-thirds of patients presenting with symptoms of chronic venous insufficiency, including lipodermatosclerosis, ulceration and dermatitis, had only superficial venous incompetence. These duplex studies of venous insufficiency reported on both sides of the Atlantic and as far away as Melbourne confirm the fact that severe chronic venous insufficiency may be treated effectively by attention to the superficial venous abnormalities. If these are corrected, the results are salutory and this has been reported.[40] Thus, the potential for curing the abnormality which is related to the venous ulceration ranges from 16.8% in the study by Hanrahan[41] at the Boston University to 53% in the study at the Middlesex Hospital by Shami.[42] As indicated, the Middlesex group does not routinely map perforator veins. If in the study by Hanrahan, the limbs with perforator reflux and those with only superficial reflux were summed, the potential for cure was present in 45.2% of limbs, a figure which is not dissimilar from the 53% of Shami.

Several workers have confirmed the possibility of correcting deep venous reflux by superficial venous surgery.[43–48]

Conclusion

Pathophysiology of chronic venous insufficiency suggests that venous hypertension which is linked to the severe changes of severe chronic venous insufficiency can be favorably modified by ablation of superficial venous reflux. Further, if this is done in combination with interruption of perforating veins, then water hammer outward flow through these veins will be halted. Presumably, the leukocyte trapping and activation which is favored by venous hypertension and the pulsatile effect of muscular contraction transmitted through incompetent perforator valves will be halted. It may very well be that the favorable observations of ulcer healing and correction of lipodermatosclerosis as well as fading of hyperpigmentation are related to correction of the causes of the changes by surgical maneuvers.

References

1. Douglas WS, Simpson NB (1995) Guidelines for the management of chronic venous leg ulceration. Report of a multidisciplinary workshop. Br J Dermatol 132:446–452
2. Blalock A (1929) Oxygen content of blood in patients with varicose veins. Arch Surg 19:898–905
3. Shami SK, Scurr JH, Coleridge Smith PD (1993) Skin blood flow in chronic venous insufficiency. Phlebology 8:72–76
4. Shami SK, Cheatle TR, Chittenden SJ, Scurr JH, Coleridge Smith PD (1993) Hyperaemic response in the skin microcirculation of patients with chronic venous insufficiency. Br J Surg 80:433–435
5. Anning JT (1954) Leg ulcers: their cause and treatment. Churchill Livingstone, London
6. Debure C. (1993) La maladie post-phlebitique des membres inferieurs: Quoi de neuf en 1993? Actualites D'Angiologie 18;147–150
7. Owens JC (1981) Management of postphlebitic syndrome. Vasc Diagnosis Therapy 3:34–40
8. Mudge M, Leinster SJ, Hughes LE (1988) A prospective 10-year study of the post-thrombotic syndrome in a surgical population. Ann Roy Coll Surg Engl 70:249–252
9. Ludbrook J (1973) Postthrombotic venous obstruction in the lower limb. Editorial. Arch Surg 106:11–12
10. Payne SPK, London NJM, Newland CJ, et al. (1996) Ambulatory venous pressure: Correlation with skin condition and role in identifying surgically correctable disease. Eur J Vasc Endovasc Surg 11:195–200
11. Gourdin FW, Smith Jr J (1993) Etiology of venous ulceration. So Med J 86:1142–1146
12. van Bemmelen PS (1992) In: quantitative measurement of venous incompetence. R.G. Landes Co, Austin p 29
13. Taheri SA, Pendergast D, Lazar E, et al. (1985). Continuous ambulatory venous pressure for diagnosis of venous insufficiency. Am J Surg 150:203–206
14. Raju S, Fredericks R (1991) Hemodynamic basis of stasis ulceration: A hypothesis. J Vasc Surg 13:491–495
15. Negus D (1985) In: Bergan JJ, Yao JST (eds) Surgery of the veins. Grune & Stratton, Orlando, p 196
16. Homans J (1917) The etiology and treatment of varicose ulcer of the leg. Surg Gynecol Obstet 24:300–311
17. Linton RR (1938) The communicating veins of the lower leg and the operative technique for their ligation. Ann Surg 107:582–593
18. Brewer AC (1950) Varicose ulceration. Br Med J ii: 270
19. Bjordal RI (1972) Circulation patterns in incompetent perforating veins in the calf and in the saphenous system to primary varicose veins. Acta Chir Scand 138:251–261
20. Whimster I (1956) Cited in: Dodd H, Cockett FB The pathology and surgery of the veins of the lower limb. Churchill Livingstone London pp 262–266
21. Fearnley G (1965) Fibrinolysis Edward Arnold, London
22. Browse NL, Gray L, Jarrett PEM, Morland M (1977) Blood and vein wall fibrinolytic activity in health and vascular disease. Br Med J i:478–481
23. Wolfe JHN, Morland M, Browse NL (1979) The fibrinolytic activity of varicose veins. Br J Surg 66:185–187
24. Browse NL (1983) Venous ulceration. Br Med J 286:1920–1922
25. Burnand KG (1990) Aetiology of venous ulceration. Br J Surg 77:483–484
26. Michel CC (1990) Aetiology of venous ulceration. Letter to the Editor. Br J Surg 77:1071
27. Coleridge Smith PD, Scurr JH (1990) Aetiology of venous ulceration. Letter to the Editor. Br J Surg 77:1071–1072
28. Layer GT, Stacey MC, Burnand KG (1986) Stanozolol and the treatment of venous ulceration: An interim report. Phlebology 1:197–203
29. Moyses C, Cederholm-Williams SA, Michel CC (1987) Haemoconcentration and the accumulation of white cells in the feet during venous stasis. Int J Microcirc; Clin Exp 5:311–320
30. Coleridge Smith PD (1994) Microcirculation in venous disease. R. G. Landes Co., Austin, pp 192–194
31. Coleridge Smith PD Etiology and pathophysiology of chronic venous insufficiency. http://www.ucl.ac.uk/~rehk999/pdcs htm
32. Wilkinson LS, Bunker C, Edwards JCW, Scurr JH, Coleridge Smith DP (1993) Leukocytes: their role in the etiopathogenesis of skin damage in venous disease. J Vasc Surg 17:669–675
33. Coleridge Smith PD (1994) Venous ulcer. Br J Surg 81:1404–1405
34. Leu AJ, Leu H-J, Franzeck UK, Bollinger A (1995) Microvascular changes in chronic venous insufficiency: A review. Cardiovasc Surg 3:237–245
35. Bradbury AW, Ruckley CV (1993) Role of the leucocyte in the pathogenesis of vascular disease. Br J Surg 80:1503–1512
36. Christopoulos D, Nicolaides AN, Cook A, Irvine A, Galloway JMD, Wilkinson A (1989) Pathogenesis of venous

ulceration in relation to the calf muscle pump function. Surgery 106:829–835

37. Myers KA, Ziegenbein W, Zeng GE, Matthews PG (1995) Duplex ultrasonography scanning for chronic venous disease: Patterns of venous reflux. J Vasc Surg 21:605–612

38. Shami SK, Sarin S, Cheatle TR, Scurr JH, Coleridge Smith PD (1993) Venous ulcers and the superficial venous system. J Vasc Surg 17:487–490

39. Sarin S, Scurr JH, Coleridge Smith PD (1992) Medial calf perforators in venous disease: The significance of outward flow. J Vasc Surg 16:40–46

40. Lees TA, Lambert D (1993) Patterns of venous reflux in limbs with skin changes associated with chronic venous insufficiency. Br J Surg 80:725–728

41. McMullin GM, Scott HJ, Coleridge Smith PD, Scurr JH (1989) A comparison of photoplethysmography, Doppler, and duplex in the assessment of venous insufficiency. Phlebology 4:75–82

42. Darke SG, Penfold C (1992) Venous ulceration and saphenous ligation. Eur J Vasc Surg 6:4–9

43. Hanrahan LM, Araki CT, Rodriguez AA, et al. (1991) Distribution of valvular incompetence in patients with venous stasis ulceration. J Vasc Surg 13:805–812

44. Shami SK, Sarin S, Cheatle TR, Scurr JH, Coleridge Smith PD (1993) Venous ulcers and the superficial venous system. J Vasc Surg 17:487–490

45. Walsh JC, Bergan, Beeman S, Comer TP (1994) Femoral venous reflux abolished by greater saphenous vein stripping. Ann Vasc Surg 8:566–570

46. Goren G (1996) Letter to the Editor – Regarding venous ulcers and the superficial venous system. J Vasc Surg 18:716–719

47. Sales CM, Bilof ML, Petrillo KA, Luka NL (1996) Correction of lower extremity deep venous incompetence by ablation of superficial venous reflux. Ann Vasc Surg 10:186–190

48. Pedberg Jr FT, Pappas PJ, Araki CT, Back TL, Hobson II RW (1996) Hemodynamic and clinical improvement after superficial vein ablation in primary combined venous insufficiency with ulceration. J Vasc Surg 24:711–719

SECTION 2
Clinical Features

Profile 5

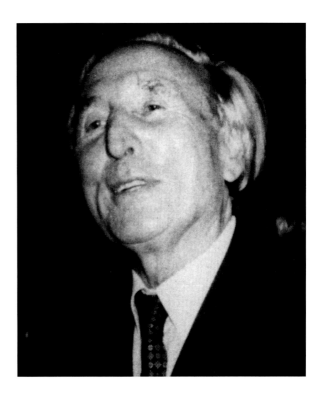

Robert May
1915–1984

The prominent Austrian vascular surgeon Robert May was the leading personality and the grand old man in the German speaking Cosmos of Angiology for decades, until his death in 1984. Almost all of his 230 publications were on venous disease. He authored more than 40 book chapters on evaluation and treatment of venous disorders, and his name is attached to four important textbooks that he co-authored or co-edited with Gottlob (*Venous valves*), with Weber (*Pelvic and abdominal veins* and *Functional phlebology*) and with Nissl (*Phlebography of the lower extremities*).

His experimental work on venous problems started in 1954 in the laboratory of Gottlob in Vienna. In 1956 he was the first, with Thurner, to describe the left iliac vein compression syndrome ("pelvic vein spur"), known in the English literature as Cockett's compression syndrome. He recognized that narrowing or occlusion at the origin of the left common iliac vein is an important cause of left sided "spontaneous" deep venous thrombosis.

His book with Nissl on phlebography, published in 1959, discussed the technical details and importance of ascending and descending phlebography and pelvic phlebography and greatly improved our understanding of deep venous thrombosis and lower extremity varicosity. May's textbook on pelvic and abdominal veins has been for many years the bible of vascular surgeons on how to perform venous thrombectomy, high ligation of the saphenous vein, excision of varicose veins or venous reconstruction for occlusive disease. He pioneered the concept of atraumatic technique.

With his Austrian charm, hard work and enormous productivity, May maintained contact with leading phlebologists and vascular surgeons all over the world, and introduced many new ideas during the 1970s, and 1980s, that became part of our daily work in treating patients suffering from venous disease.

Clinical Presentation and Classification of Chronic Venous Disease 5

Robert L. Kistner and Bo Eklof

Effective communication about diseases of the blood vessels requires a classification that categorizes patients into well-defined groups which can be reliably reproduced. The classification needs to be capable of distinguishing two dissimilar conditions which have the same external appearance by elements in the classification other than the appearance. This is particularly important in chronic venous disease where similar external features, such as discoloration, skin changes, and even ulceration are found in individuals with widely divergent venous pathology. Consider the extremities pictured in Fig. 5.1 and Fig. 5.2. The limb in Fig. 5.1 bears the appearance of the classical "post-phlebitic" leg so often discussed in the literature. This diagnosis when made by external appearance indicates that the patient has had previous deep venous thrombosis followed by some degree of recanalization with the subsequent slow development of discoloration, thickening and ulceration of the skin, and with the probability of swelling and pain as part of the clinical picture. The fact is that a thorough laboratory and phlebographic evaluation, including duplex scanning and ascending phlebography, revealed an absolutely normal venous system. There are no findings of either obstruction or reflux, and no traces of previous superficial or deep venous disease in this patient. The skin changes in this diabetic patient were due to repeated trauma from striking his leg against the rungs of a ladder in his occupation, followed by contusion and scarring over time.

A more frequent example of "mistaken identity" is found in the extremity of the patient in Fig. 5.2.

Again, this extremity has the external manifestations of the advanced post-phlebitic, or post-thrombotic, leg with stasis discoloration, thickening, inflammation and ulceration. Thorough laboratory and phlebographic diagnosis of this patient, including duplex scan, air plethysmography, ascending and descending phlebography, proved the veins to be extensively involved with reflux in the deep, perforator and saphenous distribution but the entire process was due to primary reflux. The saphenous vein had been recently stripped. There was no trace of post-thrombotic disease anywhere in the extremity. The surgical implications and the prognosis are materially different because it is primary rather than secondary post-thrombotic disease in this case.

These are just two examples that could be cited to prove that interpretation based on external appearance alone is bound to contain significant error, and conclusions based upon this type of data will be wrong. Still, external appearance persists as the standard upon which many chronic venous diagnoses are based. With this in mind an international group of experts in chronic venous disease acting as an ad hoc committee of the American Venous Forum devised the CEAP classification in 1994 and have promulgated its adoption around the world.[1,2] The need for this classification grew from the confusion that exists about chronic venous disease because prior methods of classification addressed the clinical appearance in detail, but failed to require definitive evaluation of the Etiology (primary, secondary, or congenital), the Anatomic distribution of the disease in the superficial, perforator, and deep veins, or the Pathophysiologic

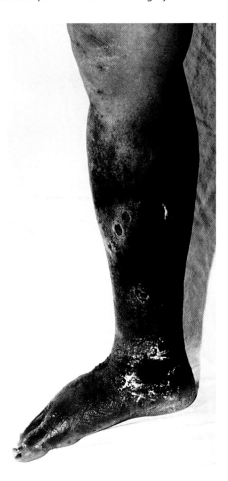

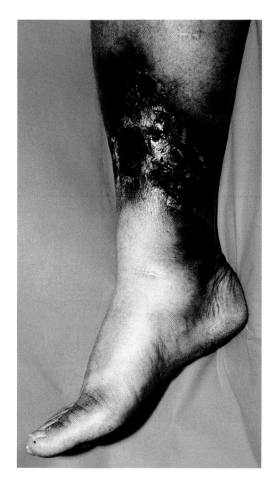

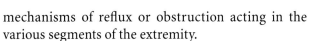

Fig. 5.1. This limb bears the appearance of the "post-phlebitic" extremity but normal veins were found on definitive testing by duplex scan and ascending phlebography. ($C_{4, b-S-}$ E_O A_O P_O)

Fig. 5.2. This limb bears the appearance of the "post-phlebitic" limb but definitive testing of the veins revealed all of the changes were due to primary reflux (non-thrombotic). ($C_{3, 4, 5, 6-S-}$ E_{P-} $A_{S, D, P-}$ $P_{R2, 3, 13, 14, 15, 18}$; disability score, 2; severity score, $19(C_{11}-A_6-D_2.)$

mechanisms of reflux or obstruction acting in the various segments of the extremity.

The concept of a formal venous classification is not new. Prior efforts have consisted of ways to categorize the superficial effects of chronic venous disease, such as varicose veins, skin changes and ulcers. The major venous classifications used in the Western Hemisphere have been those of Widmer[3] in Europe and that which was contained in the Reporting Standards in Venous Disease of the Joint Council of the SVS/ISCVS (Society of Vascular Surgery/International Society of Cardiovascular Surgery) authored by an ad hoc committee under the leadership of John Porter in 1988.[4] Widmer's contribution is a clinical classification of varicose veins and chronic venous insufficiency which offers a visual separation of superficial manifestations but lacks the definitive studies of the deep and

perforator veins to identify etiology, distribution and pathophysiology. The SVS/ISCVS committee's method adds more detail by addressing aspects of the etiology and anatomic distribution of the disease but it does not codify them, nor does it require separation of obstructive from reflux problems; it has been a widely used clinical classification that improved upon previous methods. There was a more detailed classification reported by Sytchev[5] which recognizes each of the four aspects of clinical, etiologic, anatomic, and pathophysiologic mechanisms of venous insufficiency, but it did not achieve wide recognition. In South America there has been an intense interest in classification and there are important contributions, especially in the classification of perforator disease, available in the Spanish language.[6]

Table 5.1. Elements of vascular diagnoses classification

Arterial	Venous	Element
foot ulcer	leg ulcer	C (clinical appearance)
atherosclerosis vs embolic	primary vs post-thrombotic	E (etiology)
femoral-popliteal	deep (fem-pop-tib)	A (anatomic distribution)
stenosis/occlusion	reflux/obstruction	P (pathophysiologic mechanisms)

Requirements for Classification

The elements necessary for a reliable classification of venous disease can be compared to those needed in arterial disease (Table 5.1). For an arterial diagnosis it is customary and routine to identify: the **C**linical problem, e.g., claudication, ulceration, etc.; the **E**tiology of the problem, e.g., arteriosclerosis, arteritis, vasospastic, etc.; the **A**natomic location and its segmental involvement; and the **P**athophysiology, e.g., stenosis/occlusion, aneurysm, embolism, etc. These same elements (CEAP) are needed in the classification of chronic venous disease to facilitate progress toward a scientific analysis of the natural history and the impact of various treatment modalities in chronic venous disease states.

Adoption of a system that requires this amount of detail for venous diagnosis represents a major change in the approach to chronic venous disease and will have to be deemed worthwhile to justify the extra effort involved. The simple fact is that the venous system is at least as complex as the arterial system and requires accurate data if it is to be understood enough to allow definitive surgical therapies to emerge. The choice is to continue to accept the confusion that presently exists from diagnosis based upon visual classification in the interest of keeping the process simple, or to adopt the habit of carefully documenting chronic venous entities with objective testing methods sufficient to satisfy the CEAP requirements because the complexities of the venous system require accurate and reproducible detail to support scientific analysis.

The CEAP Classification

The CEAP classification consists of four elements:

Clinical presentation: classes 1–6 (Table 5.2)

Etiologic basis: primary, secondary, congenital (Table 5.3)

Anatomic distribution: superficial, perforator, deep (Table 5.4A)

The veins are divided into 18 anatomic segments in Table 5.4B

Pathophysiologic basis: reflux, obstruction, both (Table 5.5)

These four elements may be written in shorthand for quick recognition:

$$C_{(1-6)-(S \text{ or } A)}E_{(P,S \text{ or } C)} \ A_{(S,P \text{ and/or } D)}P_{(R,O \text{ or both, with}}$$

affected segments)

Table 5.2. Clinical classification (C_{0-6})

Class 0	No signs of venous disease
Class 1	Telangiectases or reticular veins
Class 2	Varicose veins
Class 3	Edema
Class 4	Skin changes
Class 5	Healed ulceration
Class 6	Active ulceration

Table 5.3. Etiologic classification (E_C, E_P, E_S)

Congenital (E_C)
Primary (E_P) – with undetermined cause
Secondary (E_S) – with known cause, e.g. post-thrombotic

Table 5.4. Anatomic classification (A) and segments (B)

A. Classification

	Superficial Veins (A$_S$)
	Deep Veins (A$_D$)
	Perforating Veins (A$_P$)

B. Eighteen anatomic segments

Segment number	
	Superficial veins (AS)
1	Telangiectases/reticular veins
	Greater (long) saphenous (GSV)
2	Above knee
3	Below knee
4	Lesser (short) saphenous (LSV)
5	Non-saphenous
	Deep veins (AD)
6	Inferior vena cava
	Iliac
7	Common
8	Internal
9	External
10	Pelvic-gonadal, broad ligament, other
	Femoral
11	Common
12	Deep
13	Superficial
14	Popliteal
15	Crural-Anterior tibial, posterior tibial, peroneal (all paired)
16	Muscular-Gastrocnemial, soleal, other
	Perforating veins (AP)
17	Thigh
18	Calf

Table 5.5. Pathophysiologic classification (P$_{R, O}$)

Reflux	(P$_R$)
Obstruction	(P$_O$)
Reflux and obstruction	(P$_{R, O}$)

Table 5.6. Diagnostic methods

Phase 1: history and physical examination
   O.D. = office (hand-held) Doppler
Phase 2: vascular laboratory examination
   D.S. = duplex scan
   APG / PPG = air or photo plethysmography
Phase 3: radiologic examination
   A.P. = ascending phlebography
   D.P. = descending phlebography

Table 5.7. Disability scale

0	Asymptomatic
1	Symptomatic – without support
2	Symptomatic – with support
3	Unable to work – even with support

When the CEAP classification was designed, two rating methods, a disability scale (Table 5.7) and a severity scoring scale (Table 5.8) were devised to aid in estimating the impact of the disease on the life of the patient. These scales are useful adjuncts but are not basic to the CEAP classification itself. The disability scale (Table 5.7) was intended to address the impact the venous problem had on the patient, while the severity scale was devised to gauge the overall clinical and physiologic severity of the problem (Table 5.8). By calculating the severity score which consists of the numerical sum of the clinical severity scale (C#) plus the number of anatomic segments (A#) plus the disability score, it is possible to estimate the relative severity of the clinical problem and to observe changes in the severity with new treatments or new complications.

Table 5.8. Clinical severity scale

Pain	0 = none; 1 = moderate, not requiring analgesics; 2 = severe, requiring analgesics
Edema	0 = none; 1 = mild/moderate; 2 = severe
Venous Claudication	0 = none; 1 = mild/moderate; 2 = severe
Pigmentation	0 = none; 1 = localized; 2 = extensive
Lipodermatosclerosis	0 = none; 1 = localized; 2 = extensive
Ulcer – Size (largest ulcer)	0 = none; 1 = <2 cm diameter; 2 = <2 cm diameter
Ulcer – Duration	0 = none; 1 = <3 months; 2 = >3 months
Ulcer – Recurrence	0 = none; 1 = once; 2 = more than once
Ulcer – Number	0 = none; 1 = single; 2 = multiple

The total severity score (s.s.) is the numerical sum of the clinical severity scale (C) plus the number of anatomic segments (A) plus the disability score (D). (C# + A# + D# = S.S.)

Fig. 5.4. Telangiectasia without other venous disease does not ▶ require more than the simple clinical classification of C_1 and a designation of presence or absence of pain. $C_{1(A/S)}$; disability score, 0; severity score, 0–1

CEAP Examples

1. The CEAP of a typical varicose vein patient is shown in Fig. 5.3

2. The most frequent complaint, that of telangiectasis, is the simplest to classify (Fig. 5.4)

3. A more complicated case of advanced post-thrombotic disease (Fig. 5.5)

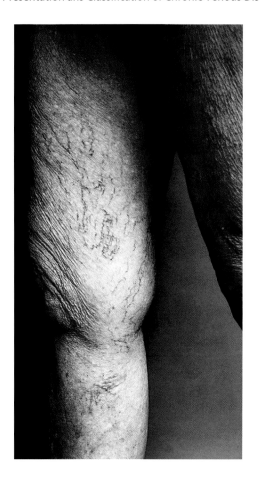

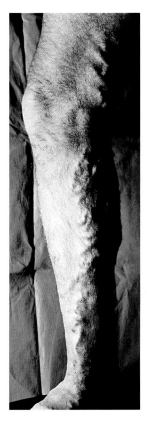

Fig. 5.3. Patient with postural discomfort due to varicose veins and an incompetent greater saphenous vein in an otherwise normal venous system. (C_{2-S} E_{P-} A_{S-} $P_{R2, 3}$; disability score, 0; severity score, $3(C_1–A_2–D_0.)$

Fig. 5.5. Patient with true post-thrombotic extremity including ▶ a history of previous ulceration. Presented with partially disabling aching and swelling and external manifestations of varicose veins and stasis discoloration and thickening of the skin. Work-up revealed post-thrombotic obstruction in the iliac vein and post-thrombotic reflux in the femoral, popliteal, tibial, perforator and saphenous veins. ($C_{2, 3, 4, 5-S-}$ E_{S-} $A_{S, D, P-}$ $P_{R2, 3, 11, 12, 13, 14, 15, O-7, 9}$; disability score, 2; severity score, $18(C_6–A_{10}–D_2)$.

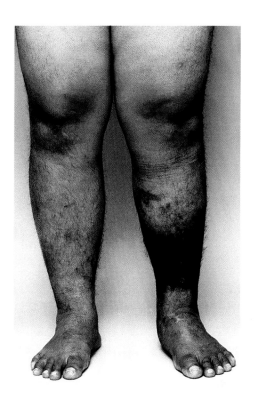

Clinical Use of the CEAP Classification

In diagnosing and formulating treatment for a new case of chronic venous disease a logical sequence is one which begins with identification of the clinical problem and an estimate of its severity, and proceeds by choosing objective tests appropriate to the clinical state, after which the CEAP classification emerges. Treatment alternatives arise from knowledge of the entire venous system taken in context with the individual's way of life and personal needs (Fig. 5.6).

The diagnostic work-up needed for CEAP classification can be conceived as three phases: phase 1 is the office phase and includes history, physical examination, and hand-held Doppler examination; phase 2 is in the vascular laboratory which includes duplex scanning and plethysmography, and the occasional case that requires venous pressure; and phase 3 is radiologic which includes ascending and descending phlebography. These testing levels can be applied to each case according to its complexity and the amount of surgical treatment that might be offered. Phase 1 applies to all chronic venous cases; phase 2 applies to cases that could benefit from individualized treatment; phase 3 is reserved

for surgical cases as preoperative studies to guide the surgeon's choices, and for diagnostic problems that remain after the phase 2 studies.

When reporting the classification it is helpful to know which testing methods were used to make the diagnoses because a different degree of reliability and objectivity belongs to different tests, e.g., duplex scans are more reliable than the hand-held Doppler, and both are different from phlebographic data. This can be achieved by appending abbreviations in Table 5.6 for the diagnostic method(s) used to arrive at a particular CEAP determination and denoting the phase (office, laboratory, radiologic) of diagnostic testing used to determine the CEAP.

It also helps to record the date that the CEAP was determined with the diagnostic method(s) upon which it is based. If additional testing is performed later that changes the diagnosis, the new CEAP can be recorded with a new date, or if a new complication develops it can be recorded with its new date, and in this way a longitudinal record of the disease process develops.

The full presentation of the CEAP classification may appear like this:

CEAP   :   Dx Method   :   Date
                  Disability Score
                  Severity Score

An example from Fig. 5.3:

$C_{2-S}E_{P-}A_{S-}P_{R2,3}$:   Duplex Scan   : 1/4/96
                          Disability Score: 0
                          Severity Score : 3

An example of the CEAP findings of a consecutive series of cases that presented to our clinical practice is illustrated in Fig. 5.7.[7] There was a dominance of primary venous disease and a large number of varicose veins, but still there were 14% with venous ulceration. Reflux clearly is the dominant pathophysiologic problem and the superficial veins are the anatomic site involved in the vast majority of cases. A myriad of additional data about the series and about the individual cases is available in the accumulated data from the CEAP records in these cases.

As a contrast to the findings in the consecutive series of cases with chronic venous insufficiency, Fig. 5.8 depicts the findings in 56 cases of venous ulcer.[8] There is a higher frequency of secondary disease than in the consecutive cases and much more perforator and deep disease. Reflux remains dominant. The superficial veins are involved in most

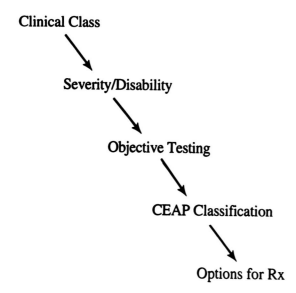

Clinical Class

Severity/Disability

Objective Testing

CEAP Classification

Options for Rx

Fig. 5.6. Practical approach to clinical decision-making in chronic venous disease.

cases while the perforator and deep veins are far more involved than they were in the consecutive cases.

These graphs are presented only as examples of the type of data that accrue from use of the CEAP approach. The data are a true illustration of the precise nature of the vein cases seen in that fragment of the author's practice, but do not constitute a prediction of the distribution in any other series.

Advantages of the CEAP Classification

Through the use of the CEAP classification a number of important advantages accrue:

Accurate, thorough and reproducible diagnoses are obtained. The detail demanded by the classification renders a complete diagnosis of the entire venous tree. Inclusion of the diagnostic method and the date delineates the statistical reliability of the CEAP at a given time. Inclusion of the disability and severity scores delineates the impact of the disease process on that individual.

The method is readily programmed into a format suitable for a data base that facilitates analysis of a series of cases. In our clinical practice two series were analyzed to show the general description of our patient experience over a stretch of 102 consecutive cases (Fig. 5.7) and a separate group to detail the types of cases that constituted a consecutive series of 56 venous ulcer cases (Fig. 5.8). These are small data bases and do not constitute a statistically important experience from which to draw conclusions about the general nature of chronic venous disease, but they do allow specific analysis of our cases that can easily be compared to cases from any other institution. With similar analyses from multiple institutions it would soon be possible to analyze a large experience of venous cases and begin to formulate statistically significant observations. The CEAP approach can become the basis for reliable inter-institutional communication.

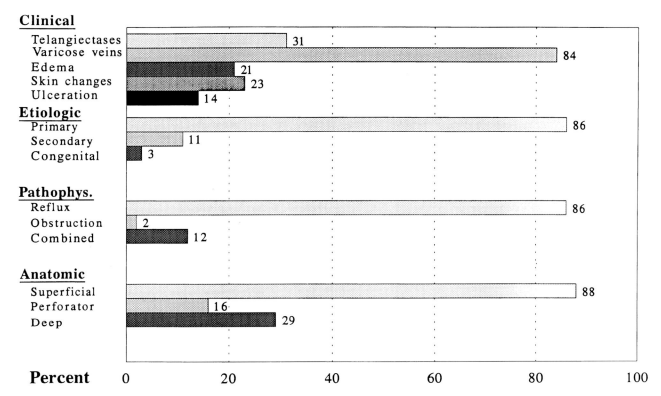

Fig. 5.7. Clinical, etiologic, anatomic, and pathophysiologic (CEAP) data for the total series (102 extremities) in this study. (Reprinted from: Kistner RL, Eklof B, Masuda EM Diagnosis of chronic venous disease of the lower extremities: The "CEAP" classification. Mayo Clinic Proceedings 1996;71:338–345.)

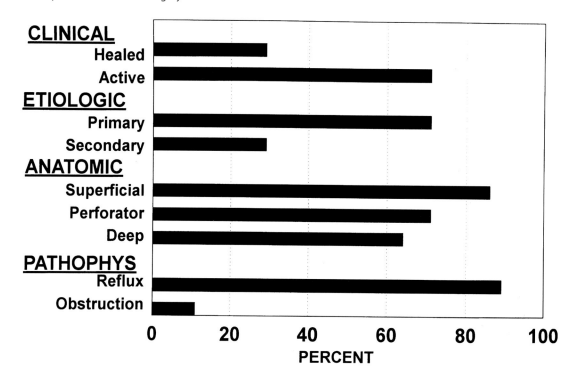

Fig. 5.8. The CEAP classification in 56 cases of venous ulceration. (Reprinted from: Kistner RL Definitive diagnosis and definitive treatment in chronic venous disease: A concept whose time has come. J Vasc. Surg 1996;24:703–710.)

Longitudinal observation of the patients is facilitated to observe the clinical course and learn the natural history in an individual or in any category such as primary reflux, secondary reflux or obstruction, reflux in the thigh *vs* the calf, and any other combination of the many variables in the classification.

Communication between individuals and institutions alike is readily achieved, bound only by the limitations of the diagnostic methods used to create diagnoses.

References

1. American Venous Forum (1996) Classification and grading of chronic venous disease in the lower limb. A consensus statement. Vasc Surg 30:5–11

2. Prepared by an Ad Hoc Committee at the American Venous Forum 6th Annual Meeting in February 1994 (1995) Classification and grading of chronic venous disease in the lower limbs: A consensus statement. Phlebology 10:42–45

3. Widmer LK (1978) Classification of venous disorders. Peripheral Venous Disorders Basel III. Hans Huber, Bern

4. Porter JM, Rutherford RB, Claggett GP et al. (1988) NA-ISCVS/SVS Ad Hoc Committee on Reporting Standards in Venous Disease. R. Rutherford, Chairman Ad Hoc Committee. Reporting standards in venous disease. J Vasc Surg 8:172–181

5. Sytchev GG (1985) Classification of chronic venous disorders of lower extremities and pelvis. International Angiology 4:203–206

6. Enrici EA, Caldevilla HS (1992) Classificacion de la Insuficiencia venosa cronica. In: Enrici EA, Caldevilla HS (eds) Insuficiencia Venosa Cronica de los Miembros Inferiores. Editorial Celcius, pp 107–114

7. Kistner RL et al. (1996) Diagnosis of chronic venous disease of the lower extremities: The "CEAP" classification. Mayo Clinic Proceedings 71:338–345

8. Kistner RL (1996) Definitive diagnosis and definitive treatment in chronic venous disease: A concept whose time has come. J Vasc Surg 24:703–10

Profile

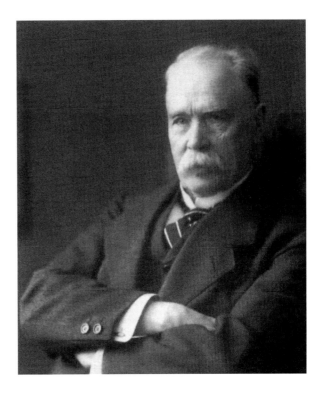

Friedrich Trendelenburg
1844–1924

Best known for the "Trendelenburg position" to everyone in medicine, Friedrich Trendelenburg personified the master surgeon, scholar and teacher. He was born in Berlin on 24 May, 1844 into a family of educators and spent his formative years in Scotland. It was during this time that he became acquainted with James Simpson, who had introduced chloroform as an anesthetic agent in 1847, and with Joseph Lister, the father of antisepsis, who had a profound influence upon him.

He received his medical degree from the University of Berlin at age 22. Following submission of his inaugural thesis on Ancient Indian Surgery he was appointed first assistant to the world renowned surgeon von Langenbeck. At the age of 31, Trendelenburg was invited to the University of Rostock as professor of surgery. This period served as a beginning for his later contributions to vascular and general surgery. It was the true origin of his prolific career which was continued by his appoint-

ment at the University of Bonn at the age of 38.

Friedrich Trendelenburg's works include observations on varicose veins, thrombophlebitis, esophageal stricture, ectropy of the bladder, diseases of the bones and joints, vesicovaginal fistula, and plastic repair of the ureter for hydronephrosis. One test and three operations that bear his name have greatest meaning in the field of vascular diseases. Trendelenburg's test determines insufficiency of the valves in varicose veins and the superficial and the deep systems. The first Trendelenburg operation was for the excision of varicose veins; the second for ligation of the greater saphenous vein to prevent reflux into varicose veins. However, the most dramatic procedure of all that bears his name is pulmonary embolectomy. Friedrich Trendelenburg reported this in 1908 while he worked at the University of Leipzig. Although none of his three operated patients survived, credit belongs to him for his conceptualization and daring attempt at this still difficult procedure.

Plethysmographic Evaluation of Venous Function

6

Clifford T. Araki, Atsushi Seyama and Robert W. Hobson II

Introduction

It is widely recognized that venous hypertension is generated by a combination of valvular incompetence, venous obstruction, and calf muscle pump dysfunction. The status of the deep and superficial veins in both the proximal and distal segments can have significant impact on the success of perforator vein surgery. Prior to operation, detailed knowledge of the pattern of venous obstruction and incompetence can help establish the likelihood of successful treatment. Postoperative assessment may uncover the changes in limb hemodynamics affected by perforator ligation.

With the current state of technology, much of this information can be obtained non-invasively through a combination of ultrasound and plethysmographic testing. Ultrasound provides its best data on the hemodynamics in specific vein segments. Plethymography extends the information to overall leg hemodynamics in a fashion complementary to ultrasound. Because plethysmographic measurements tend to be more objective, data on the changes in the hemodynamic status of the insufficient limb with perforator ligation may be best obtained through plethysmography.

Diagnostic protocols using plethysmographic equipment are based on inducing transitory changes in venous volume and thus venous flow. Because the measurement of volume changes is common to all methods, there are protocol similarities.

To review the role of plethysmographic testing prior to and following endoscopic perforator vein surgery, we describe the modalities which can be applied. The major concentration of the chapter is on the descriptive correlation of plethysmographic results with the underlying hemodynamic pathophysiology.

One particular advantage of plethysmography lies in its ability to quantitatively evaluate the short and long term effects of surgery. By plotting capacitance and outflow over time, the degree of recanalization can be determined by its relationship to the discriminant line. To date, no other method quantitates the changes in insufficiency afforded by surgery.

Instrumentation

Plethsmography for venous disease addresses the diagnosis of outflow obstruction, valvular incompetence, and calf muscle pump dysfunction. The major forms of clinically applied plethysmography include air plethysmography, photoplethysmography and impedance plethysmography, with air plethysmography currently the most popular.

Air Plethysmography. The air plethysmograph (APG) measures volume displacement as a change in pressure of an air filled plastic sleeve encasing the limb segment (typically the calf). The sleeve is inflated to 6 mmHg which is just sufficient to hold it securely in place. The system is calibrated to limb volume with the injection of a known volume of air into the sleeve and the measurement of the resultant increase in pressure.

Photoelectric Plethysmography. Photoplethysmography (PPG) is used to qualitatively assess the change in blood volume in cutaneous tissue. The PPG electrode is composed of an infrared light emitting diode and a photosensor. Light transmitted into the skin is absorbed and scattered by tissues in the illuminated field. Blood, being more opaque than surrounding tissue, attenuates the reflected light in greater proportion. The intensity of reflected light changes with tissue blood density.

Impedance Plethysmography. Impedance plethysmography (IPG) is performed by measuring the resistance to a weak electrical current passed through the limb. As limb venous volume increases, electrical resistance decreases. Typically, the IPG measurement is made for midcalf volume changes. Four circumferential electrode bands are placed around each calf. The outer pair of electrodes applies a weak alternating current. The inner electrode pair is used to determine the electrical resistance offered by the limb segment. Because the IPG passes an alternating current through the limb, the flow of electrons is impeded by resistive, capacitive and inductive elements. The latter two are reactive to the alternating current but the major portion of the impedance is resistive. Results are quantified in resistive units which are not easily translated into volume. Still, when short duration volume changes are induced, limb impedance changes are mainly caused by shifts in venous blood volume.

All forms of plethysmography applied to chronic venous insufficiency (CVI) testing provide some form of quantitative information. Plethysmography is used to evaluate venous outflow, overall venous incompetence, and calf muscle pump function. Quantifiable data allow statistical comparisons among limbs and serial evaluation of the same limb. Results can be used to observe the effects of treatment and to follow disease progression or recanalization. While invasive, ultrasonographic, and plethysmographic testing have been criticized for not being able to fully account for the severity of venous disorder, this may be a result of the uncertainty associated with the pathophysiology of CVI.

Venous Outflow Obstruction

An assessment of the venous outflow status of the limb should be made prior to any venous surgery, since any ablative procedure may be to the detriment of the limb if venous outflow is impaired. Plethysmography provides the best objective measure of outflow obstruction.

Plethysmography techniques assess the degree of obstruction by measuring the maximal rate of venous outflow from a calf with full venous engorgement. The lower extremity is elevated above heart level, with knees flexed and the hips externally rotated. A pneumatic cuff, placed around the thigh, is inflated to a pressure of 50 mmHg to 80 mmHg. This compression maintains arterial inflow while occluding venous outflow. Calf venous volume increases until distal venous pressure equals the cuff pressure. Once venous volume reaches a stable plateau, the thigh cuff is rapidly vented. The entire duration of calf volume changes is traced from pre-occlusive baseline, through plateau, to the decrease in calf volume with cuff venting, to its return to baseline.

Two measurements are extracted from the tracing: (1) venous volume or capacitance, as the difference between the volume plateau and baseline and (2) the rate of venous outflow, as the volume or resistance measured at 1 to 3 sec after the release of the thigh cuff (Fig. 6.1). Venous volume or capacitance is used as a correction which standardizes outflow among limbs. Assuming no increase in central venous pressure, the rate of outflow is then determined by the resistance to flow offered by the venous outflow channels of the limb. Normality is depicted graphically using an empirically derived discriminant line, which separates normal outflow rates relative to venous volume (Outflow *vs* Capacitance) from the abnormally reduced outflow.[1,2]

The general protocol developed for the IPG was modified for the APG which is used for CVI testing.[3] APG measurements of capacitance and outflow are used to calculate an index called Outflow Fraction (OF) which is the outflow volume at 1 sec divided by the total volume. Venous outflow is considered unobstructed if 40% or more of the retained venous volume is drained from the calf within one second of the release of the thigh cuff pressure.

Venous outflow measurements have a relatively high false-positive rate which can be reduced by patient positioning, the use of longer filling intervals, and by repetitive testing at each examination.[4]

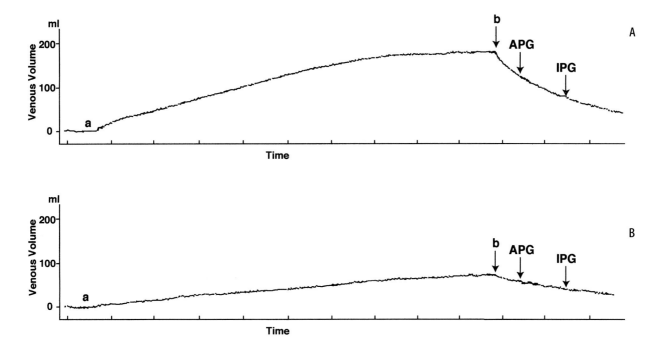

Fig. 6.1. Venous obstruction is measured through a function which combines venous capacitance and venous outflow. **A** depicts the normal outflow pattern. With thigh cuff venous occlusion (a) venous filling is allowed to continue to full or near full capacitance. Release of cuff pressure (b) provokes venous outflow from the calf. Outflow volume is determined as the difference between plateau and outflow at 1 second (APG) or at 3 seconds (IPG). Capacitance is determined as the difference in volume between plateau (b) and baseline (a). In **B** acute or chronic obstruction can cause a reduction in both capacitance and outflow.

Valvular Incompetence

Plethysmographic testing for incompetence and calf muscle pump function have been developed to duplicate the measurement of ambulatory venous pressure (AVP) non-invasively. Techniques used to measure AVP have long been considered the gold standard by which a limb should be evaluated for chronic venous insufficiency. In past decades, assessment for calf pump function were only available invasively through AVP measurements. This was measured using a needle inserted into a vein in the dorsum of the foot. The effectiveness of the calf muscle pump is determined by the reduction in foot venous pressure brought on by exercise. An efficient calf pump will reduce AVP to below 40 mmHg.[5] A second measurement, obtained in the immediate post-exercise period, is found in the return of foot venous pressure to a normal baseline standing pressure of greater than 80 mmHg. With competent valves, the return of venous pressure to baseline takes longer than 20 sec.[6] With valvular incompetence, venous reflux overwhelms the relatively slow refill through the arterial

system, leading to shorter refill times which are consistent with greater incompetence.

Since the early 1970s there have been numerous attempts to replace invasive AVP measurement with non-invasive methods. APG testing provides the most comprehensive plethysmographic assessment for CVI (Fig. 6.2). Through the calculation of venous refill time, ejection fraction, and residual volume fraction, plethysmography offers the best quantitation of calf hemodynamics for CVI assessment.

Venous Refill Time

If calf veins are emptied of blood by elevation or calf exercise, the time to complete venous filling is determined by the rate of arterial inflow and by the ability of venous valves to prevent the backflow of blood into the calf. This timed measurement is found in the return of venous pressure to the foot with AVP measurement and is also seen in the return to a stable venous volume in the calf through plethysmography.

Several plethysmographic modalities can be adapted to measure the rate of venous filling in the

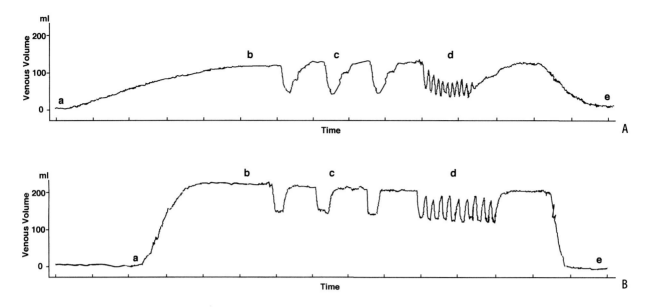

Fig. 6.2. An APG examination for insufficiency has three components. **A** displays the results of a normal APG examination. The tracing begins with the patient in supine position with leg elevated. The minimum calf volume obtained (a) serves as baseline. The patient shifts to a standing position to determine the maximum calf volume (b). After a period of quiet standing, patient is asked to perform three separate standing tip-toe maneuvers (c). This is followed by 10 tip-toes, in one second intervals (d). After the APG volume stabilizes, the patient returns to the supine position with leg elevated (e) to re-establish baseline. In **B** are the results of an APG examination performed on a CVI limb. Compared to the normal limb (**A**), venous incompetence allows a rapid increase in calf venous volume when the patient switches from supine to standing (interval a–b). In single standing tip-toe maneuvers (c), the CVI limb ejects less venous volume from the limb. Repetitive tip-toe exercise (d), demonstrates that a greater than normal blood volume remains in the calf in the CVI limb throughout a maximal exercise.

calf. In many techniques, the patient is tested while sitting or standing. The patient performs a repetitive, stationary calf exercise using knee bends or ankle flexions. The most common protocol, described for the PPG,[7] is performed with the patient sitting, with legs dependent, and feet non-weight-bearing. The PPG electrode is taped to the ankle, 10 cm above the medial malleolus. The patient is asked to perform plantar/dorsiflexion maneuvers at 1 sec intervals for 5 repetitions, then to relax and allow the passive refilling of calf veins.

Using the APG, venous reflux is determined by the rate of refill rather than refill time. The patient is made to shift from a supine position with the leg elevated to a standing position with the leg unweighted.[3] The air pressure in the APG pneumatic sleeve is recorded throughout the maneuver. Normal (Fig. 6.3) venous filling can be distinguished from abnormal (Figs 6.4 and 6.5) by the swiftness with which a venous volume plateau is reached.

A 90% of total venous volume is used to aid in the determination of the venous filling time endpoint. Not infrequently, the volume tracing incorporates a drift which obscures the venous volume plateau.

This is often true in PPG tracings. By using the 90% venous volume, the volume endpoint is shifted to a steeper portion of the filling curve and the error associated with locating the endpoint in filling time is reduced.

If PPG is used to determine incompetence, the PPG electrode should be placed distally in the leg. Published reports have demonstrated that regional venous dysfunction exists and distal valvular incompetence appeared important. Shorter refill times have been demonstrated in normal limbs at midcalf than at the ankle. Ankle refill times also appeared more strongly affected by incompetence and may be more clinically relevant measures of incompetence.[8,9]

The use of a tourniquet to exclude superficial reflux and to evaluate the deep system separately appears to have unpredictable results. Many have found the technique unreliable.[10,11] A major problem lies in the lack of an empirically derived standard for the application of a tourniquet. Tourniquets have taken the form of pneumatic cuffs, latex ligatures, or wedged velcro straps applied at different known or unknown tensions. Tourniquets have been applied above knee, below knee and segmentally to isolate

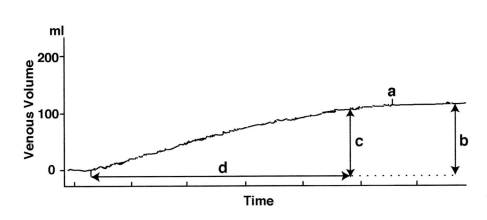

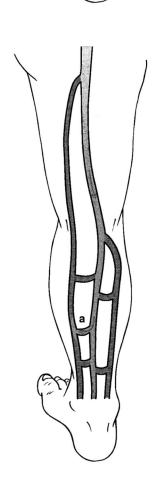

Fig. 6.3. After venous emptying, refilling of normal calf veins is primarily determined by arterial inflow. The slow inflow into the venous system lengthens the time before venous volume and pressure reach a plateau. The venous filling tracing can be obtained through PPG using a series of foot dorsiflexions. A venous refill time (a) greater than 23 sec is considered evidence of a competent venous system (blue). Using APG, a Venous Filling Index (VFI) is calculated. The total venous volume (b) is determined to calculate the 90% total venous volume (c). The time to reach 90% of total venous volume is then determined from the tracing (d). VFI is then calculated as: VFI = c/d ml/sec).

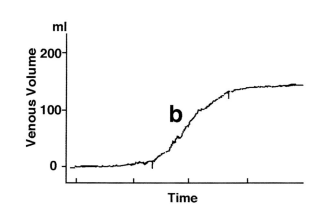

Fig. 6.4. Deep vein incompetence can greatly increase the rate of venous filling. Retrograde flow through the deep system fills the incompetent deep segments (green). With a competent superficial system (blue), reflux into the superficial system requires one or more incompetent perforators (a). Venous incompetence is indicated by a VFI greater than 2 ml/sec. A steep slope (b) in the venous filling curve is associated with a greater level of incompetence. By PPG, a venous refill time less than 20 sec is consistent with venous valvular incompetence.

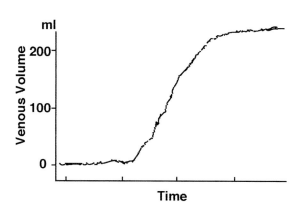

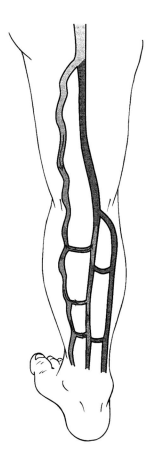

Fig. 6.5. Calf venous filling index in a limb with superficial vein incompetence. With normal perforator flow from superficial to deep, retrograde flow through an incompetent superficial vein (green) will also fill the deep system through competent perforators. In a limb with extensive superficial incompetence, both deep and superficial systems will fill rapidly. Large increases in venous volume will also be evident with the presence of vein varicosities. The magnitude of this effect may be particularly evident when switching from supine to standing.

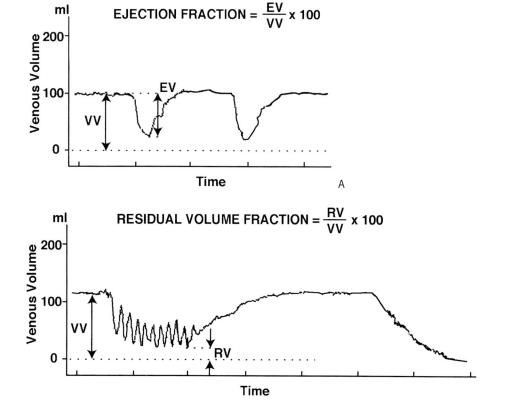

$$\text{EJECTION FRACTION} = \frac{EV}{VV} \times 100$$

A

$$\text{RESIDUAL VOLUME FRACTION} = \frac{RV}{VV} \times 100$$

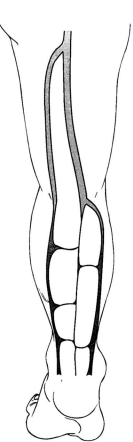

B

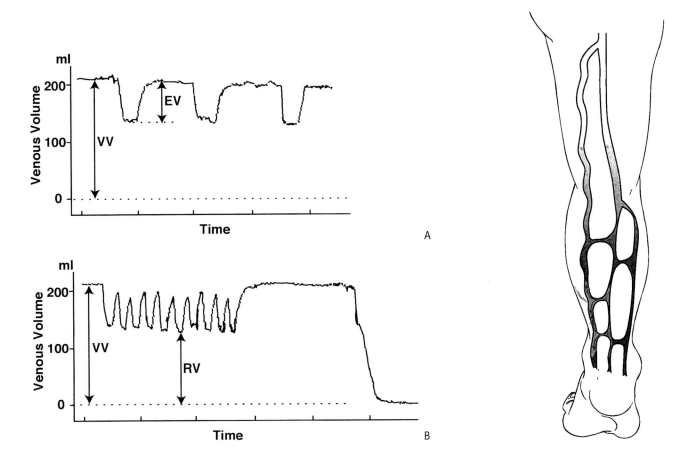

A

B

the level of incompetence. In most applications, the actual impact of the tourniquet on the underlying deep and superficial vasculature while the test was being performed was not known.

Calf Muscle Pump Function

Plethysmographic testing for venous refill time has been extensively researched. While various reports have evaluated expelled volumes from the calf to

---

Fig. 6.6. With a good calf muscle pump, most of the venous blood in the calf is ejected during maximal exercise. The percentage of blood volume ejected with calf contraction can be determined through plethysmography. As shown in **A**, Ejection Fraction is determined from a single maximal calf muscle contraction by having the patient stand on tiptoes. A normal calf muscle pump should be able to eject more than 60% of the venous volume (green). The percentage of venous volume which cannot be extracted from the leg (blue) is determined as the Residual Volume Fraction (**B**). This retained volume is determined through a series of 10 standing tiptoe maneuvers.

Fig. 6.7. In a limb with a poor calf muscle pump, EF is reduced (**A**) and RVF is increased (**B**). Superficial varicosities, lacking skeletal muscle investments, are not completely compressed. Their contribution increases total venous volume (VV) and residual volume (RV) but decreases ejection volume (EV). Calf muscle pump efficiency is also limited by inadequate ankle flexion and perforator incompetence (green). As drawn, superficial varicosities, incompetent perforators, and reduced ankle flexion will increase the residual volume (blue) and diminish the ejection volume (light blue).

explain calf pump action, until recently non-invasive testing of the calf muscle pump has not been well addressed. The best non-invasive evaluation of calf muscle pump function has been through the APG measurement (Fig. 6.6) of ejection fraction (EF) and residual volume fraction (RVF).[3]

Using the APG protocol, once the total venous volume in the calf is determined, the effectiveness of the calf muscle pump can be determined by weighing the percentage of venous volume ejected by the calf against the percent venous volume which cannot be expelled. For this assessment, the Ejection Volume of the calf is measured as the volume of blood ejected by a single maximal calf muscle contraction when the patient is standing on tiptoes. The

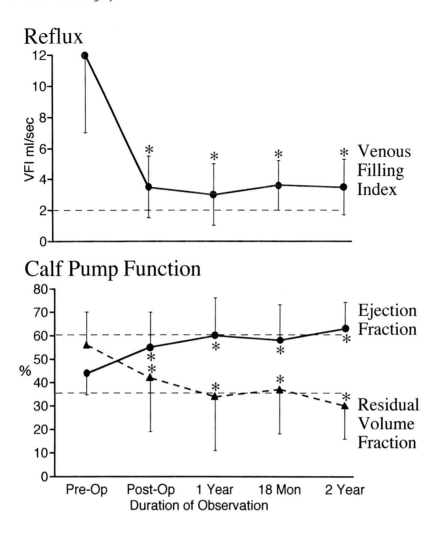

Fig. 6.8. Perforator ligation accompanied by superficial vein stripping and ligation resulted in a significant improvement in calf muscle pump function and a reduction in venous reflex in eleven limbs with venous ulcerations. Serial plethysmographic testing was performed with up to 2 years of post-operative follow-up (5 limbs). Comparisons with preoperative values demonstrated the effects of venous ablation to be significant and long lasting (means + SD; * P <0.05 compared to pre-op). (From Padberg FT, Pappas PJ, Araki CT, Back TL, Hobson RW (1996) Hemodynamic and clinical improvement after superficial vein ablation in primary combined venous insufficiency with ulceration. J Vasc Surg, 1996; 24: 711–8, with permission)

venous volume retained in the calf during contraction is determined through a series of 10 standing tiptoe maneuvers. This volume is called Residual Volume. Chronic venous insufficiency tends to be accompanied by a decrease in calf muscle pump efficiency (Fig. 6.7). Studies have shown a clinically relevant relationship between venous ulceration, calf muscle pump dysfunction, and restricted ankle range of motion (Fig. 6.8).[14,15]

The protocol for measuring residual volume was developed as the plethysmographic equivalent to the AVP measurement. Presumably, the lowest residual venous volume retained in the calf during exercise corresponds to the lowest ambulatory venous pressure attained when walking. A linear correlation between AVP and RVF of $r = 0.83$ has been reported and other forms of plethysmography have shown similar correlation with AVP and AVP-venous refill time.[13]

While non-invasive volumetric testing is used as an alternative to invasive pressure measurement, substitution assumes a linear correlation between pressure and volume. There are significant departures from linearity at both ends of the pressure-volume curve. When the calf veins are emptied and venous volume is low, large increases in volume may not be associated with significant increases in pressure. On the other end of the curve, with extensive incompetence and increased venous pressure, venous volume may be near full capacitance. Increases in venous pressure may not be reflected in increases in volume. This has been shown with a distinct nonlinear relationship between venous refill time and AVP.[12]

In APG testing, important measurements are indexed to total venous volume. OF, VFI, EF, and RVF are all affected by the venous volume contained in a leg. Volume measurements are highly variable, particularly between patients with and without CVI.[3] Indexing, notably in the calculation of EF and RVF, greatly improves the comparability of data among limbs.

Conclusion

While duplex ultrasound provides good segmental assessment of venous reflux, it is yet unable to quantify total limb hemodynamics. Plethysmography continues to have an important role in the assessment of chronic venous insufficiency. Furthermore, its use is complementary to ultrasound testing. Ultrasound provides direct information on the distribution of valvular reflux. However, its assessment of outflow obstruction and the severity of incompetence is qualitative and suggestive. Plethysmographic testing has provided and will continue to provide reliable quantitative information on overall venous insufficiency. Serial use of plethysmography has confirmed significant improvements in limb hemodynamics following perforator ligation and superficial vein stripping[16] which are otherwise difficult to demonstrate. It may prove to be the most reliable means for evaluating the hemodynamic effect of perforator surgery.

References

1. Wheeler HB, O'Donnell JA, Anderson FA, Benedict K (1974) Occlusive impedance phlebography: a diagnostic procedure for venous thrombosis and pulmonary embolism. Prog Cardiovasc Dis 17:199–205
2. Hull R, van Aken WG, Hirsh J, Gallus AS, Hoicka G, et al. (1976) Impedance plethysmography using the occlusive cuff technique in the diagnosis of venous thrombosis Circulation 53:696–700
3. Christopoulos DG, Nicolaides AN, Szendro G, Irvine AT, Bull M, Eastcott HHG (1987) Air-plethysmography and the effect of elastic compression on venous hemodynamics of the leg. J Vasc Surg 5:148–159
4. Hull R, Taylor DW, Hirsh J, Sackett DL, Powers P, Turpie AGG, Walker I (1978) Impedance Plethysmography: the relationship between venous filling and sensitivity and specificity for proximal vein thrombosis. Circulation 58:898–902
5. Christopoulos D, Nicolaides AN, Cook A, Irvine A, Galloway JMD, Wilkinson A (1989) Pathogenesis of venous ulceration in relation to the calf muscle pump function. Surgery 106:829–835
6. Schanzer H, Peirce EC (1982) A rational approach to the chronic venous stasis syndrome. Ann Surg 195:25–29
7. Abramowitz HB, Queral LA, Flinn WR, Nora PF, Peterson LK, Bergan JJ, et al. (1979) The use of photoplethysmography in the assessment of venous insufficiency: A comparison to venous pressure measurements. Surgery 86:434–441
8. Struckman JR, Mathiesen FR (1985) A noninvasive plethysmographic method for evaluation of the musculovenous pump in the lower extremities. Acta Chir Scand 151:235–240
9. Rosfors S, Lamke LO, Nordstrom E, Bygdeman S (1990) Severity and location of venous valvular insufficiency: The importance of distal valve function. Acta Chir Scand 156:689–694
10. Neglen P, Raju S (1993) A rational approach to detection of significant reflux with duplex Doppler scanning and air plethysmography. J Vasc Surg 17:590–595
11. van Bemmelen PS, Mattos MA, Hodgson KJ, Barkmeier LD, Ramsey DE, Faught WE, et al. (1993) Does air plethysmography correlate with duplex scanning patients with chronic venous insufficiency? J Vasc Surg 18:796–807
12. Nicolaides AN, Miles C (1987) Photoplethysmography in the assessment of venous insufficiency. J Vasc Surg 5:405–412
13. Araki CT, Back TL, Meyers MG, Hobson RW (1995) Indirect Noninvasive Tests (Plethysmography). In: Gloviczki P, Yao SJT (eds) The Handbook of Venous Disorders, Guidelines of The American Venous Forum. Chapman & Hall, London, pp 97–111
14. Araki CT, Back TL, Padberg FT, Thompson PN, Duran WN, Jamil Z, et al. (1994) The significance of calf muscle pump function in venous ulceration. J Vasc Surg 20:872–879
15. Back TL, Padberg FT, Araki CT, Thompson PN, Hobson RW (1995) Limited range of motion is a significant factor in venous ulceration. J Vasc Surg 22:519–523
16. Padberg FT, Pappas PJ, Araki CT, Back TL, Hobson RW (1996) Hemodynamic and clinical improvement after superficial vein ablation in primary combined venous insufficiency with ulceration. J Vasc Surg, 24:711–718

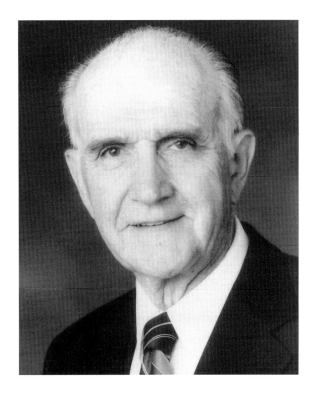

John J. Cranley Jr.
b. 1918

Although coming from a New York City background, Jack Cranley's interest in vascular surgery in general, and venous pathophysiology in particular, was shaped by his experience in the institution of the Massachusetts General Hospital and the personal influence of Robert R. Linton.

By the time Cranley was assigned to the vascular service of Dr Linton, he had completed education at Boston College and Columbia University. His internship was at the Boston City Hospital but in the United States Navy he served at the San Diego Naval Hospital and then on an animal research ship at the time of the first peace-time atom explosion at the Bikini atoll. Cranley's two-year fellowship at the Massachusetts. General Hospital following surgical training included the development of the vascular laboratory with Dr F. A. Simeone and Dr Linton. At the end of the first year of the fellowship, Simeone left for obligations in Cleveland and thus Dr Jack Cranley became the first director of a vascular laboratory in the United States.

After establishing his vascular practice in Cincinnati in association with Dr Louis G. Herrmann, he founded a vascular laboratory at the University of Cincinnati in 1952. Subspecialization in vascular surgery was not consonant with the surgical philosophies of the chief of surgery at the University of Cincinnati, Dr William Altemeier. Therefore, Cranley established his vascular service at the Good Samaritan Hospital and once again set up his vascular laboratory there. He continued as a University professor, heading the vascular clinic for a number of years and continuing classroom teaching of medical students. Very rapidly, under Cranley's direction, vascular surgery flourished in Cincinnati and at the Good Samaritan Hospital. The vascular laboratory grew to become a 17-room suite. Soon a vascular fellowship was established, and proved to be one of the first in this country. A privately funded varicose vein clinic was established under the direction of the Kachelmacher Foundation in Logan, Ohio.

Cranley's interest in venous ulcers is credited to Dr Linton and the vascular clinic at the Massachusetts General Hospital. During his entire 35 years of private practice, this interest continued. This had led to the well-known Cranley dicta that all venous ulcers will heal, 95% can be healed in an ambulatory program with pressure bandages, and that superficial venous incompetence can cause a number of venous ulcers which can be healed by radical removal of the superficial reflux. Very few recurrences will occur in such patients but the results are not as good if the patient's ulcer is derived from deep venous thrombosis or if the patient has an episode of deep venous thrombosis.

Cranley's experience with over 300 subfascial perforator vein ligations stands as one of the largest in the world. He has documented a 66% rate of permanent cure and feels that 33% recurrences were associated with deep venous insufficiency. Of some interest is his prescient observation that complete disappearance of the heavy brown pigmentation may occur in long-term follow-up of patients whose perforator vein incompetence has been eliminated by subfascial interruption.

Cranley says, "I think that the most important development in my surgical lifetime has been duplex scanning. Before that, we only had functional tests. Although the mainstay of diagnosis of deep venous thrombosis has been phleborheography even this was discouraged as soon as duplex scanning became available."

Preoperative Evaluation of Chronic Venous Insufficiency with Duplex Scanning and Venography

7

Peter Gloviczki, Bradley D. Lewis, John R. Lindsey and Michael A. McKusick

Preoperative evaluation of patients who suffer from chronic venous disease due to previous deep venous thrombosis or primary valvular incompetence has substantially changed in the last decade. Color duplex scanning is now widely available, and it has become the most useful preoperative test for evaluation of chronic venous insufficiency. We reserve contrast venography for those patients who have evidence of significant deep venous occlusion or for those who are potential candidates for deep vein reconstructions. In this chapter we will discuss advantages of duplex scanning over other diagnostic tests and present techniques of duplex examination we use to confirm valvular incompetence in leg veins. We also discuss current indications and technical details of ascending and descending contrast venography.

Duplex Scanning

The combination of B-mode ultrasound imaging with pulsed Doppler is an excellent non-invasive technique to evaluate valvular incompetence of the superficial, deep and perforating veins of the leg. Although real time B-mode imaging alone is able to diagnose venous obstruction, duplex scanning is required to establish the presence of bidirectional flow in the venous system. Spectral analysis confirms presence or absence of venous flow, it demonstrates direction of flow, and confirms flow patterns.[1-3] The addition of color Doppler to imaging has simplified the examination, shortened its time and made localization of blood vessels and recognition of both venous obstruction and valvular incompetence easier.[4-6] Color Doppler permits rapid determination of flow direction even in small or tortuous perforating veins, where the use of pulsed Doppler may be more difficult and time consuming. The information provided is mostly qualitative, although attempts to quantitate both valvular reflux and obstruction have been published in recent years.[2,4,6-8] The anatomic details provided by duplex scanning may be inferior to those rendered by contrast venography, but the test is non-invasive, free of complications, repeatable and provides sufficient information to indicate appropriate surgical intervention in most patients with chronic venous disease. It is also suitable to follow patients postoperatively to identify acute venous thrombosis, to confirm missed or newly developed incompetent perforators and to study changes in valvular incompetence of the deep veins as a result of ablation of an incompetent superficial and perforator system. Since isolated venous segments are studied, duplex scanning does not define global venous function of the limb. Therefore, we continue to use plethysmographic tests in addition to duplex scanning for preoperative evaluation of calf pump function, global superficial and deep venous incompetence and to exclude functional venous outflow obstruction, using techniques detailed in the previous chapter of this volume.

Technique of Examination

Patient Positioning

During the examination the patient stands in a 60° to 80° near upright position on a tilted examination table with the extremity to be examined abducted and externally rotated, with weight-bearing on the opposite extremity (Fig. 7.1A). A pneumatic cuff, connected to an automatic inflator is placed on the calf of the patient (Fig. 7.1B). The examination is performed with a 5 or 7 MHz linear array transducer.

Venous Flow Augmentation

To ascertain valvular incompetence, venous flow must be augmented and prolonged retrograde flow confirmed during the relaxation phase. Incompetence is confirmed if the duration of retrograde flow exceeds 1.0 sec.[1] Competence of proximal valves can be evaluated using the Valsalva maneuver, but with this technique normal deep vein valves do not close at all levels.[8] Flow can also be augmented manually, compressing the calf or thigh of the patient, distal to the probe. However, an automatic pneumatic cuff placed on the calf is the best technique

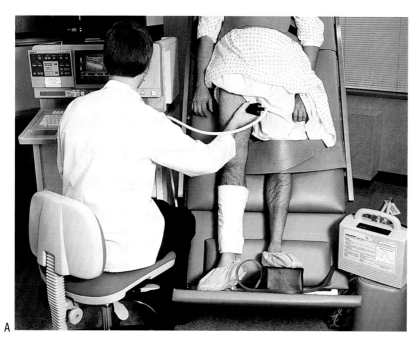

A

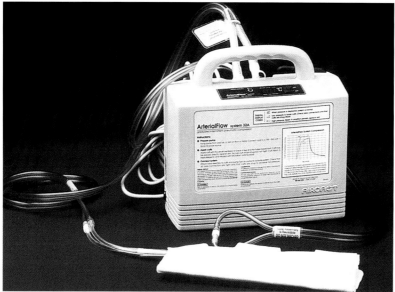

B

Fig. 7.1. Duplex examination for venous valvular incompetence. **A** The patient is in a 60–80° near upright position bearing weight on the contralateral extremity studied. **B** Automatic cuff inflator to investigate venous valve incompetence. Inflation of the cuff occurs in 0.3 sec.

available, and its use is recommended (Fig. 7.1B). Compression with the pneumatic cuff is standardized, more reproducible, and eliminates variability related to the limb size and to the sonographer's efforts.[8–11] A cuff pressure of 100 mmHg can be reached with automatic insufflators within 0.3 sec.[2]

Duplex Scanning of Superficial and Deep Veins

The examination begins at the groin by identifying the saphenofemoral junction in the longitudinal plane (Fig. 7.2). A sample volume is then placed in the common femoral vein 2–3 cm superior to the saphenofemoral junction (Fig. 7.3A). The patient is instructed to perform the Valsalva maneuver or flow is augmented using a pneumatic cuff connected to the automatic inflator. Color duplex images and the Doppler spectrum in the compression and relaxation phases are recorded (Fig. 7.3B). Reflux at the common femoral vein level may be a normal variant.

The examination is repeated by placing the sample volume in the greater saphenous vein 2–3 cm inferior to the saphenofemoral junction. Competence of the greater saphenous vein is evaluated the same way as with the common femoral vein. The examination continues caudally with longitudinal

imaging of the greater saphenous vein at the level of the mid femur and knee (Fig. 7.4A,B). At mid-thigh, the Hunterian and Dodd perforators[12] can be imaged and their valvular competence evaluated. The examination is continued, and patency and competence of the mid and lower superficial femoral vein and of the popliteal vein is studied (Fig. 7.5A,B, 7.6A,B). Valvular incompetence of the tibial veins and of the lesser saphenous vein can also be evaluated in a similar matter, although these vessels are not routinely studied in all patients. At each of these venous segments Doppler sampling is performed as the calf is compressed, augmenting cephalad flow, and then released.

Duplex Imaging of Calf Perforator Veins

The medial aspect of the leg is surveyed routinely from the knee to the malleolus. The examination begins near the paired posterior tibial veins at the level of the medial malleolus. B-mode imaging is used to survey the fascia and identify perforators, connecting the posterior arch vein, the greater saphenous vein or one of its tributaries with the posterior tibial veins. A spectral tracing within the perforator is obtained during and following augmentation of venous flow above or below the sampling site using manual compression (Fig. 7.7A,B). Color duplex is most helpful to confirm bidirectional flow even in smaller perforators as color changes by reversal of flow (Fig. 7.8A,B). The skin is marked at the site of the perforators with a permanent marker: an X represents incompetence, an O if the vein is competent and the duration of retrograde flow is shorter than 0.3 sec. In patients with lateral ankle ulcers the examination is continued to identify incompetent lateral calf perforators.

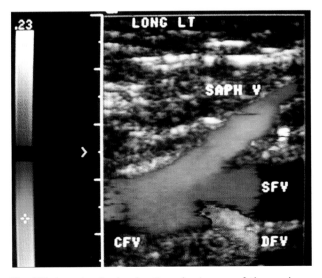

Fig. 7.2. Longitudinal color Doppler image of the saphenofemoral junction. Flow in the deep femoral vein is directed toward the probe, it is imaged therefore in red color. SAPH V = saphenous veins

Contrast Venography

While ascending and descending venography was used in every patient in the first part of our experience with endoscopic perforator division,[13] we now reserve venography for those relatively few patients who have significant deep venous occlusion, identified by duplex scanning or by plethysmography.

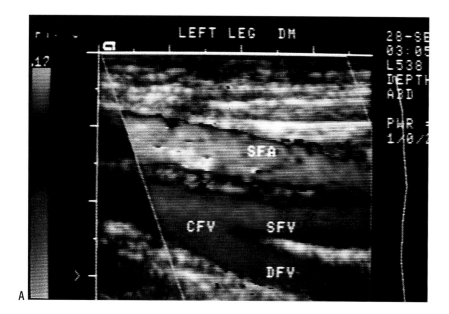

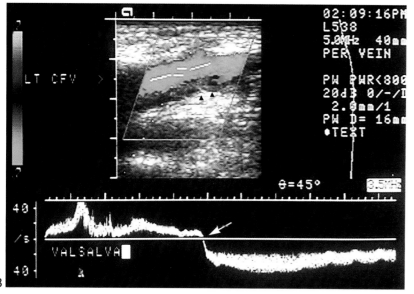

Fig. 7.3. A Color Doppler image of the femoral vessels at the groin. CFV = common femoral vein; SFV = superficial femoral vein; DFV = deep femoral vein; SFA = superficial femoral artery. **B** Post-thrombotic changes including valvular incompetence and residual old venous thrombus, partially occluding the lumen of the common femoral vein. Duplex spectral analysis demonstrates reversal of flow during the Valsalva maneuver and return of normal cephalad flow (arrow) with release of Valsalva. Note thick, adherent, old thrombus along the posterior wall of the common femoral vein (arrowheads).

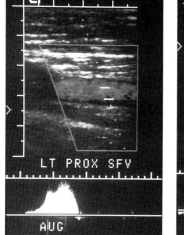
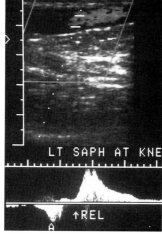

Fig. 7.4. A Spectral analysis in the proximal saphenous vein confirms valvular competence. **B** Longitudinal image of the left greater saphenous vein at the level of the knee. Duplex spectral analysis shows significant reversal of blood flow with release of distal augmentation. A = augmentation; REL = release of distal augmentation.

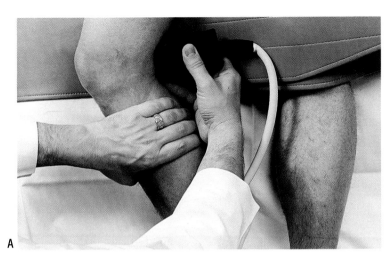

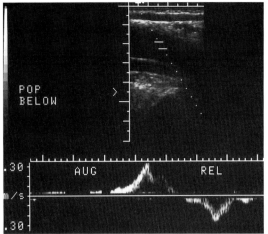

▲

Fig. 7.5. A Positioning of the transducer during evaluation of the popliteal vein for valvular incompetence, using manual distal augmentation in this patient. **B** Longitudinal image Duplex and spectral analysis of the popliteal vein with distal augmentation demonstrates significant flow reversal in the relaxation phase confirming valvular incompetence. AUG = augmentation; REL = relaxation.

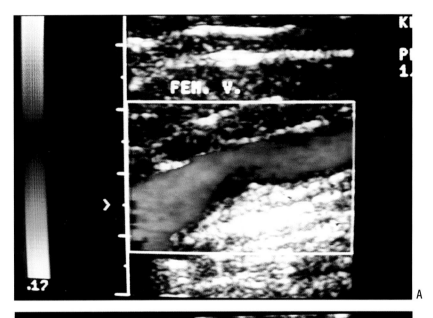

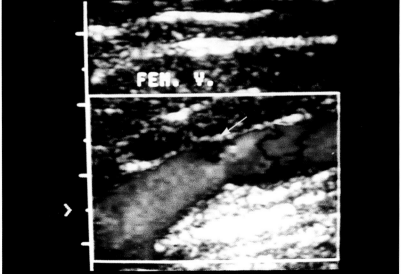

Fig. 7.6. A Longitudinal color Doppler image of the superficial femoral vein. Blue indicates cephalad flow direction. **B** With release of augmentation, there is reversal of flow depicted in red. Flow turbulence is demonstrated below the level of an abnormal incompetent valve (arrow).

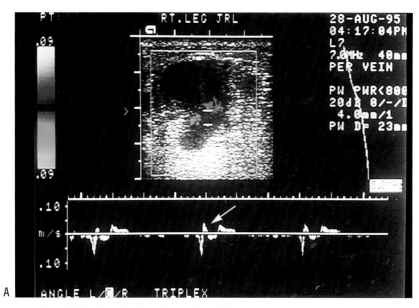

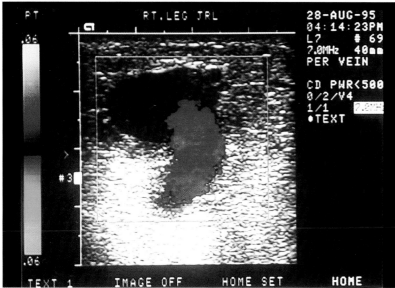

Fig. 7.7. A Color Doppler and spectral tracing of an enlarged incompetent perforating vein. Spectral analysis demonstrates bidirectional flow (arrow). Color Doppler image shows blue indicating superficial to deep flow with augmentation. **B** With release of augmentation perforator valve incompetence is shown by the color change to red.

However, we continue to use contrast venography in patients who are potential candidates for venous reconstruction either for obstruction or for valvular incompetence of the deep veins.[14,15] Contrast venography is the best test to distinguish primary valvular incompetence from post-thrombotic venous disease.[16] Ascending venography is optimal to document acute or chronic venous obstruction and is suitable to demonstrate perforator incompetence. The purpose of descending venography is to identify deep vein reflux and to define the site of vein valves and define morphologic changes in the valve cusps. Depending on the level of deep venous incompetence, thigh or even calf perforators can be imaged with descending venography. Venographic studies in deep venous obstruction are complemented by direct venous pressure measurements to help to assess collateral circulation and ascertain functional venous outflow obstruction.

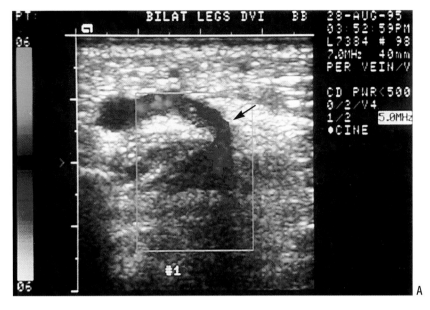

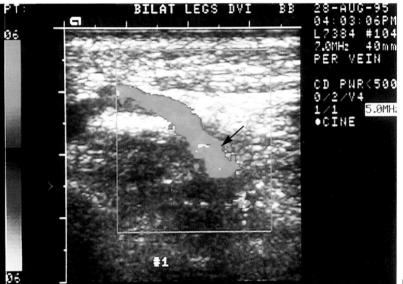

Fig. 7.8. A Color Doppler of a large perforator vein demonstrates predominantly red with distal augmentation. With this color orientation, this indicates superficial to deep flow. **B** With release of augmentation, there is flow reversal indicating an incompetent perforating vein.

Ascending Venography

The venogram is performed on a radiographic table with tilt capability to enable filming in about a 30–40° upright as well as in the supine position. The contralateral foot is supported with a purpose-built platform so that in the upright position weight is not borne on the leg to be examined. Intravenous access is obtained with a 22 gauge needle placed into a superficial vein on the dorsum of the foot in a position as lateral as possible. A 100 cm ruler with opaque markers is placed along the medial aspect of the leg to enable us to determine the correct distance of perforating veins on the film from the ankle (Fig.

7.9). Scout films are taken in the supine position to verify correct radiographic technique. An overhead tube and Bucky grid are used with a 14″ by 17″ film properly coned for maximum detail. Fluoroscopic spot films are taken as needed.

The examination is begun in the 30–40° upright position to allow contrast filling of the dependent venous structures. Intravenous contrast material with an organically bound iodine concentration of approximately 200 mg/ml is used to prevent over opacification of the venous structures that can make film interpretation difficult. A tourniquet is applied above the ankle to drive contrast material into the deep veins. This best allows the identification of incompe-

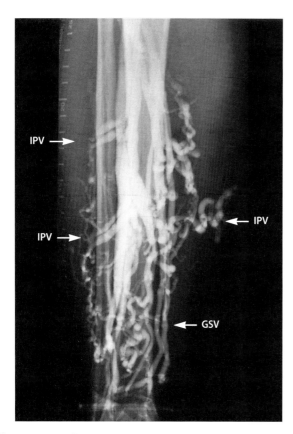

Fig. 7.9. Ascending venogram in anteroposterior projection of the right calf of a 41-year-old female with non-healing venous ulcer due to primary valvular incompetence. Note medial and lateral incompetent perforators (IPV) filling the superficial system with contrast. GSV = greater saphenous vein.

tent perforating veins (Figs 7.10, 7.11, 7.12, 7.13 and 7.14). The contrast material is injected slowly, with careful observation to ensure against extravasation. After 50 ml have been given, the tourniquet is removed and filming is begun. A total of four antero-posterior and external rotation oblique images are taken from the ankle to the mid-thigh. An additional 50 ml of contrast is injected while the filming is being done, and then a single anteroposterior image is taken of the common and superficial femoral vein region. The table is then slowly lowered to the flat position, and the patient is asked to hold breathing while the affected leg is elevated by the operator about 6″ from the table top. After a second or two, an image of the pelvis and lower abdomen is obtained to outline the iliac veins and inferior vena cava. When filming is completed, the intravenous line is flushed with 50 ml of 0.45 N saline to prevent prolonged contact of the contrast material with venous endothe-lium. With practice, this technique gives beautiful

images of the deep veins of the leg and identifies incompetent perforating veins, that fill the superficial system with contrast coming from the deep calf veins.

Descending Venography

This examination is also performed on a tilt radio-graphic table to enable filming in 30–40° upright and supine positions, and the contralateral foot is sup-ported in the fashion noted above. An opaque marker ruler is positioned medially. The groin of the leg to be examined is shaved, scrubbed, and draped for sterile percutaneous access to the common femoral vein. Lidocaine (2%) is used for local anes-thesia and with Seldinger technique a 4 or 5 French short straight catheter with several side holes is positioned in the external iliac vein. Images of the iliac system and inferior vena cava can be obtained in the supine position if necessary with a brisk hand injection of contrast and fluoroscopic spot films are taken. Contrast material with an iodine concentra-tion of 200 mg/ml is used.

The table is then positioned upright 30–40° and the descending portion of the examination is begun. Imaging is obtained in real-time using videotape recording of the fluoroscopic image, as recommended by Kistner et al.[17] Contrast material, 30–50 ml, is hand

Fig. 7.10. Ascending venogram of a 74-year-old female with ▶ venous stasis ulcers due to primary valvular incompetence. Note medial varicosity filling through incompetent perforating veins from the posterior tibial system. VV = varicosity; IPV = incompetent perforating vein; PT = posterior tibial veins; GVS = greater saphenous vein.

Fig. 7.11. Ascending venogram with anteroposterior projection ▶ of the left lower calf in a 59-year-old female with chronic venous insufficiency. Note two large medial incompetent per-forating veins filling the greater saphenous vein (GSV) and its tributaries.

Fig. 7.12. Anteroposterior projection of a left leg venogram in a ▶ 32-year-old male with chronic venous insufficiency due to primary valvular incompetence. Note several incompetent proximal paratibial perforating veins (IPV) filling the superficial system. This patient has multiple lateral incompetent perforat-ing veins (PV) as well. Faint filling of the greater saphenous vein (GSV) is visible. PTV = posterior tibial vein.

Fig. 7.13. Lateral projection of ascending venogram of a ▶ 39-year-old male with huge bilateral venous ulcers due to post-thrombotic syndrome. This patient has large incompetent greater saphenous vein (GSV) and lesser saphenous vein (LSV). There are several incompetent medial posterior and lateral perforators.

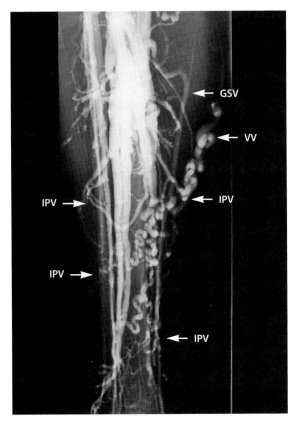

Fig. 7.10

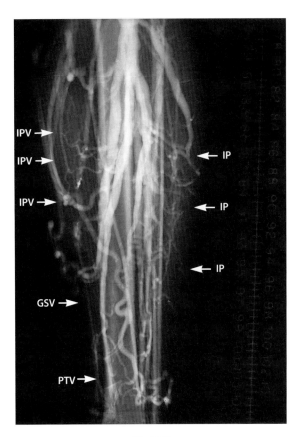

Fig. 7.12

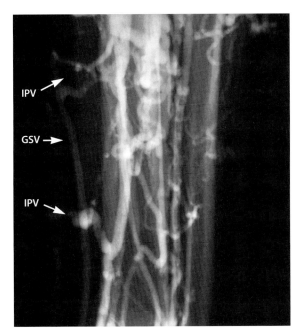

Fig. 7.11

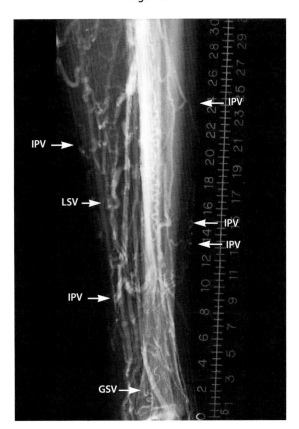

Fig. 7.13

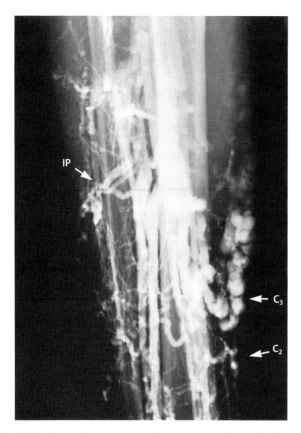

Fig. 7.14. Ascending venogram in anteroposterior projection of the right lower calf of a 64-year-old male. Note huge Cockett II and very large Cockett III perforators filling medal varicose veins. C₂ = Cockett II perforator; C₃ = Cockett III perforator

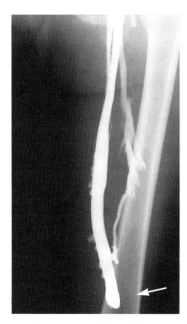

Fig. 7.15. Descending venography confirms significant reflux in the superficial femoral and profunda femoris veins (Grade 2), with a competent valve in the proximal popliteal vein (arrow).

injected and observed fluoroscopically. The common femoral vein area is carefully evaluated for contrast reflux into deep and superficial femoral veins as well as the greater saphenous vein. Incompetent thigh perforators are easily imaged with this technique. Imaging documents the extent of distal reflux into the popliteal region and below, confirming severe deep venous reflux. Reflux is enhanced by having the patient perform a Valsalva maneuver while contrast material is injected. When imaging is complete the venous catheter is removed and hemostasis achieved with manual compression. The patient is observed for about an hour in the supine position and then asked to ambulate briefly. If no bleeding problems are detected the patient is discharged.

Venous valvular function can easily be studied with descending venography and as the test is recorded on videotape, it can later be reviewed by the radiologist and the surgeon. Using information obtained with descending venography, the severity of venous valvular incompetence can be established according to the classification of Kistner et al.[17] Grade 1 reflux is limited to the upper thigh, Grade 2 to the lower thigh (Fig. 7.15), Grade 3 involves the popliteal veins and Grade 4 is severe infrapopliteal reflux, including frequently incompetence of calf perforators. In patients who have Grade 3 or 4 reflux and have recurrent symptoms in spite of treatment of superficial and perforator incompetence, reconstruction of the incompetent deep system with direct valve repair or valve transplantation should be considered.

References

1. Sumner DS (1996) Direct noninvasive tests for the evaluation of chronic venous obstruction and valvular incompetence. In: Gloviczki P, Yao J. S. T. (eds) Handbook of Venous Disorders. Chapman and Hall, London pp 130–151
2. van Bemmelen PS, Bergan JJ (eds) (1992) Quantitative Measurement of Venous Incompetence., R.G. Landes Company, Georgetown, TX
3. Nicolaides AN, Sumner DS (eds) (1991) Investigation of Patients With Deep Vein Thrombosis and Chronic Venous Insufficiency. Med-Orion Publishing Company, London
4. Weingarten MS, Branas CC, Czeredarczuk M et al. (1993) Distribution and quantification of venous reflux in lower extremity chronic venous stasis disease with duplex scanning. J Vasc Surg 18:753–759
5. Magnusson M, Kalebo P, Lukes P et al. (1996) Colour Doppler ultrasound in diagnosing venous insufficiency, A comparison to descending phlebography. Eur J Vasc Endovasc Surg 9:437–443

6. van Bemmelen PS, Bedford G, Beach K, Strandness DE (1989) Quantitative segmental evaluation of venous valvular reflux with duplex ultrasound scanning. J Vasc Surg 10:425–431
7. Vasdekis SN, Clarke GH, Nicolaides AN (1989) Quantification of venous reflux by means of duplex scanning. J Vasc Surg 10:670–677
8. van Bemmelen PS, Beach K, Bedford G, Strandness DE (1990) The mechanism of venous valve closure. Its relationship to the velocity of reverse flow. Arch Surg 125:617–619
9. Masuda EM, Kistner RL, Eklof B (1994) Prospective study of duplex scanning for venous reflux: Comparison of Valsalva and pneumatic cuff techniques in the reverse Trendelenburg and standing positions. J Vasc Surg 20:711–720
10. Markel A, Meissner MH, Manzo RA et al. (1994) Comparison of the cuff deflation method with Valsalva's maneuver and limb compression in detecting venous valvular reflux. Arch Surg 129:701–705
11. Myers KA, Ziegenbein RW, Zeng GH, Mathews PG (1995) Duplex ultrasonography scanning for chronic venous disease: Patterns of venous reflux. J Vasc Surg 21:605–612
12. Mozes G, Gloviczki P, Menawat SS, Fisher DR, Carmichael SW, Kadar A (1996) Surgical anatomy for endoscopic subfascial division of perforating veins. J Vasc Surg 24:800–808
13. Gloviczki P, Cambria RA, Rhee RY, Canton LG, McKusick MA (1996) Surgical technique and preliminary results of endoscopic subfascial division of perforating veins. J Vasc Surg 23:517–523
14. Gloviczki P, Pairolero PC, Toomey BJ, Bower TC, Rooke TW, Stanson AW, Hallett JW Jr, Cherry KJ Jr (1992) Reconstruction of large veins for nonmalignant venous occlusive disease. J Vasc Surg 16:750–761
15. Gloviczki P, Merrell SW, Bower TC (1991) Femoral vein valve repair under direct vision without venotomy: A modified technique using angioscopy. J Vasc Surg 14:645–648
16. Kamida CB, Kistner RL, Eklof B, Masuda EM: (1996) Lower extremity phlebography. In: Gloviczki P, Yao JST (eds) Handbook of Venous Disorders. Chapman and Hall, London, pp 152–167
17. Kistner RL, Ferris EB, Randhawa G, Kamida CB (1996) A method of performing descending venography. J Vasc Surg 4:464–8

SECTION 3
Surgical Interventions

Profile

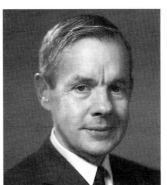

Karl A. Lofgren

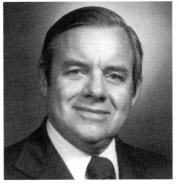

Eric P. Lofgren

Karl A. Lofgren and Eric P. Lofgren
b. 1915 and 1919

Contributions of brothers to medicine were exemplified by great physicians and surgeons such as John and William Hunter and William and Charles Mayo. In the world of venous diseases, the Lofgren brothers gained recognition through their prolific career as vein surgeons at the Mayo Clinic for more than three decades. Their services were distinguished by unfaltering devotion to the care of patients with venous disorders. Together with Dr Thomas T. Myers, within the Section of Peripheral Vein Surgery, they provided compassionate and expert care to those who suffered from venous diseases; they performed approximately 14,000 vein stripping operations and had seen nearly 140,000 patients in consultation.

Born in Sweden, Dr Karl Lofgren received his education at the Northwestern University in Chicago and at the Harvard University in Boston. His surgical training was completed at the Mayo Clinic. After a short period with the Royal Academic Hospital,

Sweden, he joined the Mayo Clinic in 1950. He advanced through the academic ranks to become professor of surgery in 1960.

Dr Eric Lofgren, also born in Sweden, was educated at the University of Illinois at Urbana and in medicine in Chicago. After a period of private practice, he joined his brother at the Mayo Clinic in 1964 to combine their efforts in the treatment of venous disorders.

The leadership of the Section of Peripheral Vein Surgery was passed from Dr Thomas T. Myers to Karl Lofgren in 1966. In 1979 Eric Lofgren became the head of the section. It was during these years that they refined diagnostic evaluation and treatment modalities for many aspects of venous disease, including telangiectasias, primary and postthrombotic varicosities, superficial thrombophlebitis and venous malformations. Their landmark study on one thousand consecutive patients, who underwent operation for treatment of varicose veins, was published in 1974 by Karl A. Lofgren. This report with more than 10 years follow-up established the role of vein stripping for treatment of varicosity. Much credit for improvement in the management of hypertensive and venous ulcerations belong to the Lofgren brothers. They studied the effects of vein stripping on venous physiology by comparing ambu-latory venous pressure measurements before and after operation. Their report on perforating veins in 1968 was important, since it called attention to the reversed orientation of valves in foot perforators.

Dr Karl Lofgren retired in 1981 and Dr Eric Lofgren in 1984. They presently reside in Rochester, Minnesota, enjoying their retirement lives.

Correction of Superficial Reflux

8

John J. Bergan and Jeffrey L. Ballard

Neglected, incompetent superficial or saphenous veins alone can produce stasis changes in the leg, not unlike those of incompetent deep veins.

TT Myers

The observation by Myers[1] 40 years ago has stood the test of time and there is abundant evidence which shows that superficial venous reflux is an important component of the syndrome of chronic venous insufficiency (CVI). In studying limbs with established deep venous thrombosis, Browse concluded that, "the development of a postphlebitic leg does not depend solely on the extent of the initial thrombosis and can apparently develop in the absence of thrombosis."[2] In a very wise analysis of the situation, he concluded that, "the lack of a simple correlation between the extent of thrombosis and the symptoms can be explained in two ways." One was that the thrombus, its location, and extent did not highlight the critical aspect of the pathophysiology or that another factor was implicated. Today, we know that the other factor in addition to venous hypertension caused by superficial and deep reflux is adherence and activation of leukocytes in the area of most severe venous hypertension.

Elimination of the factor of superficial reflux becomes as important as perforator interruption in limbs with severe chronic venous insufficiency. In order to determine the importance of superficial venous insufficiency alone, Hansson's group in Göteborg studied 114 consecutive patients with a clinical picture of venous leg ulcer.[3] Limbs were studied with the mercury strain gauge technique with and without application of a 1 cm tourniquet applied just below the knee. Efficacy of the tourniquet was tested in patients by color duplex ultrasound and reproducibility of strain gauge plethysmography was confirmed. This study demonstrated that 10% of the limbs with active ulcers had isolated superficial venous incompetence as the only pathologic feature. Only 22% of the limbs carried a diagnosis of previous venous thrombosis.

In an equally important study, van Bemmelen, working in Strandness's laboratory in Seattle, investigated the relationship of deep and superficial venous insufficiency in 42 patients.[4] Twenty five of these had venous ulcers. There were 22 patients who had a history of deep venous thrombosis, 12 of whom developed a venous ulcer, and there were 20 patients who denied a previous history of deep venous thrombosis, 13 of whom developed ulceration van Bemmelen summarized the results of his study saying, "a surprising finding was the very high prevalence of incompetence of the greater and lesser saphenous veins. The greater and lesser saphenous veins showed reflux in 15 of the 25 limbs with ulcers." The importance of this finding was summarized by Hansson in his report when he said that, "in patients with superficial venous incompetence alone, surgery can achieve normalization of venous function with the prospect of reducing symptoms and accelerating ulcer healing."[3]

In our own study of 58 limbs with the former Class 3 venous insufficiency (these would be classified as 4, 5 and 6 today), 10 limbs (17%) exhibited only superficial reflux. Thus, a significant percentage of patients could have been operated upon for cure of their venous stasis disease even though their limbs would have been classified as postphlebitic and incurable as recently as 10 years ago. Equally important is the fact that superficial reflux was a major contributor to the chronic venous dysfunction in another 17 limbs (29%). Thus, ablation of superficial reflux alone would make a major contribution to bettering of limbs with chronic venous dysfunction in nearly 60% of cases studied by us.

Another fact learned more recently is also of great importance. This is that some deep venous reflux is cured by removing superficial reflux alone. Two studies have documented this fact.[5,6] Goren, in documenting this phenomenon by APG measurements, explained ablation of deep venous reflux by superficial venous stripping as follows: "… in long-standing varicose disease presenting with the clinical picture of CVI, a concomitant Doppler or duplex scanning detectable deep vein incompetence and reflux is, in many cases, secondary to deep vein dilation. Increased superficial reflux volumes passing through the existing retrograde circuit have to be accommodated by the deep venous system, causing deep vein dilation and secondary valvular incompetence and reflux."[7]

For the most part, the observation of ablation of deep venous reflux by superficial venous stripping has been made in limbs without long-standing chronic venous insufficiency. However, it is clear that procedures designed to correct deep vein incompetence such as valveplasty or venous transposition should be postponed until some time after the superficial reflux has been controlled and the limb observed for recurrence of venous ulceration.

Among the first to emphasize the superficial venous system as a cause of chronic venous insufficiency was Simon Darke of Bournemouth. Over an 8-year period, Darke identified 213 patients with venous ulceration in 232 limbs.[8] These patients were studied by ascending and descending phlebography in addition to hand-held, continuous-wave Doppler ultrasound. Darke found that 39% of the limbs demonstrated ankle perforator and saphenous incompetence, an additional 35% of limbs had primary deep incompetence, usually associated with perforator and saphenous incompetence, and only 22% of limbs demonstrated post-thrombotic damage. Significantly, 4% of the limbs showed perforator incompetence alone.

Darke's observations made prior to 1992 were remarkably similar to the report of the North American Registry of Endoscopic Perforator Surgery.[9] In that report, incompetence of the superficial and perforator system was documented in 98 of 145 limbs (66%). Actual isolated incompetence of the superficial system was present in 14% of limbs, a figure similar to those cited above.

Finally, in a particularly well-done study, the Middlesex group reported on duplex ultrasound examination of 59 consecutive patients with venous ulcers.[10] This demonstrated that in 42 limbs (53%) there was superficial venous reflux alone. In all cases, the reflux was either in the greater or lesser saphenous system. In 25 limbs (32%), both superficial and deep venous reflux was present and, as indicated above, those limbs without previous deep venous thrombosis might be expected to have a bettering of the deep venous reflux by ablation of the superficial venous incompetence. In this study, there were only 12 limbs (15%) in which deep venous reflux was the only finding.

All of these findings make a strong case for ablation of superficial reflux in conjunction with subfascial endoscopic interruption of perforating veins.

In the past, limbs with obstruction as a cause of chronic venous insufficiency were thought to employ the superficial venous system as collateral blood flow. This logic, derived from observation of arterial obstruction and collateral flow, appears to be erroneous with reference to the venous system. Raju was able to examine 137 limbs with venous obstruction. He found that extensive proximal obstructive lesions could be hemodynamically quite mild. He said, "skin ulceration in the presence of venous obstruction was related to the associated reflux rather than to the hemodynamic severity of the obstruction itself."[1] The old-fashioned Linton procedure was done by Raju in 25 limbs with severe venous obstruction. After operation with an average follow-up of 15 months, no worsening of the hemodynamic grade of obstruction occurred. Raju commented on this saying, "thus, disruption of perforator collateral vessels did not result in a worsening of grade of obstruction." As the Linton procedure invariably corrected superficial venous reflux as well as perforator incompetence, there is now hemodynamic proof that ablation of superficial reflux does not worsen limbs with venous obstruction.

Surgical Procedure

Fig. 8.1 shows the position of the limb prior to skin preparation, exsanguination of the limb by Esmarch bandage, and application of the hemostatic tourni-

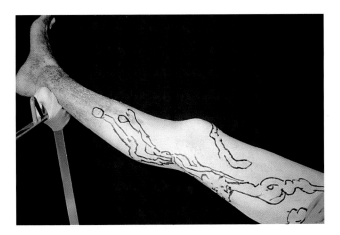

Fig. 8.1. Position of the leg to be operated upon prior to exsanguination and application of the hemostatic tourniquet.

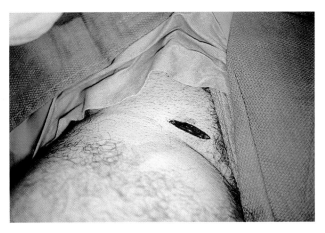

Fig. 8.2. Exposure of the saphenofemoral junction requires that the incision be placed above the inguinal skin crease as shown in this photograph.

quet. In this instance, identified perforating veins are marked with a circle and the diameter of the refluxing superficial veins is indicated by the width of the markings. The markings were accomplished with the patient standing.

Fig. 8.2 shows the placement of the proximal incision. This is made obliquely in skin lines approximately 1 cm above the inguinal skin crease. The traditionally taught incision placed in the inguinal

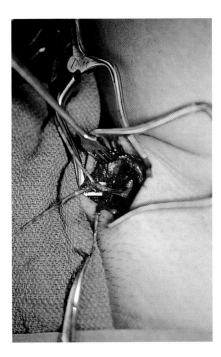

Fig. 8.3. Excision of saphenous tributaries should be done rather than simple ligation and division at their junction at the saphenous vein. Removing the primary and secondary tributaries will ablate the network of residual veins which allows recurrent reflux.

skin crease or more distally has been found to lack correlation with the actual saphenofemoral junction. Placing the incision in its proper location, proximal to the inguinal skin crease, allows a shorter incision to be made.

Fig. 8.3 shows the extent of removal of tributary veins. These are pulled into the incision beyond their primary and secondary tributaries. The reason for doing this is that simple flush ligation of the tributaries at the saphenous vein will allow a profuse network of refluxing tributaries to remain. Fig. 8.4 illustrates the recurrences according to the classification of Ruckley. This classification is useful because it clarifies thinking, not only for the primary operation but also for the treatment of recurrent venous insufficiency after proximal saphenous surgery. In treating recurrent venous insufficiency the Type I recurrences would call for a repeat groin exploration while the Type 2 recurrences would only require distal surgery.

In the Edinburgh study by Ruckley, there were 86 of 128 limbs in which there was persistence of a connection around the saphenofemoral junction.[12] In 17 limbs, the greater saphenous vein was completely intact despite the presence of a groin wound. This indicated that the primary operator had missed the saphenous vein and had instead presumably ligated one of its major tributaries. Of importance to performance of the primary operation itself was the fact that in 55 of the 86 limbs, there was a residual saphenofemoral complex in which tributaries connected the deep and superficial systems. This is displayed as the Type 1B recurrence and emphasizes the need for removing the tributary veins beyond their primary

TYPE I

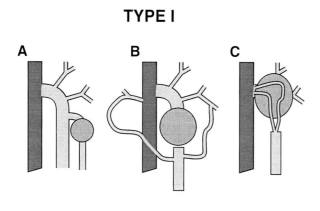

TYPE II

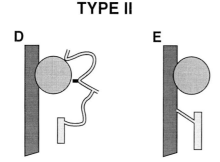

Fig. 8.4. This diagrammatic representation of Type 1 and Type 2 recurrent varicosities explains why the network of residual varicosities left in the groin can contribute to reflux in a retained saphenous vein. Simple ligation of the saphenous vein rather than stripping it out in the thigh is a major cause of recurrent varicosities and venous stasis.

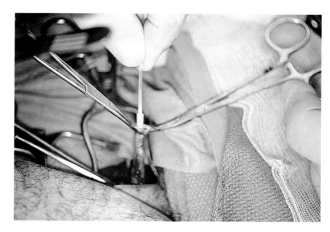

Fig. 8.5. The endoluminal stripper can be introduced from above in the patient requiring removal of the saphenous vein. Doppler and duplex ultrasonography will have proven that reflux extends throughout the saphenous vein in its thigh portion.

and secondary tributaries as shown in Fig. 8.3. Here one can see that the epigastric tributary has been extensively exposed as have the pudendal and medial posterior tributaries. These have been drawn into the wound by traction and divided after control of the distal venous segment by electrocoagulation, clipping or ligation.

After complete exposure of the tributaries to the saphenous vein, the femoral vein is exposed proximal and distal to the junction in order to ascertain that there are no major tributaries which enter the saphenofemoral junction or the femoral vein itself. The saphenous vein is divided and suture ligated flush with the femoral vein. As shown in Fig. 8.5, the intraluminal stripper can be placed from above because saphenous vein in limbs which require correction of superficial reflux has few valves. This has been confirmed angioscopically.[13] This retrograde introduction of the stripper has the advantage of minimizing the distal incision needed to retrieve the stripper.

Introduction of the stripping device from the ankle has the disadvantage of missing the posterior arch vein and allows the stripping device to enter the deep venous system by way of the angulated perforating veins in the thigh. When introduced from above, the stripping device can be identified when it stops at the first competent valve, usually in the upper anteromedial calf. After it is exposed and pulled down, the vein can be attached to the stripper by heavy ligature and a hemostatic pack affixed to the same location. The hemostatic pack is a two-inch (10 cm) roller gauze (Fig. 8.6) which has been soaked in lidocaine, 0.5%, with added epinephrine. This is a standard local anesthetic solution available in most operating rooms.

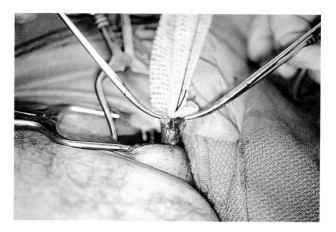

Fig. 8.6. Hemostatic packing of the saphenous vein tunnel is an adjunct which decreases thigh ecchymosis.

Fig. 8.7A shows the inverted and packed saphenous vein emerging from a short incision in the anteromedial calf. The intraluminal stripper can be seen exiting to the right in the photograph. Fig. 8.7B illustrates this maneuver diagramatically. Artist's license has exaggerated the size of the incisions and of the saphenous vein but makes the point that saphenous stripping removes veins tributary to the greater saphenous system. These tributaries can be communicating veins or perforating veins but either will preserve patency of the saphenous vein and preserve reflux within it if the saphenous vein is treated by proximal ligation alone. Note the inset in the figure which shows inversion of the saphenous vein into itself as part of the stripping maneuver. Also note the posterior arch vein which is regularly a tributary to the greater saphenous vein in the region of Boyd's perforating vein.

Fig. 8.8 shows the hemostatic pack in place and the elongated saphenous vein filled internally with its portion of the hemostatic pack. This internal packing has no function but allows the trailing gauze to pass through the thigh with minimal trauma.

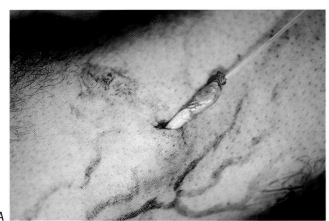

Fig. 8.7. A Inversion stripping and hemostatic packing is illustrated in this photograph which shows the endoluminal stripper exiting to the right followed by the inverted and internally packed saphenous vein. The internal pack adds its strength to the saphenous vein, allowing removal of the vein without tearing. **B** In this diagram, artist's license has exaggerated the size of the incisions and of the saphenous vein but makes the point that saphenous stripping removes veins tributary to the greater saphenous system.

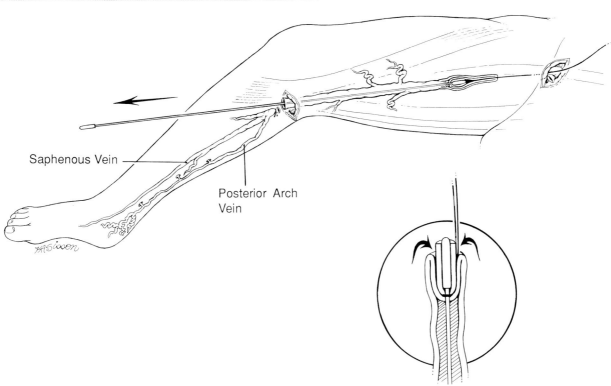

Saphenous Vein

Posterior Arch Vein

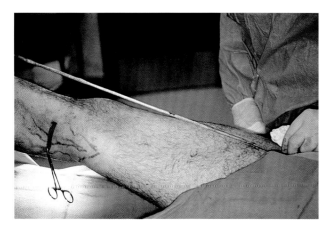

Fig. 8.8. The removal saphenous vein is longer than its tunnel in the thigh because it is elongated and tortuous in its refluxing state. Note the hemostatic pack exiting in the anteromedial calf.

Secondary Greater Saphenous Surgery

Type I reflux recurrence will demand a re-exploration of the groin incision. Very often, the scar will be low-lying and will indicate that the greater saphenous vein has been approached well below the saphenofemoral junction. In this situation, the operation may be simple. However, scar of the original operation may be dense and very difficult to manage, especially for the inexperienced. If the scar tissue proves to be dense, then the standard approach should be abandoned and dissection aimed directly at the femoral artery. Its pulsations will be obvious and the wise surgeon will expose the femoral artery without progressing laterally into the region of the femoral nerve. After the femoral sheath is opened, the dissection can proceed medially to the femoral vein. Exposure of the lateral border of the femoral vein will lead to the saphenofemoral junction which can be ligated and the stump of the vein excised with all of its tributaries without having to enter the caput medusa of recurrent high-pressure venous collaterals.[14,15]

Surgery of the Lesser Saphenous Vein

Preoperative location of the termination of the lesser saphenous vein by duplex scanning must precede surgery of the saphenopopliteal junction. Location of the termination of the lesser saphenous vein is marked on the skin with an indelible marker. Preoperative marking of the varicosities is carried out just as is done for the greater saphenous vein varicosities. For surgery of the saphenopopliteal junction, the patient is intubated and prone. A generous incision is made, superficial vessels controlled by electrocoagulation, and the deep fascia opened in the line of the incision. The sural nerve is identified, preserved, and the lesser saphenous vein identified between the two heads of the gastrocnemius muscle. At this time, the knee should be flexed and placed on a pillow or sandbag. This maneuver allows popliteal fossa exploration by relaxing the fascia lata and the gastrocnemius muscles. The vein of Giacomini will be a constant tributary and this vessel should be not only ligated and divided but excised as far as is allowed by the popliteal incision. Similarly, the gastrocnemius veins are sought for, ligated, and divided.

Opinion is divided on whether the lesser saphenous vein should be stripped or simply ligated, and the reason for disagreement is that there is no lesser saphenous vein equivalent to the mid-thigh Hunterian perforating vein of the greater saphenous system. It is our preference to strip the vein at least to mid-calf using the Oesch technique.[16,17]

Surgery of Recurrent Lesser Saphenous Incompetence

Anatomy of the recurrent incompetence must be defined by duplex ultrasonography before attempting reexploration of the popliteal fossa. At the time of surgery, the patient is intubated and prone, and a lazy-S incision is made to expose the saphenopopliteal junction. The presence of scar tissue and high-pressure venous collaterals make the dissection difficult. However, after dividing the deep fascia, the varicose tributaries to the saphenopopliteal junction must be controlled by ligation and division as they are encountered. The popliteal vein can be approached from above and identified positively. The saphenopopliteal junction can be ligated and exposure for this is facilitated by retraction of the overlying popliteal and common peroneal nerves. Surgery of recurrent saphenopopliteal reflux is among the most difficult dissections encountered in all vascular surgery.

As recurrent varicose veins of the posterior calf as well as on the lateral surface of the calf may derive from gastrocnemius vein incompetence, these veins must be identified during surgery of recurrent saphenopopliteal incompetence. The gastrocnemius veins can be identified preoperatively by duplex scan. Exposure of the gastrocnemius veins must be done carefully in order to avoid damage to the adjacent popliteal nerve.[18]

References

1. Myers TT, Cooley JC (1954) Varicose vein surgery in the management of the postphlebitic limb. Surg Gynecol Obstet 99:733–744
2. Browse NL, Clemenson G, Lea Thomas M (1980) Is the postphlebitic leg always postphlebitic? Relation between phlebographic appearances of deep vein thrombosis and late sequelae. Br Med J 281:1167–1170
3. Hansson C, Holm J (1995) Frequency of isolated superficial venous incompetence in patients with venous ulcers as measured by ambulatory strain-gauge plethysmography. Phlebology 10:65–68
4. van Bemmelen P, Bedford G, Beach K, Strandness DE Jr (1990) Status of the valves in the superficial and deep venous system in chronic venous disease. Surgery 109:703–704
5. Walsh JC, Bergan, Beeman S, Comer TP (1994) Femoral venous reflux abolished by greater saphenous vein stripping. Ann Vasc Surg 8:566–570
6. Sales SM, Bilof ML, Petrillo KA, Luka NL (1996) Correction of lower extremity venous incompetence by ablation of superficial venous reflux. Ann Vasc Surg 10:186–190
7. Goren G (1993) Letter to the Editor. Venous ulcers and the superficial venous system. J Vasc Surg 18:716–718
8. Darke SG, Penfold C (1992) Venous ulceration and saphenous ligation. Eur J Vasc Surg 6:4–9
9. Gloviczki P, Bergan JJ, Menawat SS et al. (1997) Safety, feasibility, and early efficacy of subfascial endoscopic perforator surgery (SEPS): A preliminary report from the North American Registry. J Vasc Surg. 25:94–105.
10. Shami SK, Sarin S, Cheatle TR, Scurr JH, Coleridge Smith PD (1993) Venous ulcers and the superficial venous system. J Vasc Surg 17:487–490
11. Raju S, Fredericks R (1991) Venous obstruction: An analysis of 137 cases with hemodynamic, venographic, and clinical correlations. J Vasc Surg 14:305–313
12. Stonebridge PA, Chalmers N, Beggs I, Bradbury AW, Ruckley CV (1995) Recurrent varicose veins: A varicographic analysis leading to a new practical classification. Br J Surg 82:60–62
13. Gradman WS, Segalowitz J, Grundfest W (1993) Venoscopy in varicose vein surgery: Initial experience. Phlebology 8:145–150
14. Belardi P, Lucertini G (1994) Advantages of the lateral approach for reexploration of the saphenofemoral junction for recurrent varicose veins. Cardiovasc Surg 2:772–774
15. Li AKC (1975). A technique for reexploration of the saphenofemoral junction for recurrent varicose veins. Br J Surg 62:745–746
16. Oesch A (1988) Formen und modern therapie der varikosis Schweiz Med Wochenschr 118:1242–1247
17. Oesch A (1991) Indikationen und ergebnisse der ambulanien varizentherapie Therapeutische Umschau 48:692–696
18. Negus D (1995) Leg ulcers: A practical approach to management, 2nd Edn. Butterworth Heinemann, London

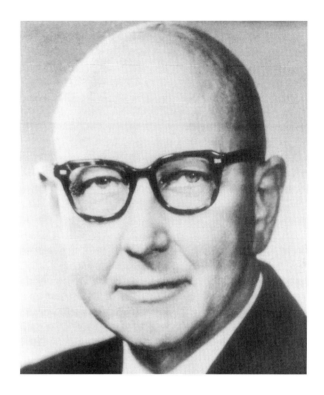

Robert R. Linton
1900–1974

On the occasion of the twentieth Annual Meeting of the New England Society for Vascular Surgery, Bruce S. Cutler, MD of Worchester, Massachusetts summarized the life and accomplishments of Robert Linton, a true pioneer in the field of modern vascular surgery. Cutler quotes Linton as saying, "at the age of 19, I witnessed a varicose vein operation at the Royal Infirmary in Edinburgh, Scotland. Many times since I have thought what a poor operation the surgeon had performed for this condition."

Linton's interest in venous disorders, stimulated by Homans, led him to the problems of severe chronic venous insufficiency, and after he had performed cadaver dissections, he was able to develop and perfect the operation of subfascial perforator vein interruption. By 1952, the Linton operation consisted of the four parts described elsewhere in this text.

Linton's lineage was unusual. He was born in Grangemouth, Scotland and, because of domestic circumstances, was reared by his father with his brother. The three emigrated to the United States where they lived on Vashon Island near Seattle, Washington. The two boys, Robert and James, matriculated in the University of Washington, and after their father's death in a motor vehicle accident, took a year off and traveled to Scotland to visit their mother. There, Robert saw operations at the Edinburgh Royal Infirmary on varicose veins, femoral hernia, nephrectomy, and drainage of a cervical abscess. The two boys graduated Cum Laude from the University of Washington and matriculated at Harvard University in the fall. Robert came under the influence of Walter B. Cannon and worked in his laboratory where he studied the physiology of sympathectomy.

At about the time he returned to the Massachusetts General Hospital from Baltimore, Robert acquired total alopecia and began his love of sailing at Isle Au Haute in Penobscot Bay. Linton was influenced strongly by E. P. Richardson at the Massachusetts General Hospital but also served under Edward D. Churchill, the John Homans' Professor of Surgery. Slowly, Linton's reputation as a vascular surgeon became established, and after 1940, he and Reginald Smithwick ran the vascular clinic at the MGH. Smithwick explored sympathectomy while Linton explored reconstructive vascular surgery. He developed the proximal portocaval shunt, performing his first operation in 1946.

After World War II, Linton was named Chief of the Peripheral Vascular Clinic and developed ideas on the training of vascular fellows long before the American Board of Surgery approved of the concept. Linton supported the development of the vascular laboratory after 1949 and accepted Kunlin's idea of a venous autograft for treatment for arterial occlusive disease. He was one of the Founding Committee of the Society for Vascular Surgery in 1946 and one of the 31 charter members of the new society when the first meeting was held the next year. His presentation at that meeting was *Post-thrombotic syndrome of the lower extremity* which was coauthored with his first vascular fellow, I. B. Hardy. Linton was the nineth president of the Society for Vascular Surgery.

Linton's career ended in 1974 because of a motor vehicle accident similar to the one which killed his father 58 years before. The accident killed his wife and delayed his acceptance of the honor of giving the John Homans' Lecture to the Society for Vascular Surgery. He finally gave the address which was entitled *John Homans' impact on diseases of the veins of the lower extremity* in June 1976.

Much credit should go to Linton for continuing an interest in venous disorders at the time when arterial surgery was flourishing and becoming dominant.

Linton's Operation and Modifications of the Open Techniques

9

Ralph G. DePalma

In his *Atlas of vascular surgery*, Linton wrote, "the post-thrombotic syndrome of the lower leg with ulceration is a condition which has plagued the human race for many centuries."[1] Linton's wisdom and thorough knowledge of chronic venous insufficiency was exemplified further as he said, "it is of extreme importance to understand that this condition is a chronic disease. Furthermore, it is not possible to restore the limb to its normal pre-thrombotic state because of the irreparable damage to the valves of the deep, communicating, and superficial system of veins. On the other hand, it is possible to cure the chronic ulcer for which the patient comes to the surgeon."

Linton's 1938 paper[2] describes the anatomy of the lower extremity veins, emphasizing interruption of incompetent communicating or perforating veins in order to mitigate transmission of venous hypertension to the skin. Linton described the more important of these as posterior tibial perforating veins saying, "they arise from either of the posterior tibial veins, the uppermost ones being found about the middle of the proximal third of the lower leg. They pass outward along the intermuscular septum between the flexor digitorum longus and the soleus muscle, passing through some of the fibers of the latter near its attachment to the posteromedial edge of the tibia. They frequently arise as double veins, and as they approach the deep fascia, may unite to form one trunk and then break up into a variable number of branches."

Linton described the distal medial perforating veins saying, "the lowest one lies at the level of the lower border of the malleolus and posterior to it.

The upper ones pass outward along the lamina profunda of the deep fascia of the leg which separates the posterior tibial vessels and nerve. Usually, they perforate the deep fascia posterior to the posteromedial edge of the tibia and pass forward to join the long saphenous vein."

Linton advocated thorough preoperative preparation of the patient. He believed that edema and infection should be controlled and the ulceration healed for at least 6 weeks before surgery. He advocated split-thickness skin grafting to close the ulcer but recognized that this was a temporary coverage. Surgery included removing the greater saphenous vein and lesser saphenous vein if it were involved. Ligation of the perforating veins was accomplished through longitudinal incisions parallel to the long axis of the leg. At first, he advocated 3 incisions but later abandoned opening the anterior and lateral compartments. He recognized that ligation of the medial group of perforating veins might be difficult because of their adherence to the periosteum of the tibia.

Linton advised excision of the deep fascia on the posteromedial aspect of the leg. By 1949, he changed the saphenous stripping to include the segment from groin to just below the knee.[3] The saphenous vein from knee to ankle was removed by developing the anterior skin flap, and the posterior skin flap allowed removal of the short saphenous vein. Linton believed that the fasciectomy reduced the amount of postoperative edema by giving better lymphatic drainage from the skin and subcutaneous tissues directly into the muscle.

Just as Linton modified his own operation,[4] others adopted differing techniques with the common

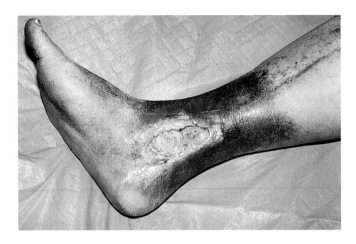

Fig. 9.1. This photograph shows a failure of the classic Linton operation done elsewhere. Note the placement of the incision and the recurrent ulceration.

objective of perforator vein interruption.[5] More recently, it has been acknowledged that important superficial reflux through incompetent greater and/or lesser saphenous veins transmit venous hypertension distally to cause skin breakdown.[6,7] As Linton said, "to effect a cure in such cases, it is necessary to interrupt the communicating veins in addition to performing a ligation … and injections … of the involved saphenous systems."[2]

Several aspects of Linton's operation proved to be unacceptable. The first was the prolonged period of bedrest, leg elevation, and hospitalization which was needed to heal the ulceration prior to surgery. Another disadvantage of his procedure was the poor healing of the longitudinal incision as it inevitably passed through markedly diseased skin. There was also disappointment that such an extensive incision was necessary to interrupt a very few perforating veins. Fig. 9.1 shows a failed Linton procedure.

Cockett's Operation

Frank Cockett, operating independent of Linton in London, recommended an extrafascial approach to perforating veins.[5] This was possible if the subcutaneous tissues were not severely effaced. He used "an accurate incision of the line of perforating veins." He also cautioned that the longitudinal incision should not be carried below the medial malleolus. His operation was based on the observation that extrafascial removal of the "enlarged … tortuous veins in the area … is really as important as tying the perforating veins from which they arise."

Fig. 9.2 illustrates the relationships of the deep and extrafascial veins before their extrafascial division. Extrafascial dissection creates a skin flap. This is quite effective in mitigating local transmission of venous hypertension. The procedure does require a period of absolute bedrest with elevation of the leg and ankle to avoid fluid accumulation beneath this flap. Fig. 9.3 shows the relationships of Fig. 9.2 after division of the perforating veins and ligation and excision of the axial veins.

Modification of the Linton and Cockett Procedures

Recognizing the problems inherent in the Linton procedure and the Cockett operation, I modified the subfascial and extrafascial dissection procedures. The objective of my technique was to interrupt transmission of venous hypertension to the skin and avoid the problem of wound healing inherent in the Linton operation.[8,9] This modified procedure had as its goal the objectives of Linton and Cockett which included complete interruption of the perforating veins, either extrafascially or subfascially and, when needed, removal of incompetent long saphenous or short saphenous veins. Ulcers were excised and grafted in one operation.

Figs 9.4 and 9.5 illustrate the concept of this operation. This shows a series of bipedicled flaps in skin lines created instead of a longitudinal incision with its medial and lateral flaps. The skin line incisions tended to heal much more readily. As indicated in

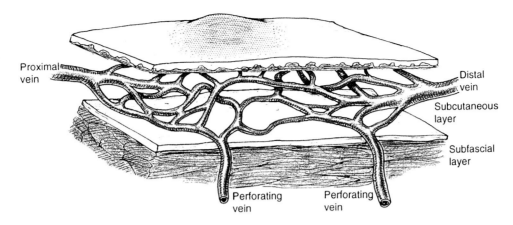

Fig. 9.2. This artist's drawing shows schematically the venous relationships to the affected skin, the fascia, and perforating veins. Note the extensiveness of the subcutaneous plexus and its relationship to proximal and distal axial veins. Note the relatively small number of perforating veins in contrast with the richness of the subcutaneous network of veins.

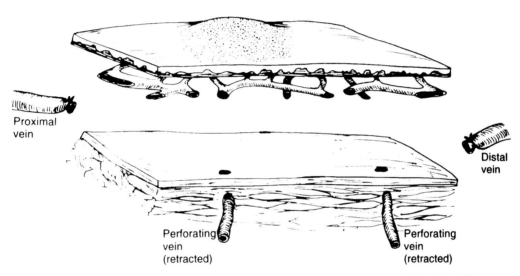

Fig. 9.3. In this diagram, the effect of extrafascial division of perforating veins and proximal and distal ligation is seen.

the diagram, the inframalleolar and foot perforating veins were also ligated through the skin line incisions. The ulcer was radically excised, down to and including fascia, with perforators passing into the ulcer bed from the posterior tibial veins ligated under direct vision. A skin graft was then applied to this defect.

The principle of using access incisions through minimally involved skin was extended further using a skin line incision over the anteromedial upper calf perforating vein (Boyd) which was also ligated[10] as shown in Fig. 9.6.

The next modification of Linton's operation was the extrafascial shearing operation.[11] The shearing portion of the procedure was considerably eased by using the phlebotome described by Simpson and Smellie.[12] Fig. 9.7 shows the phlebotome which is in current use. Figs 9.8 and 9.9 illustrate the principles of use of the phlebotome. The phlebotome is used with great caution. A single pass is made through the retromalleolar area. Fig. 9.9 illustrates the principles of the shearing procedure. Fig. 9.10 illustrates the long-term results of the shearing procedure. Fig. 9.11 illustrates the skin line incisions and the bipedicled nature of the flap.

The recurrence rate for venous ulcers in the two personal series, in which mainly the extrafascial approach was used, ranged from 9% to 10% with the

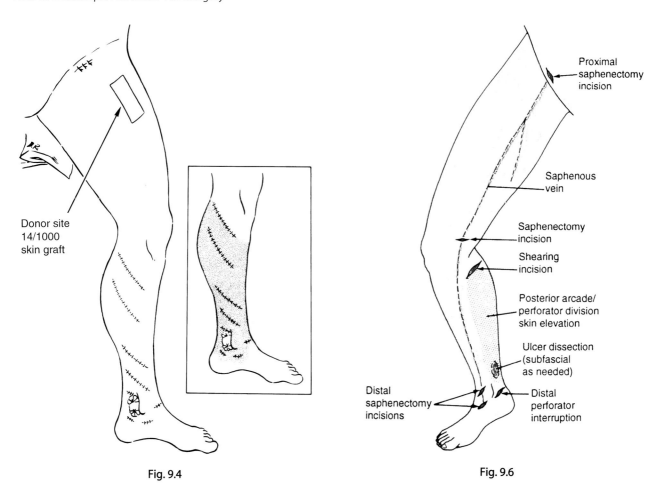

Fig. 9.4

Fig. 9.6

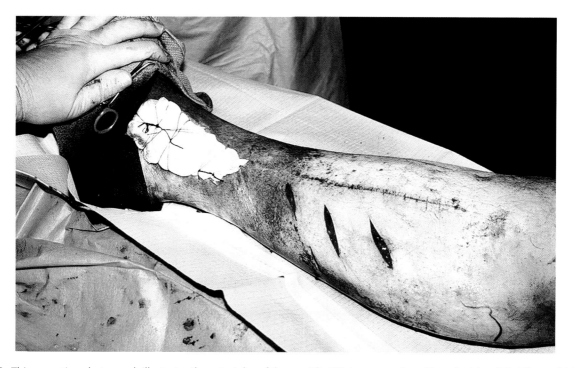

Fig. 9.5. This operative photograph illustrates the principles of the modified Linton procedure. Note the bipedicled flaps which were used to access the posterior arch vein and its perforators. The subcutaneous plexus, perforating veins, and the arch veins were found to be patent and extensive. Further, note the area of ulcer excision and skin grafting.

◀ **Fig. 9.4.** Diagrammatic representation of the original modified Linton operation for stasis ulceration due to axial reflux and medial perforator incompetence. Note the extent of the area which is dissected as shown in the shaded inset. Also note the submalleolar skin line incisions. (From DePalma RG, Surgical therapy for venous stasis surgery. Surgery 1975; 76:910–917, with permission.)

◀ **Fig. 9.6.** This diagram shows a further modification of the Linton procedure. Note the incision to expose the Boyd perforating vein and the incisions used for the shearing procedure described in the text. (From DePalma RG, Evolving approaches for venous ulceration. In: Phlébologie '95. Negus D et al. (eds). Phlébologie 1995; Suppl 1:980–82, with permission.)

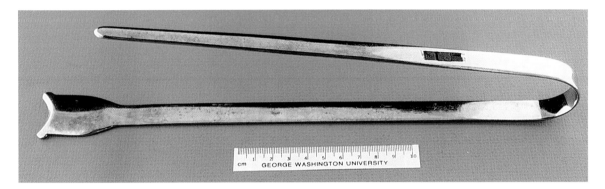

Fig. 9.7. This photograph shows the Simpson and Smellie phlebotome used for extrafascial dissection of perforating veins.

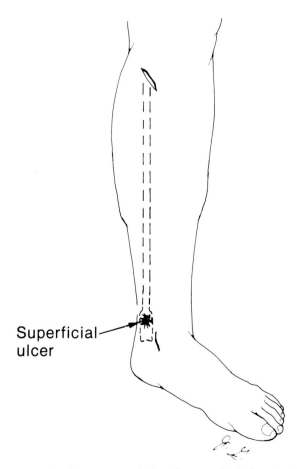

Fig. 9.8. The phlebotome allows division of perforating veins below the superficial ulceration from a remote incision which will heal without difficulty.

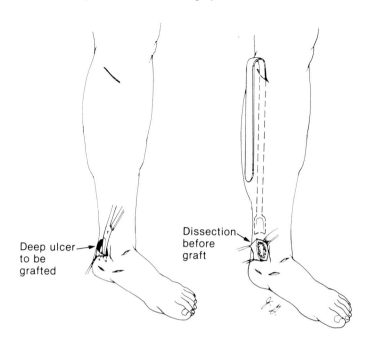

Deep ulcer
to be
grafted

Dissection
before
graft

Fig. 9.9. Excision and dissection of a deep ulcer prior to extrafascial shearing operation. Note the submalleolar access incisions which allow division of the most distal perforating veins below the malleolus.

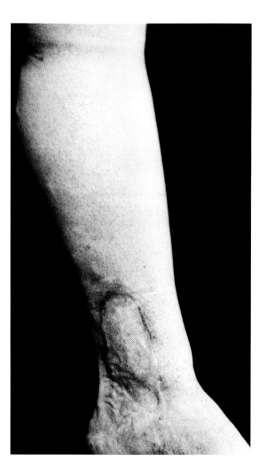

Fig. 9.10. This photograph shows the 10-year result of the shearing procedure. It was performed in a 50-year-old woman with a thrombosed superficial femoral vein, and the shearing procedure was combined with ulcer excision and skin grafting. The patient continues to wear a 30 mmHg graded support stocking.

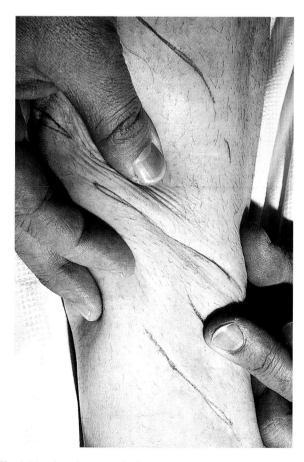

Fig. 9.11. This photograph shows how accurately the skin lines can be used to place incisions for the bipedicled flaps.

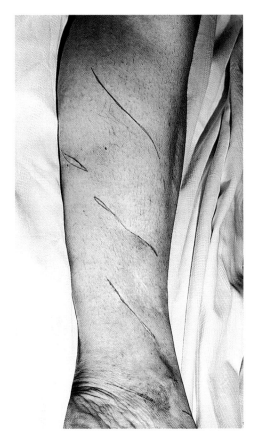

Fig. 9.12. This photograph illustrates the placement of skin line incisions, their rapid healing without excessive scarring in a limb in which skin grafting was not required, and therefore, hospitalization could be decreased. Thus, hospital time is dictated by the size of the ulcer and the need for skin graft healing.

observations extending to 10 years.[9,10,13] These modifications of the Linton procedure are especially useful to accomplish perforator interruption while reducing hospital time, especially in limbs with ulcers less than 3 cm in diameter in which skin grafts are not required (Fig. 9.12). When subcutaneous effacement is extreme or, in treatment of recurrent ulcers after previous surgery, a subfascial endoscopic perforator operation can be combined with extrafascial approaches to perforating veins.

Future Approaches

Modification of Linton's initial principles of perforator interruption are a natural outcome of modern surgical advances. Minimally invasive techniques are

an essential of modern venous surgery. Ultimately, the safety and efficacy of these procedures will make a more rational and aggressive approach to the skin changes caused by venous hypertension possible. It is anticipated that when very severe venous hypertension is present, caused by combinations of valvular reflux with and without proximal venous obstruction, perforator interruption may need to be combined with proximal venous reconstructive procedures. Nevertheless, the modifications of the Linton procedure described and illustrated in this chapter will continue to prove to be useful in severe cases.

References

1. Linton RR (1973) Atlas of Vascular Surgery. WB Saunders Co., Philadelphia, pp 127
2. Linton RR (1938) The communicating veins of the lower leg and the operative technique for their ligation. Ann Surg 107:582–593
3. Linton RR (1949) Surgery of the veins of the lower extremity. Minnesota Med 32:38–46
4. Linton RR (1953) The postthrombotic ulceration of the lower extremity: Its etiology and surgical treatment. Ann Surg 138:415–432
5. Dodd H, Cockett PR (1976) Management of venous ulcers. In: Pathology and Surgery of the Veins of the Lower Limbs. Churchill Livingston, Edinburgh pp 269–276
6. Walsh JC et al. (1994) Femoral venous reflux abolished by greater saphenous vein stripping. Ann Vasc Surg 8:566–570
7. Negus D (1992) The distal long saphenous vein in recurrent venous ulceration. In: Raymond-Martimbeau P, Prescott R, Zummo M (eds) Phlébologie. Libbey Eurotext, Paris pp 1291
8. DePalma RG (1974) Surgical therapy for venous stasis. Surgery 76:910–917
9. DePalma RG (1979) Surgical therapy for venous stasis: Results of a modified Linton operation. Am J Surg 137:810–813
10. DePalma RG (1990) Surgical treatment of chronic venous ulceration. In: Bergan JJ, Yao JST (eds) Venous Disorders. WB Saunders Co., Philadelphia pp 396–406
11. Edwards JM (1976) Shearing operation for incompetent perforating veins. Br J Surg 63:885–886
12. Simpson CJ, Smellie CD (1987) The phlebotomy in the management of incompetent perforating veins and venous ulceration. J Cardiovasc Surg 78:279–281
13. DePalma RG (1992) Surgical treatment of chronic venous ulceration. In: Raymond-Martimbeau P et al. (1992) (eds). Phlébologie. Libbey Eurotext, Paris, pp 1235–1237

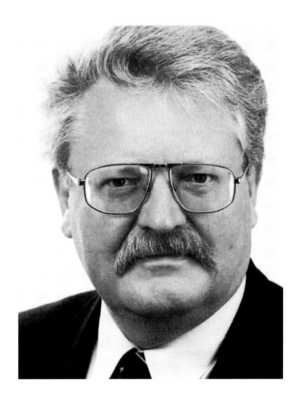

Gerald Hauer
b. 1944

After appropriate premedical preparation, Gerald Hauer graduated from the Ludwig-Maximilian University in Munich in 1969. His doctorate in medicine summarized experimental work on coronary blood flow and blood gases in the healthy human heart as influenced by insulin and glucose.

As a medical assistant, he investigated accumulated experience in treatment of venous insufficiency at the University Surgical Clinic. This stimulated him to help patients who had been labeled with the Latin phrase, *crux medicorum*. This phrase roughly described the venous ulcer as a medical cross to bear. Early on, Hauer was impressed that the standard Cockett operation had unsatisfactory cosmetic results in addition to prolonged postoperative morbidity. Very early, he began investigations "to gain optical access to the subfascial region from a healthy area in order to be able to ligate, coagulate, or clip ..." the perforating veins. From the outset, he felt that no venous ulcer could be present without incompetent associated perforating veins. The objec-

tive of the optically assisted operation was to eliminate the incompetent perforating veins to create a basis for healing ulcers.

Although the 1980s were characterized as a period of intense engagement in the treatment of perforating veins, Hauer worked as a scientific assistant at the Munich University Pathological Institute and was scientific assistant to the surgical clinic at the same University. He was registered as a surgeon in 1979 and as a specialist in accident surgery in 1977, but became a registered specialist in vascular surgery in 1987. He qualified as a lecturer at the Ludwig-Maximilian University with the theme of "the endoscopic subfascial dissection of perforating veins (ESDP)."

Since 1989, Hauer has been superintendent of the surgical department at Weilheim Hospital. He continues to be very active in demonstrating the surgical techniques of perforating vein interruption, has created a series of videos on the subject, and has published extensively, chiefly in the German language.

Technical Armamentaria for Endoscopic Perforator Vein Surgery

10

Mark J. Kulbaski and Alan B. Lumsden

Development of endoscopic perforator interruption is described fully elsewhere in this volume. In brief, in 1985, Hauer reported use of endoscopic instruments to divide perforating veins in the subfascial space of the lower extremity.[1,2] Variations of the technique were then described, including use of a mediastinoscope to access the subfascial space,[3] and distention of the subfascial space with either saline or carbon dioxide to help visualize the perforating veins.[4,5] In 1996, Gloviczki reported a patient experience in which perforating veins were divided using video-guided endoscopic instruments, subfascial carbon dioxide insufflation, and preoperative leg exsanguination to facilitate dissection.[6] The technical armamentaria which is available now to perform this type of procedure will be described in this chapter.

A typical cart containing a video monitor, carbon dioxide insufflator, light source, video recorder, and video printer is shown in Fig. 10.1. Before making the first skin incision, the leg may be exsanguinated with an Esmarch bandage followed by inflating a thigh tourniquet to 300 mmHg. Tourniquet pressure and time of inflation are monitored.

After making a 10–15 mm incision over the medial aspect of the superficial posterior compartment, a variety of instruments are available for entering the subfascial space. After identifying the fascia by blunt dissection with narrow blade retractors (e.g. Army/Navy type), a 1 cm incision in the fascia is made, through which a 10 mm trocar is placed. Disposable and reusable trocars can be used (Fig. 10.2). Alternatively, blunt dissection to find the fascia can be avoided by inserting a Visiport-type

trocar (Autosuture Company, Norwalk, CT) through the skin incision (Fig. 10.3). This device consists of a 12 mm trocar with a transparent solid end. A blade is incorporated into the end that can be advanced with a trigger control. Under direct vision, the subcutaneous fat is traversed, the fascia incised, and the trocar advanced into the subfascial space.

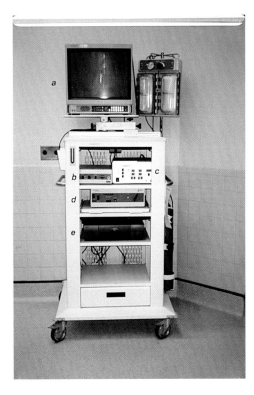

Fig. 10.1 Endoscopic cart. a: Video monitor (Sony Corp.: Tokyo, Japan), b: Insufflator (Snowden Pencer Inc.; Atlanta, GA), c: Video camera (Snowden Pencer Inc.; Atlanta, GA), d: Light source (Snowden Pencer Inc.; Atlanta, GA), e: Video (Toshiba Corp; Tokyo, Japan), f: Video printer (Sony Corp.: Tokyo, Japan).

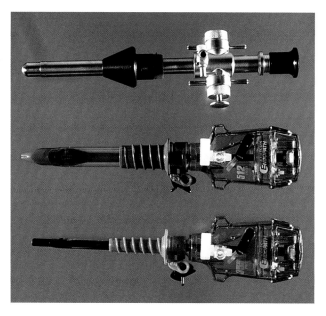

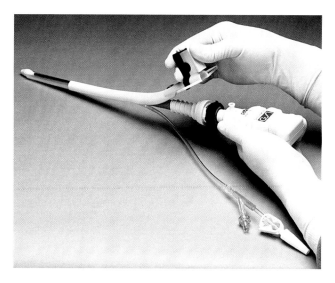

Fig. 10.5. Spacemaker Balloon Dissector with cover being removed.

Fig. 10.2. Top: 10-mm reusable trochar (Snowden Pencer Inc.; Atlanta, GA), Middle: 10-mm disposable Endopath trochar (Ethicon Eno-Surgery; Cincinnati, OH), Bottom: 5-mm disposable Endopath trochar (Ethicon Eno-Surgery; Cincinnati, OH).

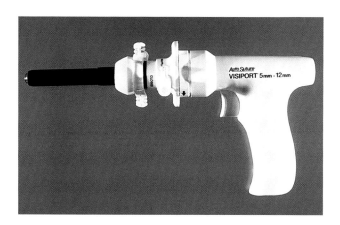

Fig. 10.3. Visiport (Auto Suture Company; Norwalk CT).

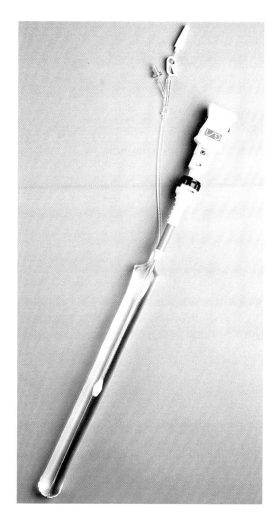

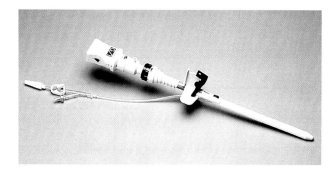

Fig. 10.4. Spacemaker Balloon Dissector (General Surgical Innovations, Inc.; Palo Alto, CA).

Fig. 10.6. Spacemaker Balloon Dissector with balloon filled with saline.

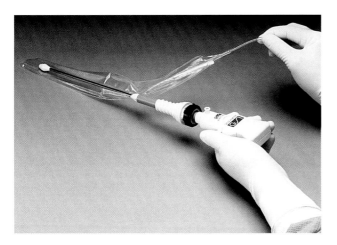

Fig. 10.7. Spacemaker Balloon Dissector with balloon being removed.

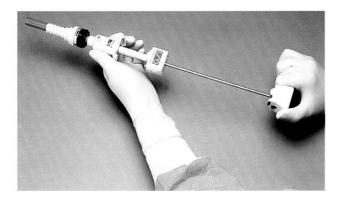

Fig. 10.8. Spacemaker Balloon Dissector with guide rod and obrurator being removed.

Enlargement of the subfascial space to visualize the perforating veins may be accomplished by connecting a carbon dioxide line to the trocar and pressurizing it to 15 to 30 mmHg. Alternatively, the spacemaker balloon dissector (General Surgical Innovations, Inc., Palo Alto, CA) may be used instead of gas insufflation to create the subfascial space (Fig. 10.4). To use this dissector, the device is inserted completely beneath the subfascial space, the balloon cover is removed (Fig. 10.5) and the balloon is filled with saline to separate the fascial from the muscle (Fig. 10.6). The saline is then evacuated and the balloon removed (Fig. 10.7). The guide rod and obturator (Fig. 10.8) are then removed, leaving a 10 mm trocar in position. A carbon dioxide line is attached and the subfascial space is maintained with insufflation to 15 to 30 mmHg.

A straight-lens, 10 mm endoscope (Olympus America, Inc., Roswell, GA), to which a videocamera is attached, is placed through the trocar to visualize the subfascial space (Fig. 10.9). A second trocar, through which operating instruments can be inserted, is placed under direct vision medial to the first trocar. If perforating veins are not immediately visible, they can be identified by blunt dissection with an endoscopic blunt cherry dissector (Ethicon Endo-Surgery, Cincinnati, OH) (Fig. 10.10). The veins can be occluded with a 5 mm. ligaclip Allport clip applier (Ethicon Endo-Surgery, Cincinnati, OH) (Figs 10.11, 10.12). Alternatively, the veins can be

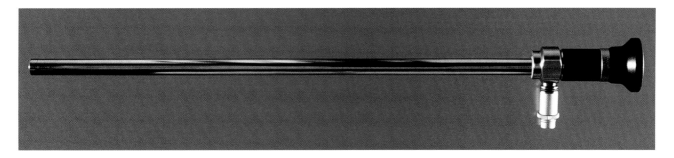

Fig. 10.9. Straight lens 10-mm endoscope (Olympus America, Inc.; Roswell, GA).

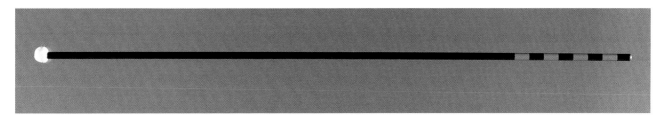

Fig. 10.10. Blunt Cherry Dissector (Ethicon Endo-Surgery; Cincinnati, OH).

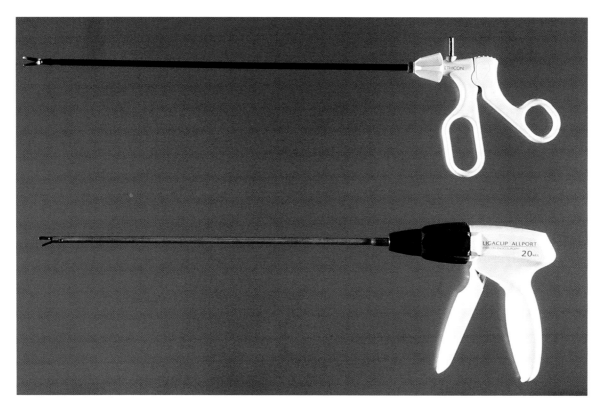

Fig. 10.11. *Top*: 5-mm curved endoscopic scissors (Ethicon Endo-Surgery; Cincinnati, OH), *Bottom*: 5-mm Ligaclip Allport clip applier (Ethicon Endo-Surgery; Cincinnati, OH).

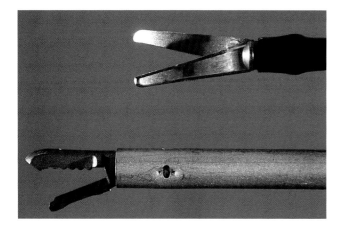

Fig. 10.12. *Top*: Close-up of 5-mm curved endoscopic scissors (Ethicon Endo-Surgery; Cincinnati, OH). *Bottom*: Close-up of 5 mm Ligaclip Allport clip applier (Ethicon Endo-Surgery; Cincinnati, OH).

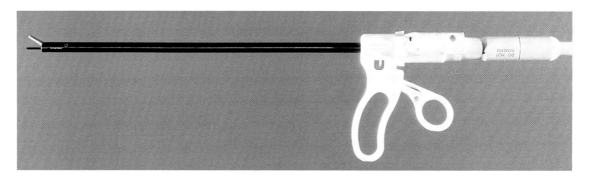

Fig. 10.13. Harmonic Scalpel (Ethicon Endo-Surgery; Cincinnati, OH).

divided hemostatically with a harmonic scalpel (Ethicon Endo-Surgery, Cincinnati, OH) which uses ultrasonic energy to seal the ends of a vessel before division (Fig. 10.13).

An alternative to the closed gas insufflation techniques is the use of open scopes. This method was pioneered and developed in Europe and is almost exclusively employed there at this time. Fig. 10.14 shows the employment of an open mediastinoscope. This method pioneered subfascial endoscopic perforator vein surgery but has been largely abandoned because of the development of specialized instrumentation.

Fig. 10.15 shows the Storz developments for endoscopic perforator vein surgery. The scope has angled optics for the videocamera and a large working

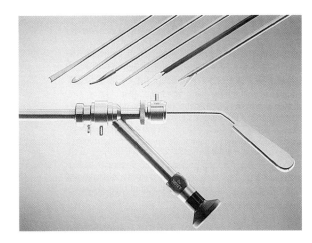

Fig. 10.16. Other instrumentation adapted to the Storz scope are illustrated in this photograph. Note the prograde and retrograde fasciotomy knives as well as the blunt dissectors.

channel. Through the working channel, the electrocoagulation clamps can be inserted and utilized. These are 1 mm and 3 mm in diameter. Further, the angulated scissors can be used to divide perforating veins after preliminary electrocoagulation.

Fig. 10.16 displays other instrumentation developed by Storz for use in the working channel of the open scope. These are modifications of Reinhard Fischer's instrumentation. The fasciotomy knives for prograde and retrograde division of the fascia are seen as well as the blunt and sharp dissecting instrumentation. These are adapted to the rather long length of the Storz scope.

Fig. 10.17 shows the open scope developed by Hauer. This instrument provides a large working channel and its relatively short length avoids prob-

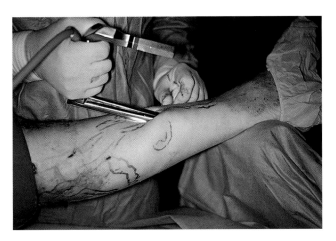

Fig. 10.14. Illustration of the open mediastinosope used in the pioneering days of subfascial endoscopic perforator vein surgery.

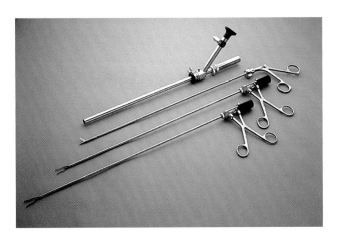

Fig. 10.15. This is a display of the early Storz instrumentation which applied video visualization to the surgical technique. The instruments shown are electrocoagulation clamps and scissors.

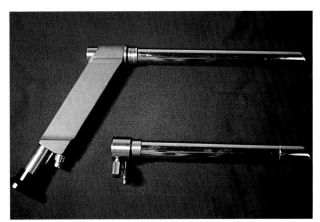

Fig. 10.17. This ETB scope is a direct descendant of the mediastinoscope. This scope was developed by Hauer for specific subfascial endoscopic perforator vein surgery.

lems of instrumental manipulation caused by the knee and by the proximal tourniquet. Electro-coagulation of perforators and clipping can be performed through the scope. Division of the perforators with angulated scissors or electrocoagulating scissors can also be accomplished.

At the end of the procedure, the fascia may be left open.[2] The trocar skin sites are closed with a subcuticular stitch and the leg is wrapped with an elastic bandage.

References

1. Hauer G (1985) The endoscopic subfascial division of the perforating veins: Preliminary report (in German). VASA 14:59–61
2. Hauer G Barkun, Wisser I, Deiler S (1988) Endoscopic subfascial dissection of perforating veins. Surg Endosc 2:5–12
3. Pierik EGJM, Wittens CHA, van Urk H (1995) Subfascial endoscopic ligation in the treatment of incompetent perforating veins. Eur J Vasc Endovasc Surg 9:38–41
4. O'Donnell TF (1992). Surgical treatment of incompetent communicating veins. In: Bergan JJ, Kistner RL (eds). Atlas of Venous Surgery. WB Saunders Co., Philadelphia pp 111–124
5. Conrad P (1994) Endoscopic exploration of the subfascial space of the lower leg with perforator vein interruption using laparoscopic equipment: A preliminary report. Phlebology 1994; 9:154–157
6. Gloviczki P, Cambria RA, Rhee RY, Canton LG, McKusick MA (1996) Surgical technique and preliminary results of endoscopic subfascial division of perforating veins. J Vasc Surg 23:517–523

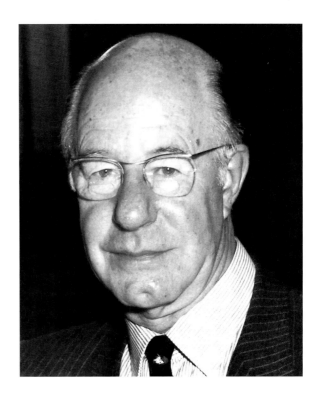

Frank Cockett
b. 1916

Although a thorough Englishman, Frank Cockett was born in Rockhampton, Queensland, Australia in 1916. His education was at the Bedford School in England and then at St Thomas's Hospital in London. His war service in 1942 led to publication of a reminiscence of the siege of Malta entitled *The Maltese Penguin*.

He was strongly dedicated to St Thomas's Hospital London where he received his training. He was appointed as consultant in 1954 on the surgical professorial unit. Cockett was also surgeon to the King Edward VII Hospital for Officers in London and his main research work throughout his active practice was on the anatomy and physiology of ankle perforating veins and the part they play in causing venous ulceration. His initial contribution on the subject, entitled "The Ankle Blowout Syndrome" was published with D. E. Elgan Jones in *Lancet* (1953) 1:17. He was also interested in venous compression syndromes, including anatomical compression of the left iliac vein published as "The Iliac Compression Syndrome" with M. Lea Thomas in the *British Journal of Surgery* (1965) 52:816.

Thoroughly respected by surgical colleagues, he served as President of the Vascular Surgical Society of Great Britain and Ireland in 1980 and was Chairman of the Venous Forum of the Royal Society of Medicine from 1985 to 1987. His volume *Pathology and Surgery of the Veins of the Lower Limb* went through two editions in 1956 and 1976 and is being revised presently. He strongly supported the historical and artistic side of St Thomas's Hospital, publishing numerous general articles in the *St Thomas's Hospital Gazette* and serving as editor of the second edition of the *History of St. Thomas's Hospital* while serving for 12 years as Chairman of the St Thomas's Hospital Works of Art and History Committee.

Cockett's main contribution to vascular surgery began in 1950 when he realized, on taking over the leg ulcer clinic at St Thomas's Hospital, that leg ulcers remained an enormous unsolved problem. During numerous painstaking dissections on cadaver limbs, including the technique of arterial and venous injections, he learned that the ankle perforating veins and not the saphenous vein were the direct venous drainage pathways of the ulcer-bearing area in the erect, exercising leg. Shortly, he studied this new concept further using the venography techniques which dos Santos had just demonstrated. He found that the ankle perforating veins were occasionally enormously enlarged, and in 1951, he operated on his first case with "great fear that the wound would not heal."

A keen athlete, Frank Cockett has always enjoyed tennis, squash, swimming and skiing but his most exciting and rewarding activity has been sailing. He has owned four boats, the second of which was not only the best, but the most famous, and this was a classic ocean racer called *Saphena*. Although he raced in early days, his later sailing experiences have involved cruising to north European coastal countries with Mrs Cockett on a seagoing yacht called *Saphena Minor*.

Mr and Mrs Cockett enjoy a productive and vigorous life based in Kensington in London where they collect marine, flower and garden pictures. They enjoy the love and affection of five children, two of whom are twins. Mrs. Cockett is currently involved in organizing the Florence Nightingale Museum at St Thomas's Hospital which Mr Cockett remarks, "I hope you will visit next time you are in London."

Subfascial Endoscopic Perforator Vein Surgery with Gas Insufflation

11

Peter Gloviczki, Linda G. Canton, Robert A. Cambria and Robert Y. Rhee

Progress in minimally invasive techniques used for abdominal surgical procedures has been primarily responsible for the renewed interest in perforator vein surgery. Initial endoscopic procedures applied single lumen endoscope or mediastinoscope for viewing and as working channel, sometimes without the benefits of video equipment and appropriate endoscopic stapling devices.[1-4] Improvement in the single scope concept adding video equipment and new instrumentation was inevitable, and currently used techniques[5-7] are discussed in detail in Chapters 12 and 15. Laparoscopic instrumentation using two ports has been the new generation of tools in the evolution of perforator surgery. Carbon-dioxide insufflation into the subfascial space was added to improve visibility and to enlarge the working space. We started the use of gas insufflation early in our experience, recognizing its advantages over infusion of water in the subfascial space as recommended initially.[8] Our team performed the first endoscopic perforator vein operation with gas insufflation on 5 August 1993, and we reported results of our first 11 procedures subsequently.[9] When we started our procedures, we were unaware of Conrad's work in Australia; he also started to use gas insufflation for his operations in 1993.[10] Unlike his technique, we have added the use of pneumatic thigh tourniquet to prevent gas embolism and more importantly, to provide bloodless field for easier dissection and division of perforating veins. In this chapter, we review our technique of subfascial endoscopic perforator vein surgery (SEPS), using laparoscopic instrumentation and gas insufflation and present early and mid-term results of the first 40 operations, performed at the Mayo Clinic.

Patient Selection

Patients with advanced chronic venous insufficiency either due to previous deep venous thrombosis or due to primary valvular incompetence are candidates for this operation. While some patients belonged to clinical Class 4 (lipodermatosclerosis, induration or eczema), most are Class 6 (active ulcer) or Class 5 (healed ulcer) patients, according to the updated classification of the Joint Vascular Societies.[11] Every patient underwent attempts to treat the ulcer non-operatively before perforator surgery, using techniques suggested elsewhere in this volume (Chapters 17, 18). The presence of active ulcer has not been a contraindication to surgical treatment. However, infected ulcers, cellulitis or eczema was first treated non-operatively to decrease chances of wound complications. Debridement and appropriate local ulcer care (Chapter 19) was complemented with graduated compression stockings, frequent elevation of the leg and in some cases, bed rest, before surgical treatment of superficial and perforating vein incompetence was undertaken.

Preoperative Evaluation

Our non-invasive venous evaluation includes strain gauge plethysmography to assess global venous function of the extremity, to confirm valvular incompetence of the superficial or deep system, and to exclude functional venous outflow obstruction (Chapter 6). However, detailed duplex scanning of the venous system of the lower extremity is the most important preoperative test of these patients, as presented in detail in Chapter 7. The test includes examination of the greater saphenous vein and deep veins for obstruction and valvular incompetence. Detailed examination of the medial perforating veins is performed on the day before surgery to establish the diagnosis of perforator vein incompetence. Incompetent perforating veins are marked on the patient leg with a permanent marker, using an X, while competent perforating veins are marked with an O. In patients who have incompetent saphenous vein or undergo avulsion of the superficial veins, careful marking of all varicose veins on the skin is also done immediately before surgery. Ascending and descending venography is now done preoperatively only in those patients who have evidence of significant deep venous occlusions on duplex scanning or plethysmography.

Surgical Technique

General or epidural anesthesia is used to perform the operation. The affected lower extremity and groin is prepared and draped in a sterile fashion and a pneumatic tourniquet placed high on the thigh.

Esmarque's bandage is wrapped around the elevated extremity (Fig. 11.1) and the tourniquet is inflated to 300 mmHg. The duration of the tourniquet inflation is continuously monitored.

The most frequent port size that we use for the operation is 10 mm, although 5 mm port is also available. The two ports have to be placed distant from the site of the ulcerations, but still close enough to reach the level of the ankle with the endoscopic instruments and the video camera. The ports should also be far away from each other to permit easy manipulation. The first incision is made about 10–12 cm distal to the level of the tibial tuberosity, about 2–3 cm medial to the medial edge of the tibia. The skin incision is limited to less than 12 mm to avoid air leak and the fascia is incised with a fine blade (Fig. 11.2A, B).

A 10-mm laparoscopic port is inserted with the help of a blunt obturator to prevent placement of the port into the calf muscles. We have used Fogarty's dissecting balloon (*see* Chapter 13) in several patients at this stage of the operation and found it helpful to enlarge the pre-existing subfascial space, that only contains very loose connective tissue. The use of balloon, however, does not obviate the need for gas insufflation. Once the port is placed under the fascia, carbon dioxide is insufflated to obtain a pressure of 30 mmHg (Fig. 11.3). A 10-mm video camera is inserted in the subfascial space to confirm correct port position. The second 10-mm port is inserted 5–6 cm more posterior and 2–3 cm more distal to the first incision into the subfascial space. We use the video camera to guide placement of the trocar which is inserted with the second laparo-

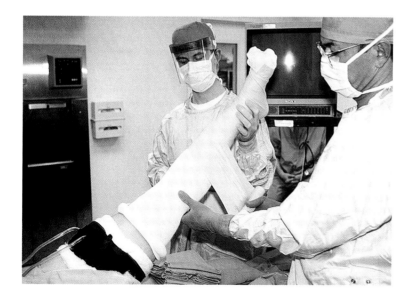

Fig. 11.1. Endoscopic perforator division is performed in a bloodless field, placing a pneumatic tourniquet on the thigh and exsanguinating the extremity with an Esmarque bandage.

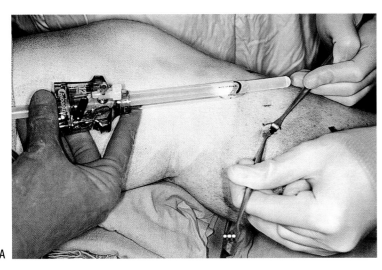
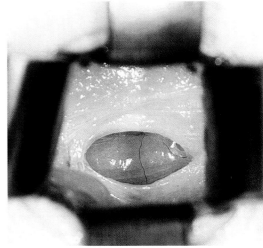

A   B

Fig. 11.2. **A** 10-mm laparoscopic port is placed with help of blunt obturator into subfascial space. **B** Incision of the fascia of the superficial posterior compartment. Note the small skin incision to permit air seal round port. (With permission from Gloviczki P, Cambria RA, Rhee YR, Canton LG, McKusick MA. Surgical technique and preliminary results with endoscopic subfascial division of perforating veins. J Vasc Surg (1966) 23:517–523.)

scopic port. If a clear view of the port placement through the video camera is not obtained, we prefer a small incision made in the fascia under direct vision, as for the first port placement, to avoid trauma by the trocar. Dissection is performed with laparoscopic forceps and scissors which are placed through the second port (Figs 11.4, 11.5).

The loose connective tissue that remains between the fascia and the calf muscles after gas insufflation is divided sharply with laparoscopic scissors. The most important veins that can be easily dissected from the superficial posterior compartment are the distal paratibial perforators, located usually just medial to the first endoscopic port, the more distally

located Cockett III and the Cockett II perforators (*see* Chapter 2).

The veins are dissected and clipped using the 10-mm or 5-mm clip applier. Since the jaws of the 10-mm clip applier (Ethicon-Endo-Surgery, Inc.) are tilted, they permit better visual control of clip placement (Fig. 11.6A). However, the 5-mm Alport clips are stronger and very reliable. After placement of clips the veins are divided with laparoscopic scissors to facilitate further dissection (Figs 11.6B, 11.7). Small arteries or small nerves may accompany some of the perforating veins. Most of the time, these structures are divided without undue consequences.

The entire subfascial space from the edge of the

Fig. 11.3. Carbon dioxide is insufflated through first port, that is used for the video camera. Placement of a second 10-mm port is performed under video control. Note that incompetent perforators were marked with an X preoperatively using duplex scanning (With permission from Gloviczki P, Cambria RA, Rhee Y R, Canton LG, McKusick MA. Surgical technique and preliminary results with endoscopic subfascial division of perforating veins. J Vasc Surg (1966) 23:517–523.)

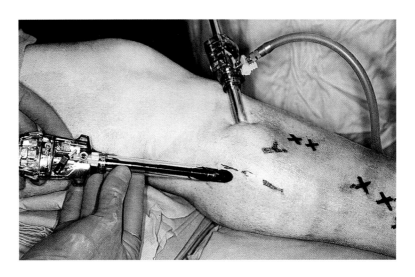

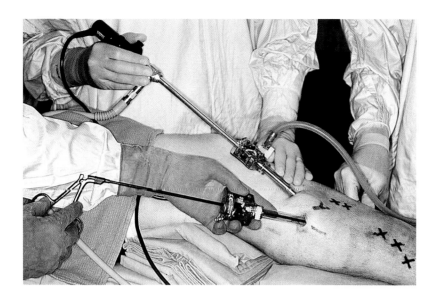

Fig. 11.4. Clipping and division of perforators is performed with laparoscopic Instruments placed through the second port; first port is used for video control. (With permission from Gloviczki P, Cambria RA, Rhe YR, Canton LG, McKusick MA. Surgical technique and preliminary results with endoscopic subfascial division of perforating veins. J Vasc Surg (1996) 23:517–523.

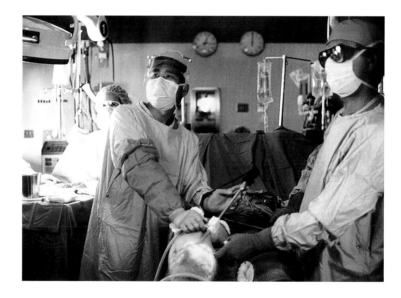

Fig. 11.5. Setup of the team for endoscopic perforator surgery. The surgeon is operating from the side opposite to the affected limb, the first assistant is standing on the ipsilateral side controlling the video port. (With permission from Gloviczki P, Cambria RA, Rhee YR, Canton LG, McKusick M A. Surgical technique and preliminary results with endoscopic subfascial division of perforating veins. J Vasc Surg (23:517–523.)

tibia to the posterior midline and down to the level of the ankle is explored and all medial perforating veins are interrupted (Fig. 11.8). There is frequently a duplication of the fascia between the superficial and deep posterior compartment (intermuscular septum) that has to be incised to uncover the Cockett II perforators. These and other perforators can also be found under the fascia of the deep posterior compartment. To access these, paratibial fasciotomy has to be performed (Fig. 11.9A, B). Attention has to be paid not to injure the posterior tibial vessels and the tibial nerve during paratibial fasciotomy. To divide more proximal paratibial perforators, the insertion of the soleus muscle on the tibia may also have to be incised (*see* Chapter 2 for details of anatomy).

Perforators proximal to the port placement can be divided by turning both ports around, and dissection continued up to the level of the knee. Distal dissection can be limited by the patient's anatomy, by the length of the leg, a thick layer of subcutaneous fat, a large knee preventing current instruments to be tilted in proper angle to reach distally or by a very rigid, liposclerotic tissue of the lower leg. Retromalleolar perforators in our experience rarely could be divided using endoscopic technique.

After completion of the procedure gas insufflation is stopped, the video camera, the dissecting instruments and ports are removed, and any residual subfascial or subcutaneous gas is manually expressed from the limb through the two small incisions. The tourniquet is then deflated. If the patient has an

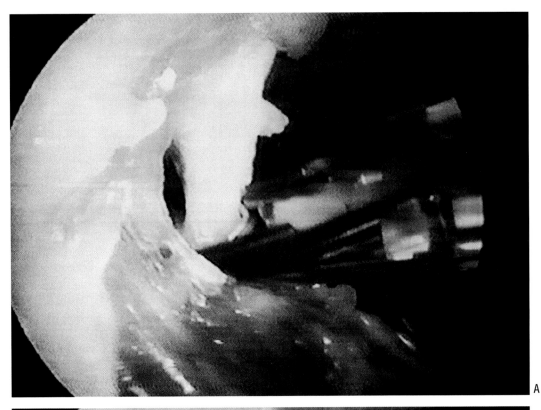

A

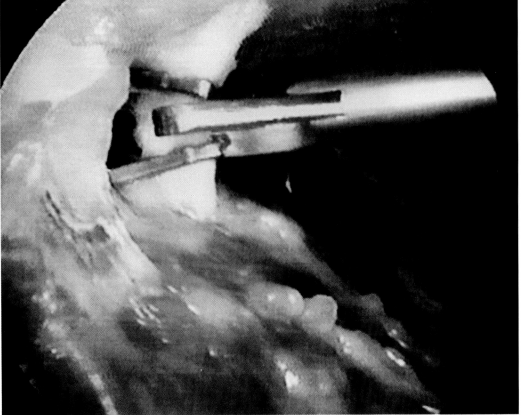

B

Fig. 11.6. A Clipping of a medial calf perforator with a 10-mm clip applier. **B** Division of the perforator with endoscopic scissors after placement of vascular clips. (With permission from Gloviczki P, Cambria RA, Rhee YR, Canton LG, McKusick MA. Surgical technique and preliminary results with endoscopic subfascial division of perforating veins. J Vasc Surg (1966) 23:517–523.)

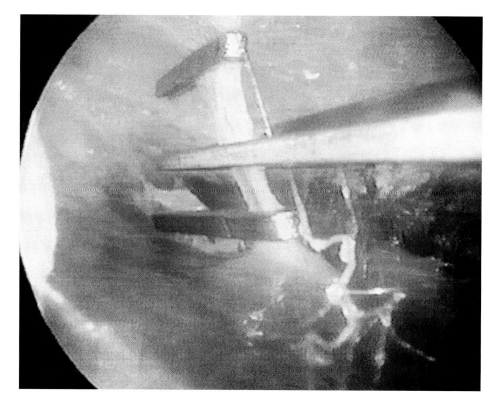

Fig. 11.7. Endoscopic division of a smaller perforator after placement of two clips on the vein.

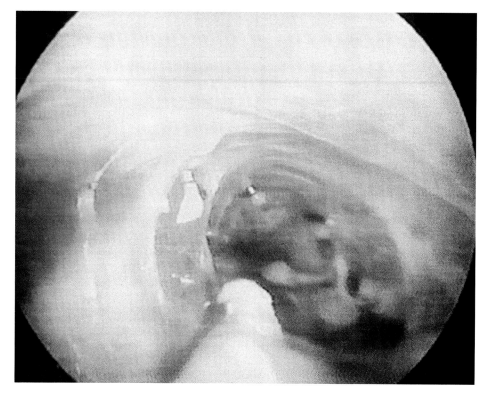

Fig. 11.8 Full view of the superficial posterior compartment after clipping and division of the medial perforating veins. (With permission from Gloviczki P, Cambria RA, Rhee YR, Canton LG, McKusick MA. Surgical technique and preliminary results with endoscopic subfascial division of perforating veins. J Vasc Surg (1996) 23:517–523.)

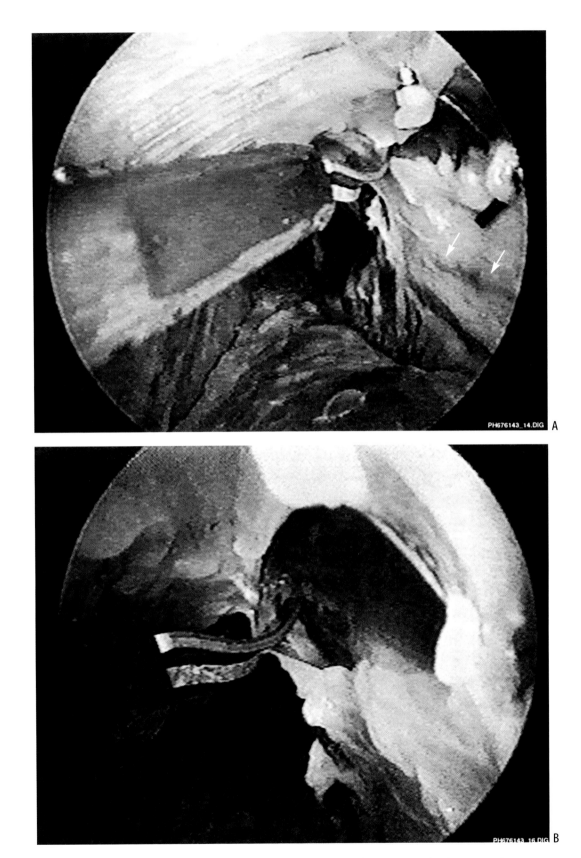

Fig. 11.9. A Paratibial fasciotomy performed with endoscopic scissors in a right leg, entering the deep posterior compartment. Note the posterior tibial vessels, transparent through the deep fascia (arrows). **B** Completion of the fasciotomy in the same patient.

Table 11.1. Signs and symptoms of chronic venous insufficiency in 40 limbs

Signs and symptoms	Limbs (%)
Pigmentation	39 (98)
Pain	35 (88)
Edema	33 (83)
Ulcer	20 (50)
Lipodermatosclerosis	21 (53)
Varicosity	36 (90)
Venous claudication	1 (3)

incompetent superficial system, high ligation and stripping of the saphenous vein is performed, together with varicose vein avulsion which is done through small stab wounds. The incision for the first port is used frequently to dissect the distal end of the saphenous vein below the knee to complete stripping of the greater saphenous vein. Longer incisions are closed with interrupted 2–0 subcutaneous Vicryl, and the skin is closed with interrupted 4–0 subcutaneous Vicryl. The extremity is wrapped with elastic bandage, the leg is elevated 30° and ambulation permitted 3 h after the operation. Most patients are discharged within 24 h after overnight observation.

Clinical Material

Between 5 August 1993, and 31 December 1996, 40 SEPS procedures were performed in 34 patients, 22 females and 12 males. Mean age of the patients was 48 years, ranging from 28 to 77 years. Twenty limbs had active ulcers (Class 6), six had healed ulcers (Class 5). Eleven limbs had lipodermatosclerosis or other skin changes of chronic venous disease (Tables 11.1 and 11.2). Sixty percent of the ulcers were greater than 2 cm in size, and 60% did not heal for more than 3 months before the operation. The etiology of chronic venous disease was previous deep venous thrombosis in 15 (38%) of the 40 limbs, in 9 limbs with a history of trauma preceding the venous thrombosis. Twenty six limbs (65%) had primary valvular incompetence. Preoperative evaluation revealed deep venous incompetence in 88% of the limb, with associated deep venous obstruction in 7 limbs. Twenty-one limbs had incompetence of the greater saphenous vein.

Results

Intraoperative Data

The number of perforating veins divided during the 30 SEPS procedures averaged 4.8, ranging from 1 to 10. Mean tourniquet time was 53 minutes, ranging from 25 to 75 min. Additional operations were performed in 35 limbs. These included stripping of the greater or lesser saphenous veins (25 limbs and 1 limb, respectively), high ligation of the greater saphenous vein (3 limbs), and avulsion of varicose veins without operation on the saphenous veins (7 limbs). In 5 limbs, procedures other than the SEPS were not performed

Clinical Results

Our follow-up averaged 14 months, ranging from 1 to 40 months. Clinical outcome was excellent in 29 patients where the ulcer either healed or did not recur and the patients had no significant residual symptoms (Figs 11.10, 11.11, 11.12 and 11.13). Most patients continued to use elastic compression. The clinical status of 9 patients improved with less symptoms and/or healing of the ulcers at last follow-up. One patient with no significant improvement had recurrent ulcers, although they were smaller and healed for longer periods of time than before surgery. Pain and swelling increased because of perioperative deep venous thrombosis in another patient resulting in worse early outcome at 4 weeks postoperatively. Clinical score of chronic venous disease improved significantly during follow-up from 7.37 to 2.26 ($P<0.005$) (Table 11.3), using a scoring system suggested by the consensus committee of the American Venous Forum.[12] Ulcers in all 20 patients healed ultimately, with recurrence occurring during follow-up in 1 patient only. Ulcer healing was rapid in most patients, with a median time from operation to ulcer healing of 36 days (mean: 106 days; range: 11–670 days). One of 6 patients who had healed ulcer at the time of SEPS had ulcer recurrence during follow-up.

Table 11.2.   Preoperative classification of chronic venous disease in 40 limbs

Category		No. of patients (%)
Clinical class (C)	C_1 = telangiectases or reticular veins	0 (0)
	C_2 = varicose veins	0 (0)
	C_3 = edema without skin changes	1 (3)
	C_4 = skin changes ascribed to venous disease (e.g. pigmentation, venous eczema, lipodermatosclerosis)	11 (28)
	C_5 = skin changes as defined above with healed ulceration	8 (20)
	C_6 = skin changes as defined above with active ulceration	20 (50)
Etiology (E)	Primary	25 (62)
	Secondary	15 (38)
Anatomy (A)	Superficial[a]	35 (88)
	Deep	35 (88)
	Perforator[b]	40 (100)
Pathophysiology (P)	Reflux only	36 (90)
	Obstruction only	0 (0)
	Reflux and obstruction	4 (10)

[a] Incompetence of greater saphenous vein was documented preoperatively in 21 patients only (53%)
[b] In 2 patients perforator incompetence was not documented by preoperative tests.

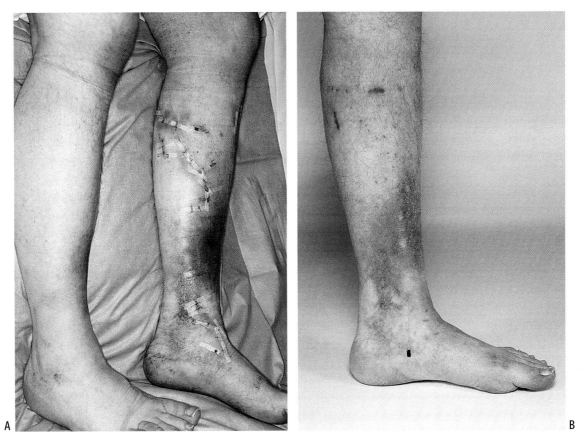

A   B

Fig. 11.10. A Intraoperative photograph of the legs of a 60-year-old male with severe left lower extremity chronic venous disease. **A** Postoperative photograph of the same leg at 3 months after endoscopic perforator vein division, saphenous vein stripping and varicose vein avulsion; early clinical result was excellent.

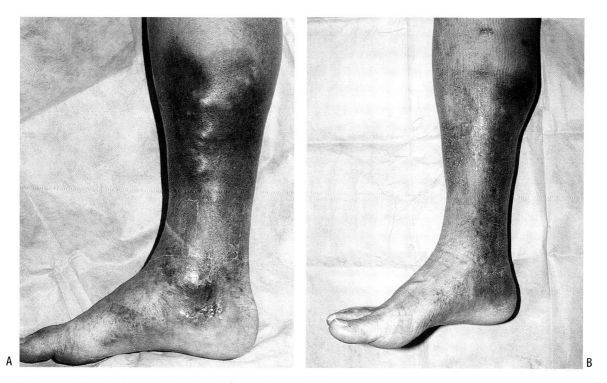

A   B

Fig. 11.11. A Right leg of a 64-year-old male with 2-year history of ulcer and severe post-thrombotic syndrome. **B** Postoperative picture at 6 weeks shows healed ulcer and incisions following SEPS, stripping and avulsion of varicose veins. Three years later the patient is asymptomatic, does not use elastic stockings and had no ulcer recurrence.

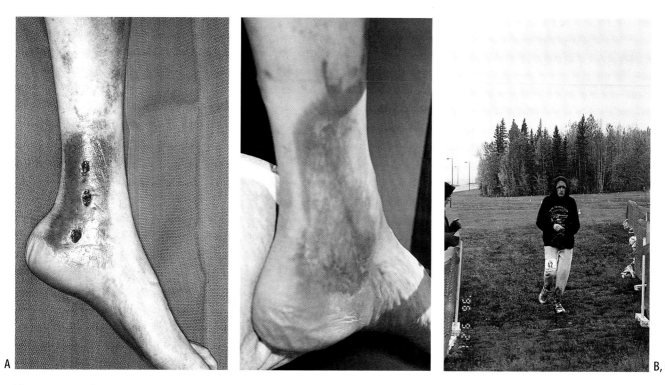

A   B, C

Fig. 11.12. A Left leg of a 39-year-old male with severe post-thrombotic syndrome and bilateral recurrent venous ulcers of 10 years duration. SEPS procedure and in a second stage skin grafting were performed. **B** Photograph of the leg 3 years later shows healed ulcers. **C** Same patient 2 years and 9 months after operation completing the 26.2 miles of the Alaska Equinox, considered to be one of the most difficult marathons in the United States.

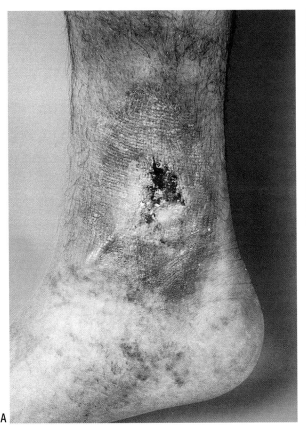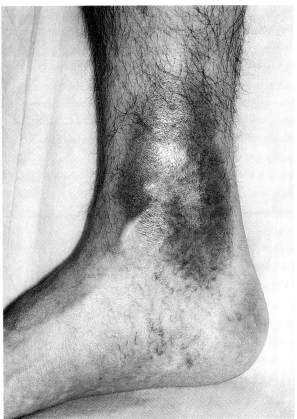

Fig. 11.13. A Thirty-six-year-old male with post-thrombotic ulcer right ankle, before endoscopic division of 6 medial perforating veins. **B** Photograph of the same leg 10 months later shows healed ulcer.

Complications

No early or late mortality occurred. One patient developed a superficial groin wound infection at the site of high ligation of the grater saphenous vein, for an incidence of wound infection of 2.5%. We did not observe wound infections at the site of the endoscopic port placement.

One patient developed iliofemoral deep venous thrombosis within 5 days after surgery, for an early incidence of 2.5% (1/40). This patient had severe post-thrombotic syndrome with chronic inferior vena cava occlusion but no evidence of functional outflow obstruction on preoperative plethysmographic studies. SEPS was combined with stripping of his grossly incompetent greater saphenous vein and avulsion of multiple, extensive varicosity. Perioperative thrombosis prophylaxis included elastic stockings and early ambulation, but heparin was not given to avoid bleeding complications due to the elevated venous pressure, observed during avulsion. This patient required hospitalization for severe pain and swelling 5 days after the operation and was treated with full anticoagulation. Four weeks later duplex scanning showed almost complete recanalization of the deep system and his clinical symptoms have markedly improved.

One patient developed superficial thrombophlebitis proximal to the area of the port placement within a few days after the operation. Postoperative duplex scanning in this patient excluded early deep venous thrombosis. However, this 46-year-old male, with a history of frequent recurrent deep venous thromboses and documented protein C deficiency, developed recurrent popliteal vein thrombosis 2 months after the operation. Overall, his clinical condition did not improve postoperatively.

Two patients developed saphenous vein neuralgia (5%, 2/40); both underwent stripping of the greater saphenous veins in addition to perforator interruption. One of our patients with preoperative episodes of cellulitis developed one additional episode 6 months postoperatively requiring hospitalization and intravenous antibiotic treatment.

Table 11.3. Mean clinical scores of chronic venous disease in 40 limbs (In patients with both preoperative and postoperative clinical scores reported)

Category	Scoring system	Mean preoperative score	Mean postoperative score

Pain	0 = none
	1 = moderate, not
	     requiring analgesics
	2 = severe, requiring
	     analgesics
		1.0	0.42

Edema	0 = none 1 = mild/moderate 2 = severe	0.78	0.31
Venous claudication	0 = none 1 = mild/moderate 2 = severe	0.03	0.03
Pigmentation	0 = none 1 = localized 2 = extensive	0.98	0.97
Lipodermatosclerosis	0 = none 1 = localized 2 = extensive	0.53	0.36
Ulcer size: (largest ulcer)	0 = none 1 <2 cm diameter 2 >2 cm diameter	0.93	0.03
Ulcer: duration	0 = none 1 _ ≤3 months 2 _ ≥3 months	0.88	0.03
Ulcer: recurrence	0 = none 1 = once 2 = more than once	0.96	0.08
Ulcer: number	0 = none 1 = single 2 = multiple	1.28	0.03
Total mean clinical score[a]		7.37	2.26

[a] $P < 0.005$

Discussion

The minimally invasive endoscopic Linton operation using carbon-dioxide insufflation is a good technique for dissection and interruption of medial incompetent perforating veins of the leg. Video-assisted visual control brings definite advantage over blind avulsion of perforators using shearing instruments[13] or over the use of small, limited incisions[14] that do not permit full exploration of the subfascial space. Wound complications of the classic or modified Linton operations[15–19] using longer skin incisions made frequently in diseased, lipodermatosclerotic skin (Fig. 11.14A) were significantly more frequent than reported wound complications of endoscopic procedures.[1–10,20] All incisions for port placement have healed by primary intention in our patients (Fig. 11.14 B,C). Endoscopic techniques have clear advantages when used for division of incompetent perforators to decrease ambulatory venous hypertension in the area of the leg most sensitive to develop venous ulcerations.

We use laparoscopic instrumentation and video equipment that is readily available in all hospitals where general surgery is performed. Although we have asked for and received approval of our

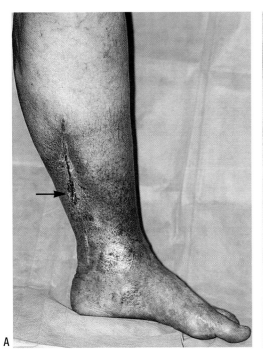
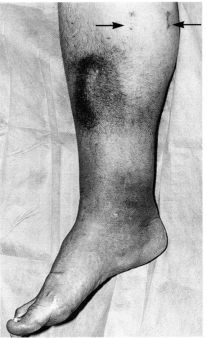
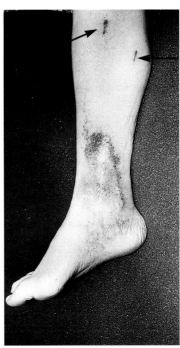

A   B,C

Fig. 11.14. A Forty-four-year-old female 3 years following modified open Linton operation for post-thrombotic left leg ulcer. Her ulcer healed early but her incision (arrow) dehisced and healed only recently by secondary intention. **B, C** Excellent wound healing (and early healing of an active ulcer) (arrows) at 5 and at 6 weeks after endoscopic procedures.

Institutional Review Board to study our first series of patients who underwent this operation, perforator ligations using open or endoscopic techniques are accepted treatment options in patients with chronic venous disease (Current Procedural Terminology code 37760).

Similar to other video-assisted endoscopic procedures, SEPS also has a learning phase, that is much shorter if the surgeon has laparoscopic experience. Anatomy in the subfascial compartments is complex and dissection of perforating vein requires skill and patience. A minimum of 5–8 operations are needed to obtain sufficient skills to accomplish this operation safely and effectively. Gas insufflation enlarges the operating space, makes recognition and dissection of perforators and incision of the deep fascia and the intermuscular septum easier. Air leak around the ports may develop if longer skin incision is made but it can be controlled easily by a purse-string skin suture placed around the port. Most technical problems can be overcome with experience. In patients with severe lipodermatosclerosis, it may be difficult to advance the endoscope all the way to the ankle. For this reason, division of the retromalleolar Cockett perforator with this technique is usually not possible. Improving current

instrumentation and increasing experience with ancillary techniques, such as the use of balloon dissectors, hold promise to facilitate dissection of most or all perforators. Sometimes a third port has to be placed to reach distal perforating veins.

The safety, early efficacy and complications of this operation is discussed in detail in Chapter 21, where we present results of the North American Subfascial Endoscopic Perforator Surgery (NASEPS) registry. Thirty of our 40 procedures were included in that report, that analyzed data of 148 SEPS procedures, performed in 17 centers in the United States and Canada. Similar to results of the registry, our data also confirmed rapid ulcer healing, high patient satisfaction and the relatively low risk of infectious complications when compared to the classic or modified Linton operations. While in the NASEPS registry no major thromboembolic complication was reported, one of our recent patients with inferior vena cava obstruction and severe post-thrombotic disease developed acute deep venous thrombosis after SEPS, stripping and avulsion of large varicosities. In this patient the proximal venous obstruction with removal of some of the venous collaterals during stripping was the presumed cause of deep venous thrombosis. In similar patients we now suggest staging the operations and perform stripping and varicose vein avulsion first, unless preoperative studies confirm significant deep venous obstruction, precluding any ablation of superficial veins. If symptoms persist, SEPS can be performed later using heparin anticoagulation during placement of the tourniquet, without the additional risk of hemorrhage that may occur at sites of stripping and avulsions due to anticoagulation. This case emphasized to us the need for perioperative thrombosis prophylaxis using subcutaneous non-fractionated or low molecular weight heparin in all patients who have evidence of residual deep venous obstruction or who have underlying coagulation abnormality (*see* Chapter 16).

Future controlled prospective trials should assess late results and focus on recurrence rate, cost savings, functional recovery, return to work and length of ulcer- and pain-free state of the patient. Clinical improvement should be supported by documented improvement in calf pump function, although the appropriate test to demonstrate effective operation and confirm the effect of perforator interruption in patients with deep vein incompetence continues to be a topic of considerable controversy (*see* Chapter 6). The need for deep vein valve reconstruction in addition to treatment of perforator and superficial reflux[21] has to be reevaluated in view of the good initial results of the endoscopic procedures. Most importantly, the need for endoscopic perforator division in addition to treatment of superficial reflux has to be addressed to establish the final role of perforator vein interruption in the treatment of chronic venous disease. Setting up the NASEPS registry to collect data on a large number of operations in a multicenter study has been the initial, major step towards the final goal to find the correct and most cost-effective way to manage this severe and debilitating chronic disease.

Acknowledgements. The authors acknowledge Michael B. Farnell, MD. for his advice and help to perform the first endoscopic procedure of this series.

References

1. Hauer G (1985) The endoscopic subfascial division of the perforating veins – preliminary report (in German) VASA 14:59–61

2. Fischer R (1989) Surgical treatment of varicose veins; endoscopic treatment of incompetent Cockett veins. Phlébologie 1040–1041

3. Fischer R, Sattler G, Vanderpuye R (1993) The current status of endoscopic treatment of perforators (In French). Phlébologie 46:701–707

4. Jugenheimer M, Junginger T (1992) Endoscopic subfascial sectioning of incompetent perforating veins in treatment of primary varicosis. World J Surg 16:971–975

5. Wittens CHA, Pierik RGJ, van Urk H (1995) The surgical treatment of incompetent perforating veins. Eur J Vasc Endovasc Surg 9:19–23

6. Pierik EGJM, Wittens CHA, van Urk H (1995) Subfascial endoscopic ligation in the treatment of incompetent perforating veins. Eur J Vasc Endovasc Surg 9:38–41

7. Bergan JJ, Murray J, Greason K (1996). Subfascial endoscopic perforator vein surgery: a preliminary report. Ann Vasc Surg 10:211–219

8. O'Donnell TF (1992) Surgical treatment of incompetent communicating veins. In: Bergan JJ, Kistner RL (eds). Atlas of Venous Surgery. W.B. Saunders, Philadelphia, pp 111–124: Linton RR (1938) The communicating veins of the lower leg and the operative technique for their ligation. Ann Surg 107:582–593

9. Gloviczki P, Cambria RA, Rhee YR, Canton LG, McKusick MA (1996) Surgical technique and preliminary results of endoscopic subfascial division of perforating veins. J Vasc Surg 23:517–523

10. Conrad P (1994) Endoscopic exploration of the subfascial space of the lower leg with perforator vein interruption using laparoscopic equipment: a preliminary report. Phlebology 9:154–157

11. Porter JM, Moneta GL and an International Consensus Committee on Chronic Venous Disease (1995) Reporting standards in venous disease: an update. J Vasc Surg 21:634–645

12. Executive Committee, American Venous Forum (1996) Classification and grading of chronic venous disease in the lower limbs: a consensus statement. In: Gloviczki P, Yao JST (eds) Handbook of Venous Disorders. Chapman & Hall, London; pp 652–660

13. Edwards JM (1976) Shearing operation for incompetent perforating vein. Br J Surg 63:885–886

14. De Palma RG (1974) Surgical therapy for venous stasis. Surgery 76:910–917

15. Hyde GL, Litton TC, Hull DA (1981) Long term results of subfascial vein ligation for venous stasis disease. Surg Gynaec Obstet 153:683–686

16. Negus D, Friedgood A (1983) The effective management of venous ulceration. Br J Surg 70:623–627

17. Johnson WC, O'Hara ET, Corey C et al. (1985) Venous stasis ulceration: Effectiveness of subfascial ligation. Arch Surg 120:797–800

18. Wilkinson GE, Maclaren IF (1986) Long-term review of procedures for venous perforator insufficiency. Surg Gynecol Obstet 163:117–120

19. Cikrit DF, Nichols QK, Silver D (1988) Surgical management of refractory venous stasis ulceration. J Vasc Surg 7:473–478

20. Gloviczki P, Bergan JJ, Menawat SS et al (1997) Safety, feasibility and early efficacy of subfascial endoscopic perforator surgery (SEPS): a preliminary report from the North American Registry. J Vasc Surg, 1997 25:94–105

21. Sotturai VS (1990) Comparison of surgical modalities in the treatment of recurrent venous ulcer. Int Angiol 9:231–235

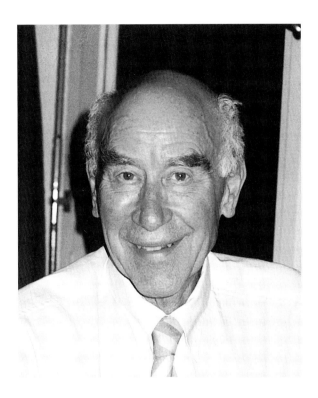

Reinhard H. Fischer
b. 1920

Always a thoughtful student of venous problems, Reinhard Fischer made fundamental contributions to the beginnings of endoscopic subfascial vein surgery. His textbook, *Surgical management of varicose veins* was published by H. Huber in 1972 but his long-lasting contributions will be the early exploration of subfascial surgery and the founding of the Association for Study of Fasciotomy and Endoscopy.

Since 1985, Fischer has been in private group practice in St Gallen, Switzerland but from 1959 on, he was Director of the Wattwil District Hospital and head of its surgical department. There, he founded a school for practical nurses and was cofounder of a school for scrub nurses. He has held offices in numerous regional and national professional organizations and is a member of the Swiss Society of Surgery as well as the North American Society of Phlebology and the of Mayo Alumni Association.

In the early 1950s, he completed a fellowship in general surgery at the Mayo Clinic in Rochester, Minnesota and there was assigned to the Section of Peripheral Vein Surgery with Drs T. T. Myers, A. K. Lofgren, and E. Lofgren. Prior to this, he had served as captain in the Medical Corps of the Swiss Army following achieving a diploma at the University of Basle and serving an internship and externship at the University of Utrecht, The Netherlands, as well as in Biel and St Gallen, Switzerland.

As a medical student, Fischer came under the influence of Dr Hildebrand who was head of a Swiss district hospital. His ambition at that time was to become head of a district hospital. The Mayo experience, he says, defined his concept of practicing medicine which included the fact that most progress in medicine is obtained in continuous international exchange of information.

Fischer's feeling about the future is that phlebology will be most successful when it is practiced in groups of several physicians together with a number of conscientious, efficient, and dedicated technicians. In these times of economic stress, phlebology groups will compete on the basis of quality, friendly service to the patient done in an economically efficient way. In doing this, phlebology may be an example for the rest of medicine in its demonstration of efficiency in a high level of specialization in medicine and surgery.

Subfascial Endoscopic Perforator Vein Surgery: the Open Technique

John J. Bergan, Jeffrey L. Ballard and Steven Sparks

Several events occurring during the 1980s encouraged exploration of video-endoscopic perforator vein interruption during the 1990s. Among these was realization that all of the severe stigmata of the "postphlebitic" leg could be caused by superficial venous reflux and varicose veins.[1,2] This meant that an operation could be offered to patients with severely changed limbs with an expectation of marked improvement of venous function, if not complete cure of the cutaneous manifestations. In addition, duplex technology had revealed that some forms of deep venous reflux could be reversed by ablation of superficial reflux from saphenous veins and varicosities.[3,4] This observation implied that removal of refluxing superficial veins improved venous function. Therefore, in limbs with obvious severely deranged venous physiology as shown by marked ankle skin pigmentation with or without ulceration, complete reversal of the pathophysiology might be anticipated. The observation that limbs with all the stigmata of the postphlebitic state could be operated upon with the single objective of ablating superficial reflux and perforator incompetence and then finding that the deep reflux was improved without valveplasty was encouraging.[5] This gave substance to the prescient question of Norman Browse in 1980, "Is the postphlebitic limb always postphlebitic?"[6]

These facts encouraged duplex study of patients with severe chronic venous insufficiency (CVI) in the hope that limbs would be uncovered in which relatively simple operations could be done with high expectation of success.

A serious problem remained: how to correct the reversal of flow caused by perforating vein check valve failure under the severely dystrophic skin of the distal leg. Experience had shown that incisions made through liposclerotic and atrophic epidermis were fraught with peril.[7] Yet knowledge that perforator interruption would prevent transmission of high exercise-induced compartmental pressures through failed perforator vein check valves to the skin provided a strong stimulus to explore ways of accomplishing this.

Subsequent investigations proceeded along two different pathways. The first was to use existing instruments designed for laparoscopic surgery and employ CO_2 gas insufflation to expand the subfascial space. This was done by Conrad in Australia[8] and by Gloviczki in Rochester.[9] Our own explorations were along another path. This was to adopt methods that had been thoroughly developed in Europe by Hauer, Sattler, and Fischer.[10,11] (Fig. 12.1) Their increasingly vast experience had proven that the open scope, non-gas-insufflating operation was effective, swift, and uncomplicated. Hauer's operation in particular had allowed two generations of endoscopes to be designed for the specific task of exploration of the potential subfascial space in the leg.[12] Our experience in applying the lessons learned from surgeons on the continent was encouraging because, for the first time, it appeared that operations in the face of an open leg ulcer were not hazardous and that perforator vein interruption appeared to accelerate ulcer healing.[13]

Rationale for performing perforator interruption was provided by knowledge that leukocyte trapping and activation could be responsible for the cutaneous changes and the ulcerations of CVI.[14] Thus, the blowout theory of Cockett[15] achieved scientific veracity. Simply stated, it was apparent that muscular contraction could force calf blood under high pres-

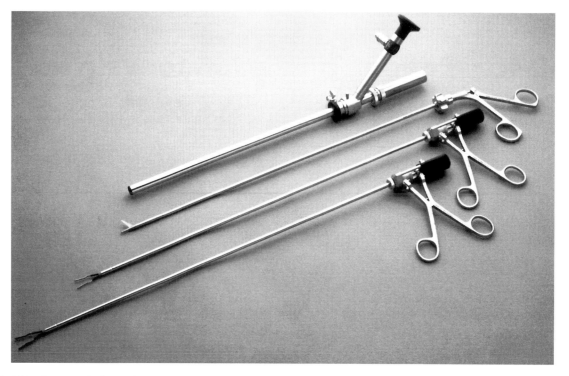

Fig. 12.1. This photograph shows the Storz instrumentation used for endoscopic perforator vein interruption. The straight tube indicates the working channel while the angulated port displays the attachment of the video camera. Instruments utilized include the angulated scissors and small and large bipolar electrocoagulation forceps.

sure through failed perforator valves directly into unsupported dermal and subdermal pre-capillary venules. There the abnormal ambulatory venous hypertension would favor leukocyte trapping and activation. Logically, perforator vein interruption could halt this process.

Preoperative Evaluation

The initial physical examination provides requisite information for arriving at a proper classification of venous insufficiency. Limbs with clinical classes 4, 5 and 6 now become candidates for SEPS. Table 12.1 displays the various examinations which might be considered in evaluating venous function in a limb which is slated for the SEPS procedure. Use of the hand-held, continuous-wave Doppler ultrasound probes confirms presence of axial reflux so that preliminary plans for surgery can be made. Further, a preliminary mapping of relevant perforating veins can be done, thereby confirming that subfascial exploration is justified. While not considered part of

the routine physical examination by some, it is our opinion that the operating surgeon should use the hand-held Doppler in examination of the limb with severe CVI.

While treatment with appropriate wound cleansing, antibiotics if necessary, and compression therapy with non-elastic compression proceeds, other testing can be ordered (Fig. 12.2). Initially, ascending and descending phlebography was done in order to obtain complete information about the status of the deep venous circulation and location of the perforating veins. This was accomplished in 20 of the first 31 limbs operated upon by us. All ascending phlebograms showed at least one, and as many as six, perforating veins, some of which were located laterally (Fig. 12.3). In three veins, a degree of proximal venous obstruction was present. This experience demonstrated that very little information was obtained that changed either the need for operation or the conduct of the procedure. In particular, descending phlebography did show deep venous reflux but duplex scanning revealed the same information. Neither affected the decision for surgical intervention. Therefore, phlebography is no longer done except in limbs with lateral leg ulceration or

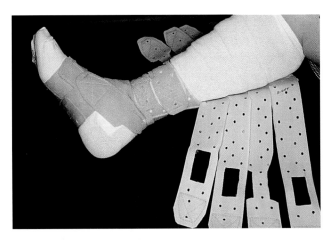

Fig. 12.2. This photograph shows the method of inelastic compression utilized after initial examination. The non-stretch dressing acts as an Unna boot and is used in situations of most severe chronic venous insufficiency (and lymphedema). The CircAid support can be removed for non-invasive testing.

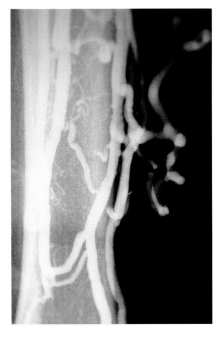

Fig. 12.3. In this preoperative phlebogram, the region of the medial leg just superior to the medial malleolus is illustrated. The perforating vein and its external arborization is probably the 12 cm Cockett II perforator.

suspected iliac venous obstruction as suggested by duplex scanning.

Duplex scanning has been done in every limb in which the SEPS procedure has been contemplated. In all instances, the technique includes the obstructive protocol, the reflux protocol, and the search for perforating veins.[16] When perforating veins were identified, they were also verified during subfascial exploration. However, apparently significant perforating veins were identified by endoscopy which were not detected by preoperative duplex examination. This is important, and suggests that subfascial exploration should not be denied to a patient with obvious venous insufficiency in whom no perforating veins are discovered by preoperative duplex ultrasound.

In developing the subfascial technique, Hauer found that of 71 endoscopically uncovered perforating veins, only 40 were precisely marked during palpation, only 43 during duplex ultrasound examination, and only 35 by phlebography. Thus, the sensitivity of available techniques is clearly inadequate.[15] Neither the presence nor absence of deep venous reflux affects the decision for performing the surgery. While this calls into question the need for, and value of, duplex scanning, it is not anticipated that it will be abandoned as part of the preoperative examination in the near future. It does provide information regarding prognosis as it is felt that presence of persistent postoperative popliteal venous reflux is an adverse prognostic finding.[17]

Since nothing found on duplex scans affects the

decision for surgery in a limb with clear-cut CVI, it may be that scans will only be done in the postoperative period in the future. Such a practice would yield prognostic information and would provide requisite information about the need for strict compliance in the wearing of post procedure support stockings. Admittedly, the hand-held, continuous-wave Doppler instrument provides the same information at lower cost.

Magnetic resonance phlebography has the advantage of providing information about anatomic venous obstruction, especially at the iliac level. Though somewhat claustrophobic, it is better accepted than ascending phlebography.

Though plethysmographic techniques are mentioned in Table 12.1, this is done chiefly to indicate their present status. Their dependence upon tourniquet application as part of the study has rendered them unreliable in separating superficial from deep reflux[18] but the quantitative PPG shows promise in providing prognostic information.

The air plethysmograph is proving to be increasingly useful. Its pre- and postoperative information is beginning to validate perforator interruption in general[5] while the information provided in a particular patient limb is a guide to prognosis and future care.[17]

Table 12.1. Procedures for preoperative assessment prior to SEPS operation

Physical examination	Essential
Doppler ultrasound	Essential
Duplex ultrasound	Essential
Reflux protocol	Essential
Obstruction protocol	Essential
Perforator examination	Essential
Ascending phlebogram	Sometimes desirable[a]
Descending phlebogram	Unnecessary[a]
Magnetic resonance phlebography[b]	Detects obstruction
Air plethysmography	Gives physiologic information[b]
Impedance plethysmography	Obsolete
Photoplethysmography	Obsolete
Mercury-strain-gauge plethysmography	Obsolete

[a] May provide interesting, sometimes useful, information
[b] Usually interesting but not essential

Operative Technique

Important but non-technical considerations attend the operation of subfascial perforator vein interruption. These include setting of the operation, choice of anesthesia, use of a tourniquet and need for antithrombotic prophylaxis.

Preliminary Considerations

Unlike the standard Linton operation, the SEPS procedure does not require hospitalization. Our preference, even in the aged, is a completely out-patient surgical event. Some may feel more comfortable observing the patient for a short time postoperatively as this allows monitoring of ambulation as well as providing some increased comfort and emotional support for the patient. Our experience suggests that neither is necessary as the troublesome postoperative subfascial hematomas induced by physical activity have occurred after 48 h postoperatively, and that the patients being young (for the most part) and vigorous, do not need hospital attendants for their care.

While both spinal and epidural regional anesthesia would be theoretically applicable to the needs of the SEPS operation, in fact neither is desirable. Increasing experience with Diprivan induction[19] and laryngeal mask control of the airway has made these our techniques of choice. Prolonged post anesthesia recovery and nausea and vomiting have not been postoperative problems. Patients are routinely discharged home within 1 hour of conclusion of application of the dressing. Of course, post spinal headache and urinary retention are not any consideration if regional anesthesia is not used.

While an orthopedic tourniquet has not proven to be essential to the performance of the operation, it has appeared to be useful. It was used in 14 of our first 31 cases and not used in the remainder. A tourniquet has been used in the subsequent operations. Ancillary use of Esmarch exsanguination or the roll-on tourniquet to accomplish the same purpose has been thought to improve subfascial visualization. Both techniques diminish the size of perforating veins and might cause an underestimation of their importance. The perforating veins appear white after limb exsanguination and no accurate estimation of their size is possible. Use of an occlusive tourniquet without preliminary limb exsanguination has allowed better estimation of perforator vein size but has also caused some bloody staining when cauterization or clipping has been incomplete before vein division. This is largely an aesthetic consideration.

At this time, prophylaxis against venous thromboembolic disease is an important consideration prior to either in-patient or out-patient operations. Patients coming to the modern SEPS procedure would have been labeled as survivors of a prior episode of deep venous thrombosis (DVT) in the past. The terms "postphlebitic" or "post-thrombotic" leg were formerly in universal use. Therefore, by definition, such patients with what is now termed "chronic venous insufficiency," would be in the category of highest risk for postoperative deep venous thrombosis and pulmonary embolization. Now, it is clear that only a fraction, though a sizable fraction, are truly post-thrombotic. The remainder have not had prior experience with DVT.

In the SEPS Registry, only one-third of patients had experienced a previous thrombotic episode.[20] These patients with proven prior DVT are those who should receive consideration for DVT prophylaxis. In such individuals, it is our current practice to administer parenteral fractionated heparin once daily, commencing before surgery and proceeding for 5 days postoperatively. Other patients without evidence of a prior episode of DVT may or may not have evidence of deep venous reflux. If DVT was not experienced in the past, it is felt that no thrombo-embolism prophylaxis is necessary. Postoperative ambulation will be dictated by the wishes of the operating surgeon.

Conduct of the Operation

In the operating suite, after induction of general anesthesia and after sterile preparation of the entire lower extremity, the limb is exsanguinated and placed on a sterile, drape-covered limb holder. The tourniquet is inflated to 250 mmHg. The time is recorded and the pressure is monitored. Using the endoscope as an indicator of distal distance to be explored, an incision site is selected. This is usually 4 cm lateral to the posterior edge of the tibia. The 25–30 mm incision is made vertically and deepened through the superficial fascia (tela aponeurotica) to expose the deep fascial which is cleared bluntly of subcutaneous fat. Saphenous tributary varicosities seen in the incision are excised but the saphenous nerve, if present, is preserved.

The fascia is incised throughout the length of the incision, separated from the underlying muscle with a finger. The open scope is inserted, having been warmed prior to insertion to minimize fogging (Fig. 12.4). The scope is passed distally to, but not below, the medial malleolus of the tibia and then is manip-

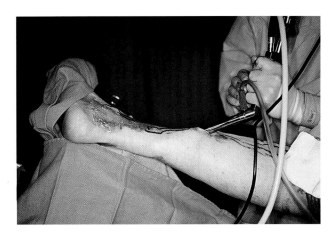

Fig. 12.5. This operative photograph illustrates distal insertion of the scope to the level of the malleolus and suggests that the scope can be manipulated as far posteriorly as the middle and as far anteriorly as the edge of the tibia to create adequate operative space.

ulated anteriorly and posteriorly in a pendulum- like action to mobilize the entire subfascial space.

After developing the entire subfascial space from the tibial edge to the midline, the scope is removed from its sheath and the distal glass cleansed with Fred solution (Betadine liquid will also serve to prevent fogging). The scope is then reinserted distally to the level of the malleolus (Fig. 12.5). While watching the monitor for any evidence of perforating veins, the scope is withdrawn using the same pendulum action as before. This now allows visualization of the entire retrotibial area. The Cockett II perforating veins cluster around 9–12 cm from the heel pad. These may be covered by the fascia of the deep posterior compartment. Exposure of these veins requires sectioning of the intermuscular septum. As the scope is withdrawn proximally above the distal one-third of the leg, the subfascial saphenous vein is searched for posteriorly. The adjacent sural nerve is seen. If obliteration of the lesser saphenous vein is required, this can be accomplished by multiple clipping and electrocoagulation and division of the vein after thorough mobilization of the vein away from the nerve. (Fig. 12.6).

As the scope is withdrawn, the paratibial fascia of the deep posterior compartment is inspected for evidence of paratibial perforating veins. These will be suspected if the preoperative clinical examination revealed pretibial ulceration or marked pigmentation and atrophic skin changes. If there are preoperative indications, the intermuscular septum is

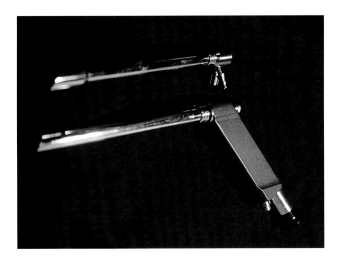

Fig. 12.4. This photograph indicates the rugged nature and short length of the Hauer endoscope. Note the angulation of the end of the sheath which creates space within which to work. The working channel and video-optics are enclosed with the handle and can be inserted or removed for cleaning and defogging.

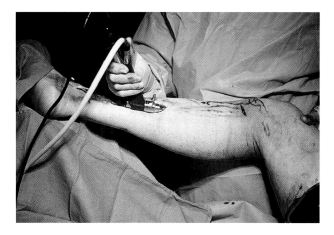

Fig. 12.6. After distal exploration, electrocoagulation, clipping, and division of perforating veins has been accomplished, the scope is reversed to inspect the proximal third of the leg where the Boyd perforating vein is expected to be found.

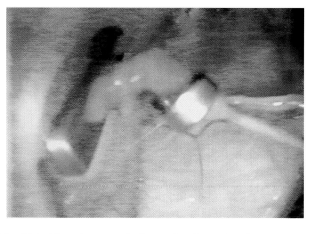

Fig. 12.8. This photograph shows the clipped perforating vein emerging from the muscle on the left and bifurcating prior to passage through the fascia to the right. The hemostatic clips in place are Ethicon 5 mm clips.

incised and the paratibial perforators mobilized and divided (Fig. 12.7).

Perforating veins in the exsanguinated limb will appear much smaller than in the non-exsanguinated limb. They will frequently appear white rather than blue. Also, the perforating veins emerging from the muscle will frequently bifurcate prior to passing through the fascia (Fig. 12.8). The perforators and branchings can be electrocoagulated prior to division or they can be controlled with the use of hemostatic clips. While actual division of the perforating vein may not be necessary, most surgeons will favor

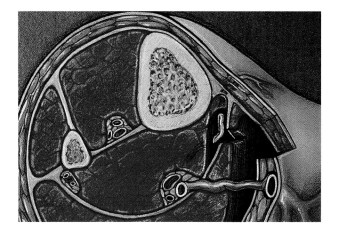

Fig. 12.7. This artist's drawing illustrates the possibility of opening the fascia of the deep posterior compartment in order to expose paratibial perforating veins. This is especially true of the very important Cockett III perforating vein. Its presence can be suggested by pretibial hyperpigmentation or paratibial ulceration.

cutting the vein as part of the subfascial perforating vein procedure (Fig. 12.9).

Likewise, at the distal most aspect of the leg, an attempt should be made to identify the Cockett I perforator in its retromalleolar location. The rigid scope allows viewing somewhat distal to the scope itself and may allow perforator clipping even though division may not be possible. Excessive force should not be used in attempting visualization of the retromalleolar perforator as there is potential for tibial nerve injury.

Order of Performance of Procedures

Clearly, in a developing operation, varying techniques will be used by various surgeons. Some principles guide the election of the order of the procedures.

First, the most limiting complication which has occurred is a subfascial hematoma. This has caused excessive pain and has limited ambulation in some patients operated on early in the experience. Second, experience with surgery of the superficial venous system has taught that stripping of the saphenous vein from groin to knee causes a tremendous proximal venospasm. This, in turn, causes distal venous hypertension and excessive bleeding during stab avulsion of varices. Third, release of tourniquet causes a hyperemia and bleeding from transected and uncontrolled vessels. Fourth, many surgeons have been taught to perform saphenous stripping as a last step prior to applying pressure dressings.

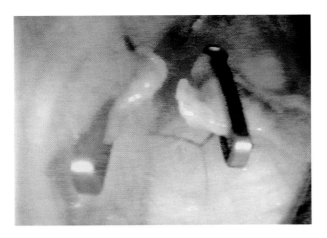

Fig. 12.9. Perforator vein clipping and cutting are illustrated here. However, electrocoagulation and cutting prove to be less expensive and useful for small veins.

With these principles in mind, we currently perform the procedures in the following order. First, the Esmarch bandage and tourniquet exsanguinate the limb and control inflow. Second, the subfascial exploration is done choosing a site for an entrance of the scope which will coincide with maximum mobility of the instrumentation and possible use of the incision for removing clusters of varicosities or terminating the saphenous stripping. After perforator interruption and fasciotomy, the subfascial exploration wound is left open and the procedure continues with ablation of superficial reflux. The groin incision and passage of the stripping device can proceed with the tourniquet in place. While this is done, the stab avulsion portion of the procedure can continue, and if necessary, the saphenous vein can be cannulated at the ankle for removal of the leg portion of the vein if it is thought to be the source of varicosities or in any way contributes to the severe chronic venous insufficiency. After all else is done, the tourniquet is released, the saphenous vein stripped, the subfascial space thoroughly irrigated, and the skin closure is begun.

Our own technique is enhanced by internally packing the saphenous stripping tunnel as described elsewhere in this volume. Wound closures are effected with monofilament adsorbable suture. The wound is reinforced with Steri-Strips and infiltrated with 0.25% marcaine local anesthesia. The local anesthesia allows comfort in the recovery room, early mobilization of the patient, and the possibility of discharge home within 1 hour of the termination of the procedure.

Surgical Dressing

The conduct of compression therapy following surgery will vary with the experience of the operating surgeon. Our own technique is to apply a pressure dressing with its overwrapped elastic bandages and remove this at 48 h following surgery. The elastic bandages are used for external support for the next 10–14 days. Local wound care will return to that used preoperatively. That is, if Unna boots were being used preoperatively, they are placed at 10–14 days postoperatively. If the CircAid support has been the mainstay of therapy, it is used from the 48-h dressing change onward. Under such compression, rapid healing of the incisions is expected and similarly, an acceleration of healing of the venous stasis ulcer is also expected.

Postoperative Medication

Patients with confirmed preoperative deep venous thrombosis are given thromboembolism prophylaxis. This takes the form of Fragmin, 5000 units administered subcutaneously on the day of surgery and for 5 days postoperatively. The patient himself can be taught to administer the drug and no anticoagulant monitoring is given. Full ambulation at 5 days is expected, and therefore, a decrease in the tendency to form new endovenous thrombosis. Antibiotics are given preoperatively and are continued postoperatively for 5 days in anticipation of possible cellulitis from bacteria in the open ulceration. While cellulitis is listed as a problem in reports of the operation, in fact this has proven to be a complication which is easy to control.

Results

It is apparent that complications of subfascial perforating vein surgery are not related to the technique employed during the procedure.[20] As in any developing surgery, there may be vast differences in performance of the operation. Tawes, for example, has illustrated his technique utilizing the balloon dissector for subfascial space expansion.[21] Although Pigott's commentary[22] supported the use of the space dissector, in fact a very large experience has accumulated in which the space dissector was not used.[10,11,23–25]

As the technique draws closer to standardization, there is no doubt that many factors will come in to play. Among these is the economic factor which dictates that reusable instrumentation will become dominant, simplicity of the procedure will become favored, and specialized instrumentation will develop to ease performance of the operation (Fig. 12.10). While results will continue to improve, it is expected that the results will be similar to those published at this time.

In our developing experience, the most serious problem was subfascial wound hematoma which occurred in 2 patients (6%). That complication has been virtually eliminated by careful attention to subfascial space irrigation, late but not delayed closure of the cutaneous incision used for endoscopic explor-

ation, and early release of the hemostatic tourniquet. The factor of cellulitis described in the registry report and noted by us will undoubtedly continue to be a problem as aggressive treatment of the venous ulcer itself will include subfascial perforator vein surgery. Nevertheless, it is not expected that the problem of cellulitis will exceed 5%. Our preliminary and explorative experience showed a cellulitis complication of 9%, a figure quite similar to that in the registry report. Unlike the problems of wound sepsis which occurred with the open Linton procedure, the cellulitis experienced after subfascial perforator vein interruption by the endoscopic technique is easily controlled on an out-patient basis by prescribing appropriate antibiotic therapy.

At present, the operation is used, for the most part, in treatment of venous ulceration but is also being used for prevention of recurrent ulceration. Early experience suggests that the findings of the Edinburgh group are correct. Those limbs that are most vulnerable to recurrent ulceration are those with persisting popliteal venous reflux. Such reflux will largely be due to previous deep venous thrombosis in limbs that are truly postphlebitic. At this time, recurrence of symptomatic chronic venous insufficiency has been in those limbs with popliteal venous reflux and the manifestations have, for the most part, consisted of dermatitis, easily controlled by appropriate prescriptions, or minor perforative ulcerations responsive to increase in local pressure. A final tabulation of results would be inaccurate at this time as it is expected that the procedure itself will improve and even the selection of patients will become better.

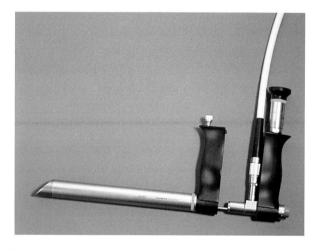

Fig. 12.10. This photograph illustrates the prototype Olympus scope which has been specially designed for the subfascial perforating vein interruption. Note the rugged handle, a portion of which is attached to the sheath and the remainder attached to the scope itself. The video camera port is on the angled portion of the instrumentation, and the handle itself is placed at a right angle in order to increase leverage. A subtle change is illustrated in the hooded end of the scope in which the instrumentation views the fascia rather than the muscle side of the exposed tissue. Not illustrated is the fact that the scope can be used with CO_2 insufflation or utilized entirely open. Experience with this instrument has shown that the CO_2 insufflation does give an improved visualization of the subfascial space. The scope has an 85° field of view and the outer sheath is either 16 to 22 mm in diameter. The working channel is a generous 6 × 8.5 mm and the overall working length of the scope is similar to the Hauer scope at 200 mm.

Conclusion

The subfascial perforator vein interruption surgery performed by the open technique has proven to be an operation well within the capabilities of general surgeons and interested vascular surgeons. Availability of non-disposable instrumentation and simplicity of the procedure itself makes the operation extremely cost effective. Because operative morbidity is decreased by the small size of the incision, the absence of serious septic complications, and the prevention of subfascial hematomas, even overnight hospitalization has been found to be unnecessary in nearly all cases.

As the procedure has proven itself to be effective in control of severe chronic venous insufficiency, it is clear that more complex procedures such as valveplasty and valve transplantation can be held in reserve for those few cases in which the ablation of superficial reflux and control of perforators has proven to be ineffective.

References

1. Shami SK, Sarin S, Cheatle TR, Scurr JH, Coleridge Smith PD (1993) Venous ulcers and the superficial venous system. J Vasc Surg 17:487–500
2. Hanrahan LM, Araki CT, Rodriguez CT et al. (1991) Distribution of valvular incompetence in patients with venous stasis ulceration. J Vasc Surg 13:805–812
3. Walsh JC, Bergan, Beeman S, Comer TP (1994) Femoral venous reflux abolished by greater saphenous vein stripping. Ann Vasc Surg 8:566–570
4. Sales CM, Bilof ML, Petrillo KA, Luka NL (1996) Correction of lower extremity deep venous incompetence by ablation of superficial varicosities. Ann Vasc Surg 10:186–190
5. Padberg FT, Pappas PJ, Araki CT, Back IL, Hobson RW (1996) Hemodynamic and clinical improvement after superficial vein ablation in primary combined venous insufficiency with ulceration. J Vasc Surg 24:711–719
6. Browse NL, Clemenson G, Lea Thomas M (1980) Is the postphlebitic limb always postphlebitic? Relation between phlebographic appearances of deep vein thrombosis and late sequelae. Br Med J 281:1167–1168
7. DePalma RG (1974) Surgical therapy for venous stasis. Surgery 76:910–917
8. Conrad P (1994) Endoscopic exploration of the lower leg with perforator vein interruption using laparoscopic equipment: A preliminary report. Phlebology 9:154–157
9. Gloviczki P, Cambria RA, Rhee RY, Canton LG, Mikusick MA (1996) Surgical technique and preliminary results of endoscopic subfascial division of perforating veins. J Vasc Surg 23:517–523
10. Hauer G (1985) Die endoskopische subfasciale diszision der perforansvenen Vorlaufige Milleilung. VASA 14:59–61
11. Fischer R, Sattler G, Vanderpuye R (1993) Le traitement endoscopique des perforantes (TEP) situation actuelle. Phlébologie 46:701–707
12. Hauer G, Bergan JJ, Werner A, Wittenhusen M, Nasralla F (1997) Development of endoscopic dissection of perforating veins and fasciotomy for treatment of chronic venous insufficiency. (Submitted for publication).
13. Bergan JJ, Murray J, Greason K (1996) Subfascial endoscopic perforator vein surgery (SEPS): A preliminary report. Ann Vasc Surg 10:211–219
14. Scott HJ, Coleridge Smith PD, Scurr JH (1991) Histological study of white blood cells and their association with lipodermatosclerosis and venous ulceration. Br J Surg 78:210–211
15. Cockett FB, Jones BE (1953) The ankle blow-out syndrome: A new approach to the varicose ulcer problem. Lancet i:17–23
16. Wittens CHA, Pierik RGMJ, van Urk H (1995) The surgical treatment of incompetent perforating veins. Eur J Vasc Endovasc Surg 9:19–23
17. Bradbury AW, Stonebridge PA, Callam MJ, Ruckley CV, Allen PL (1993) Foot volumetry can predict recurrent ulceration after subfascial ligation of perforators and saphenous ligation. Br J Surg 80:845–848
18. van Bemmelen PS, van Ramshorst B, Eikelboom B (1992) Photoplethysmography reexamined: Lack of correlation with duplex scanning. Surgery 112:544–548
19. Eledjam JJ (1994) Utilisation du Diprivan*pr en complément a l'anesthésie locorégionale. Ann Fr Anesth Réanim 13:593–597
20. Gloviczki P, Bergan JJ, Menawat SS et al. (1997) Safety, feasibility, and early efficacy of subfascial endoscopic perforator surgery (SEPS): A preliminary report from the North American Registry. J Vasc Surg 24:94–105
21. Tawes RL, Wetter A, Hermann GD, Fogarty TJ (1996) Endoscopic technique for subfascial perforating vein interruption. J Endovasc Surg 3:414–420
22. Pigott JP (1996) The space race: No clear winner yet in endoscopic perforator surgery. J Endovasc Surg 3:421–422
23. Sparks S, Ballard JL, Bergan JJ (1997) Early benefits of subfascial endoscopic perforator surgery (SEPS) in healing venous ulcers. Ann Vasc Surg 11:367–374
24. Bergan JJ, Ballard JL, Sparks S, Murray JS (1996) Subfascial surgery of perforating veins; SEPS. Phlébologie 49:467–472
25. Wolters U, Schmitz-Rixen T, Erasmi H, Lynch J (1996) Endoscopic dissection of incompetent perforating veins in the treatment of chronic venous ulcers. Vasc Surg 30:481–487

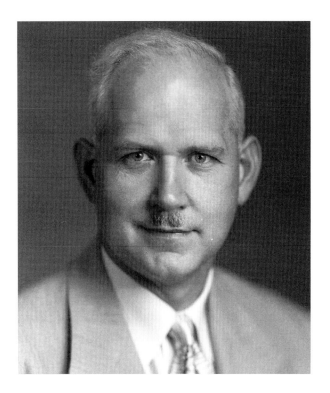

Thomas Twidwell Myers
1906–1980

It is Dr T. T. Myers to whom credit for the development of the flexible vein stripper belongs. As the head of the Section of Peripheral Vein Surgery of the Mayo Clinic for more than 20 years, he pioneered the management of many aspects of venous disease.

Born in Kansas, Dr Myers received the bachelor's degree at the University of Kansas and medical degree at the University of Chicago Rush Medical College in 1934. After a brief period of private practice, he underwent surgical training at the Mayo Clinic and was named to the staff in 1944. Dr Myers was appointed head of the Section of Peripheral Vein Surgery in 1947. This section was unique for the Mayo Clinic and also for the medical world because it specialized exclusively in the management of venous disorders. He became associate professor of surgery in 1960, and remained the head of the section until 1966. The section existed until 1984, when its surgical function was integrated into the Section of Vascular Surgery.

Myers advocated extensive operation for varicose veins and developed the modern stripping method with the invention of the flexible intraluminal stripper, the prototype of the disposable stripper that is widely used today. His innovative genius and unusual dedication to venous surgery has been appreciated by both those who have been afflicted by and those who have treated venous disease.

Endoscopic Perforator Vein Surgery: Creation of a Subfascial Space

13

Robert C. Allen, Roy L. Tawes, L. Albert Wetter and Thomas J. Fogarty

Introduction

The endoscopic treatment of incompetent perforator veins has opened a whole new era in peripheral venous surgery. This concept was introduced in 1985 by Hauer who first described the endoscopic technique for the division of perforating veins.[1] The importance of incompetent perforator veins in chronic venous insufficiency is clear as 1%–2% of the general population have or have had venous ulceration with an associated disease process that is marked by chronicity and recurrence when treated with conservative medical therapy.[2] Past conventional surgical therapy has been efficacious in the majority of cases, but complicated by a high morbidity rate.[2] This has led to a general trend toward conservative management despite the dismal course of the disease with standard compression therapy. Endoscopic modes of treatment are increasingly being applied in all fields of surgical treatment due to their decreased invasiveness and markedly reduced patient morbidity. Numerous authors have clearly demonstrated the benefits of the endoscopic modality in the treatment of incompetent perforator veins with significantly reduced morbidity rates.[3–6] The majority of these series have included patients with advanced chronic venous insufficiency manifested as severe lipodermatosclerosis and healed or open venous ulcers. Endoscopic therapy has, however, also been applied to patients with less severe chronic venous insufficiency with equally good results.[7]

Anatomy of the Subfascial Space

Most incompetent perforating veins occur on the medial aspect of the lower leg above the medial malleolus along Linton's line. These represent communication between the posterior arch veins and the posterior tibial veins. The lower leg is divided into four distinct fascial compartments including the anterior, lateral, and superficial and deep posterior compartments. The superficial posterior compartment is the most important for this discussion as it represents the best region to access communicating veins between the superficial and deep venous systems. This area is most vividly illustrated by Linton's line located on the medial aspect of the calf several centimeters posterior and medial to the tibia. The subfascial space that is crucial to the endoscopic treatment of perforating veins is located on the medial aspect of the calf deep to the fascia of the superficial posterior compartment and above the underlying muscle in the paratibial region. This is the area which is a potential space that must be adequately dissected to create a cavernous endoscopic working field.

Endoscopic Methods

Introduction

The movement toward minimally invasive techniques in peripheral venous surgery has been strengthened by recent advances in non-invasive duplex ultrasound testing, balloon dissection techniques to create an endoscopic operating field, and improvements in video endoscopic instrumentation and techniques. Creation of a subfascial space in the lower leg is the crucial step facilitating endoscopic treatment of incompetent perforator veins. Once this working space is dissected, the endoscopic procedure can be performed in an unencumbered operative field from a remote incision, to treat all perforating veins. All minimally invasive video-assisted techniques are dependent on adequate operative working space. This space may be pre-existing, as in the peritoneal or pleural cavities, or surgically created via balloon dissection. Open surgical procedures for perforator ligation in the past have created a very large subfascial space, but required lengthy incisions in diseased skin and subcutaneous tissues which resulted in unacceptable wound morbidity. The various techniques used either alone, or in combination, to create a subfascial space for the endoscopic treatment of incompetent perforators include saline infusion, carbon dioxide (CO_2) insufflation, mechanical retraction, and balloon dissection.[3–8] Although all of these modalities accomplish the goal of creating a subfascial space, each has advantages and disadvantages. The authors believe that balloon dissection followed by CO_2 insufflation, however, is the preferred modality for creating the operative field. It is the most conducive to the endoscopic approach and we utilize this technique in clinical practice.

Balloon Dissection

Balloon dissection has been shown to be an effective enabling technique for converting potential spaces into "real-time" operative fields in a variety of locations for numerous different pathologic states. It has proven to be especially useful for laparoscopic preperitoneal hernia repair and is most commonly utilized in this application. Balloon dissection has the distinct advantage of following the planes of least resistance, which results in the creation of a relatively bloodless field. The friable connective tissue planes adjacent to the fascia are separated from the underlying muscle while the stronger tissue planes, including venous structures, are left relatively undisturbed. The balloon expands in both radial and longitudinal directions to create a large subfascial space. The components of the balloon dissector are shown in Fig. 13.1. The extensive subfascial plane created by the balloon allows for the treatment of distal retromalleolar perforating veins. Saline is used as the balloon inflation media to facilitate the atraumatic dissection. The dissecting balloon inflated with saline solution is illustrated in Fig. 13.2. Saline inflation allows the operating surgeon to obtain tactile feedback at the time of balloon inflation to optimize balloon positioning and to control precisely the volume of the dissected working space. Carbon dioxide insufflation is employed after

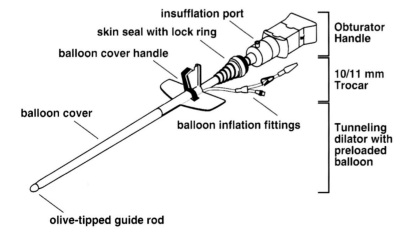

Fig. 13.1. Components of balloon dissector for creation of a large subfascial working space (General Surgical Innovations, Palo Alto, CA). An integral 10-mm endoscopic port is included.

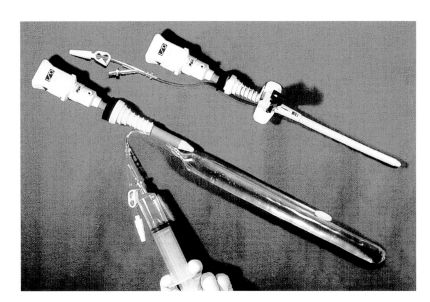

Fig. 13.2. The balloon dissector device prior to (above) and after (below) balloon cover removal. Note the degree of radial and distal balloon expansion that occurs when fully inflated with saline solution.

balloon dissection to maintain the dissected subfascial space. This approach results in a visual field that is less encumbered in comparison to dissection techniques using mechanical means alone.

Other Methods

Mechanical dissection and retraction can be accomplished with a variety of endoscopes including an arthroscope or mediastinoscope.[2–4] This technique uses one or two access incisions in the medial aspect of the upper leg and relies on blunt dissection with the instrument to create and maintain the subfascial space. The field of view with this method is typically restricted and may limit the number of perforating veins which can be treated. This blunt mechanical dissection technique may also increase the risk of bleeding complications and postoperative hematoma formation.

Gas insufflation has also been used as the principal modality in the creation of a subfascial operating space.[5,9] In this technique, a 10-mm laparoscopic port is typically placed in the subfascial space following a transverse incision. Insufflation is then instituted to a pressure of 30 mmHg in order to dissect a subfascial working space. This technique is less efficient and, in our opinion, creates a suboptimal working space. Some advocates of this technique believe these pressures may carry an attendant risk of CO_2 embolus with inadvertent venous trauma. Therefore, a proximal pneumatic tourniquet is usually employed with this approach.

Balloon Technique

The balloon technique for the creation of the subfascial space is straightforward, with the procedure easily learned by surgeons with minimal endoscopic or laparoscopic experience. Equipment necessary for this procedure is available routinely in a standard laparoscopy cart and includes a CO_2 insufflator, 10-mm endoscope, video camera with light source, and a video monitor (Fig. 13.3). Two laparoscopic ports are used – a 10-mm port for the endoscope and a 5-mm port for the instrumentation. The initial transverse skin incision is made approximately 10 cm (about one hand breadth) below the popliteal crease and 3–4 cm posterior medial to the tibia in an area of minimally diseased skin. The fascia of the superficial posterior compartment is identified and incised transversely. Blunt dissection with the surgeon's fingertip initiates the subfascial plane. The balloon dissector with attached handle, protective balloon cover, and guide rod/obturator is then advanced into the subfascial plane towards the posterior aspect of the medial malleolus (Fig. 13.4). Fig. 13.5 illustrates the cross-sectional orientation for optimal balloon positioning. Balloon insertion should proceed with minimal resistance to advancement until the balloon handle cover meets the incision. The peel-away balloon cover is then removed via its handle prior to balloon inflation (Fig. 13.6). The balloon is then inflated with 200–300 ml of saline in a gradual manner alternating two 60-ml syringes for fluid introduction. The balloon expands

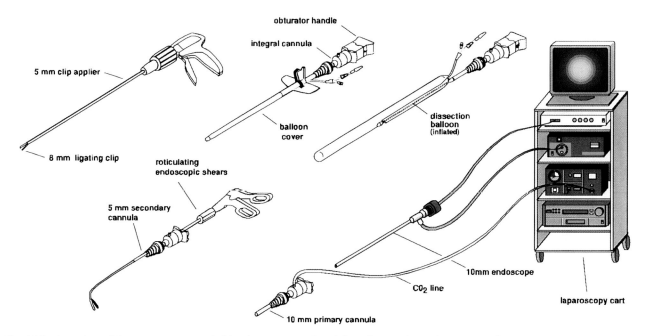

Fig. 13.3. Overview of the equipment needed for the creation of a subfascial space for endoscopic perforator vein surgery. Important elements of the system are the balloon dissector, endoscopic ports, 5-mm endoscopic clip applier (Ethicon Endosurgery, Cincinnati, OH), roticulating graspers (United States Surgical Corp., Norwalk, CT), endoscope, and CO_2 insufflation apparatus.

radially and also propagates distally with the creation of a large subfascial space (Fig. 13.7). The profile of the balloon may be palpated beneath the skin during the inflation process to track its progression. Balloon inflation is complete at 300 ml or upon feeling any undue tension on the overlying skin. The next step is deflation and removal of the balloon, followed by removal of the obturator from the 10-mm fascial port. The 10-mm fascial port is then secured to the fascia to ensure an airtight seal and CO_2 insufflation is commenced at 8–15 mmHg pressure (Fig. 13.8).

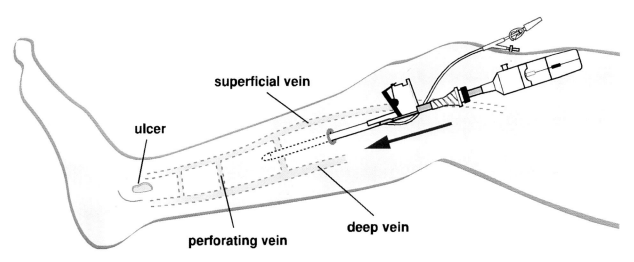

Fig. 13.4. Insertion of the balloon dissector through the initial transverse incision. The direction of insertion is subfascial posterior to the tibia and directed towards the posterior aspect of the medial malleolus.

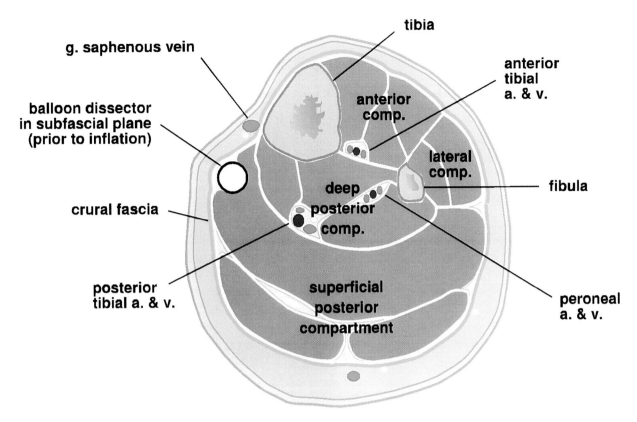

Fig. 13.5. Cross-sectional anatomy of the proximal calf demonstrates the correct positioning of the balloon dissector. The optimal location is 2–3 cm posterior medial to the tibia just below the fascia of the superficial posterior compartment.

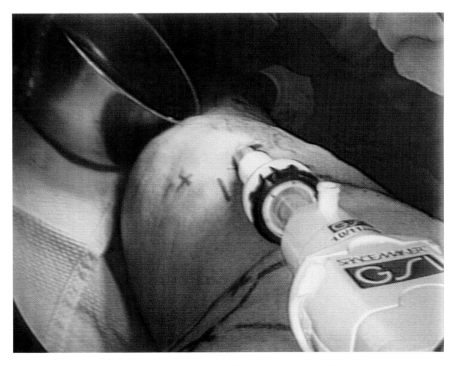

Fig. 13.6. Intraoperative view of balloon dissector after balloon cover removal, immediately prior to balloon inflation.

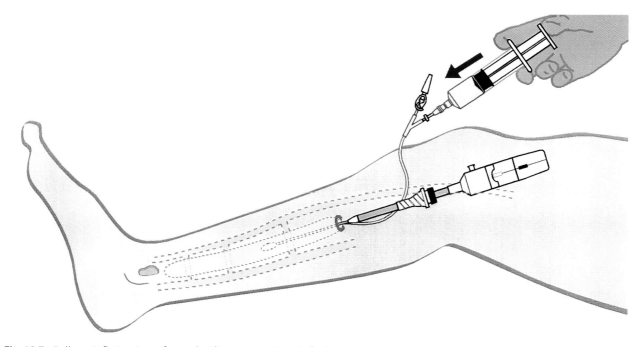

Fig. 13.7. Balloon inflation is performed utilizing 200–300 ml of saline. The balloon expands both radially and distally with minimal trauma to surrounding tissue thus creating a large bloodless working space.

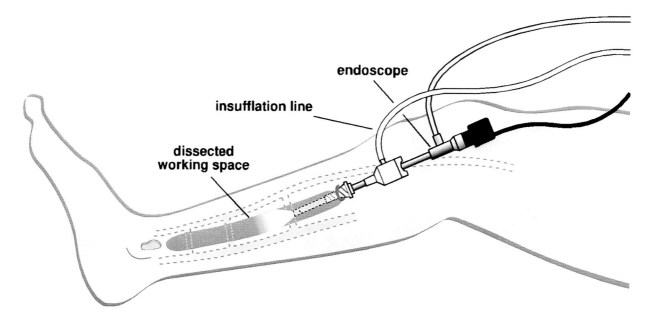

Fig. 13.8. The balloon is removed and replaced by the integral 10-mm endoscopic fascial port. The airtight fascial port permits CO_2 insufflation of the subfascial space to distend the dissected operative working space.

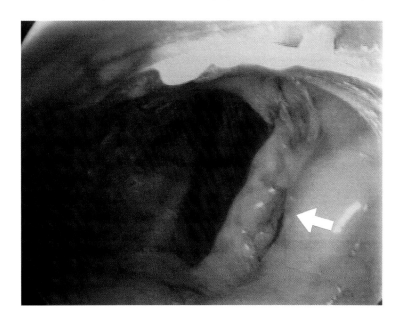

Fig. 13.9. Endoscopic view of subfascial operative space following CO_2 insufflation. Note large perforating vein on the right (arrow).

A zero degree 10-mm rigid endoscope with attached video camera and light source is then introduced through the 10-mm fascial port and into the dissected space (Fig. 13.9). Next, an incision for the 5-mm working port is made several centimeters distal to the original port, located as posterior as possible to facilitate perforator vein dissection and clipping. This 5-mm ancillary working port is placed under direct endoscopic visualization. The subfascial space is characteristically large and bloodless, with unobstructed access to the perforator veins from the upper leg towards the malleolar area. Perforating veins may be readily visible or may require a modest amount of blunt dissection for complete exposure.

Working in a proximal to distal manner, perforating veins are sequentially identified, clipped, and in some cases, divided with endoscopic scissors (Figs

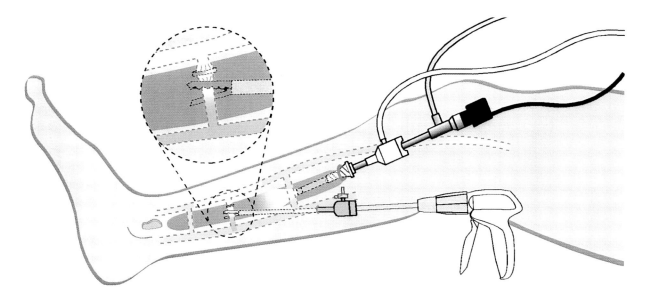

Fig. 13.10. A separate 5-mm working port, made under direct visualization, is placed in as posterior a position as possible for optimal triangulation of the instruments. The perforating veins are sequentially identified and interrupted.

13.10, 13.11, 13.12, 13.13, and 13.14). All visible perforating veins are treated and special attention is paid to perforators in the immediate vicinity of the diseased tissue, typically in the inframalleolar region (Figs 13.15 and 13.16). Also the preoperative skin markings that had been marked by duplex evaluation are addressed to insure that no important perforators are left untreated at the time of the procedure. The endoscope and fascial ports are then removed and the incision sites are checked to address any local venous pathology. Superficial venous stripping and ligation are then addressed as indicated by the preoperative duplex evaluation. The skin is closed with a subcuticular suture and steri-strips. A light compressive dressing is then applied from forefoot to upper calf. After adequate experience, the endoscopic procedure can be accomplished routinely in less than 30 min. The patient is allowed to fully recover from the anesthetic prior to ambulation. The overwhelming majority of patients can be treated as out-patients and tolerate the procedure very well. The patient is fully ambulatory the following day with compression hose and is seen for office follow-up in 1 week.

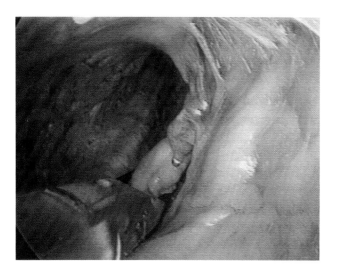

Fig. 13.11. Endoscopic clipping of perforating vein via clip applier inserted through separate 5-mm fascial port.

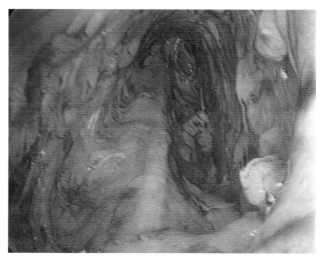

Fig. 13.13. Retraction of perforator vein after division with endoscopic shears. The full extent of the balloon-dissected subfascial space is clearly visualized, facilitating distal exploration.

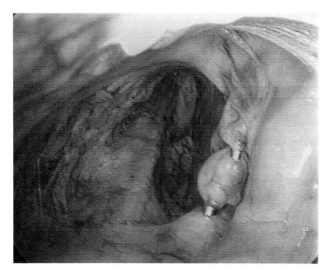

Fig. 13.12. Perforating vein after placement of hemoclips prior to division. Proper clip application and attention to all side branches is essential to maintain a clear operative field.

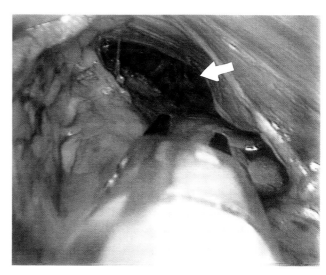

Fig. 13.14. Distal exploration of the subfascial space as a clip applier is advanced distally. Retromalleolar perforating veins are visualized at the distal region of the dissected space (arrow).

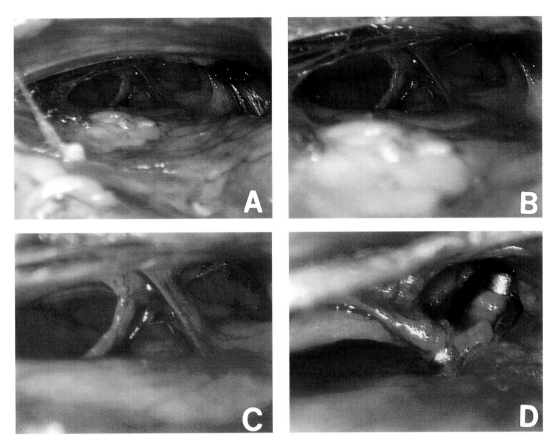

Fig. 13.15. The endoscopic procedure utilizing balloon dissection facilitates clear visualization and instrument access to distal perforators. Images **A** through **C** depict advancement of the endoscope towards retromalleolar perforators.Image **D** depicts successful endoscopic clipping of retromalleolar perforators.

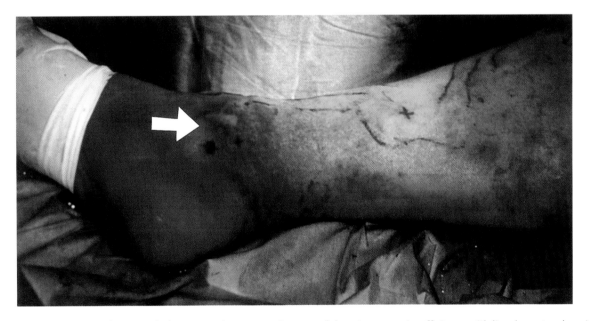

Fig. 13.16. Intraoperative photograph demonstrating severe changes of chronic venous insufficiency with lipodermatosclerosis and site of healed ulcer (arrow). Black ink markings from preoperative duplex (below arrow) show location of the retromalleolar perforators that were clipped in Fig. 13.15.

Results

Thirty patients with severe lipodermatosclerosis or open venous ulcers have been treated, with short term follow-up. Preoperative evaluation was performed using duplex scanning to locate and mark the incompetent perforating veins, and also to rule out deep venous thrombosis. An average of 4 perforators per limb were treated in this patient group. All obtained a desirable result (e.g. ulcer healing, reduced pain) with no complications.

Conclusion

The endoscopic treatment of incompetent perforating veins has brought about a new era in the surgical treatment of peripheral venous disease. Balloon dissection followed by CO_2 insufflation creates a large, bloodless subfascial operative field. Early results demonstrate relief from symptoms with minimal wound morbidity. Minimally invasive surgical techniques appear likely to play an increased role in the management of patients with chronic venous insufficiency.

References

1. Hauer G (1985) The endoscopic subfascial division of the perforating veins – preliminary report (in German). VASA 14:59–61
2. Wittens C, Pierik R, Van Urk H (1995) The surgical treatment of incompetent perforating veins. Eur J Vasc Endovasc Surg 9:19–23
3. Pierik E, Wittens C, Van Urk H (1995) Subfascial endoscopic ligation in the treatment of incompetent perforating veins. Eur J Vasc Endovasc Surg 9:38–41
4. Bergan J, Murray J, Gleason K (1996) Subfascial endoscopic perforator vein surgery: A preliminary report. Ann Vasc Surg 10:211–219
5. Gloviczki P, Cambria R, Rhee R et al. (1996) Surgical technique and preliminary results of endoscopic subfascial division of perforating veins. J Vasc Surg 23:517–523
6. Tawes R, Wetter A, Hermann G, Fogarty T. Endoscopic technique for subfascial perforating vein ligation.
7. Jugenheimer M, Junginger T (1992) Endoscopic subfascial sectioning of incompetent perforating veins in treatment of primary varicosis. World J Surg 16:971–975
8. O'Donnell T (1992) Surgical treatment of incompetent communicating veins. In: Bergan J, Kistner R, (eds) Atlas of venous surgery. WB Saunders, Philadelphia; 111–124
9. Conrad P (1994) Endoscopic exploration of the subfascial space of the lower leg with perforator vein interruption using laparoscopic equipment: A preliminary report. Phlebology 9:154–157

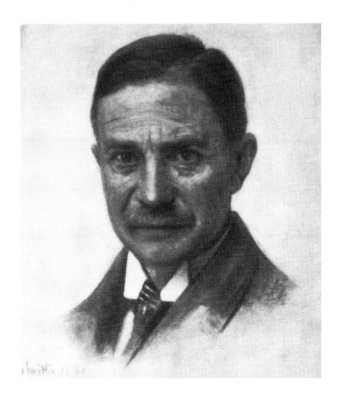

Georg Perthes
1869–1927

Born in Rheinland, Georg Perthes was orphaned at the age of fourteen and reared by his aunt, a granddaughter of a well known bookseller and patriot, Friedrich Perthes. At an early age Perthes was introduced to Friedrich Trendelenburg. This encounter played a pivotal role in Perthes' career decision and led to a life-long relationship with the master surgeon. The two complemented and influenced each other throughout their lives. Following completion of medical education he became Trendelenburg's resident and subsequently followed him to Leipzig in 1895. There he rapidly rose to the rank of professor in 1898. Subsequently was appointed the director of the surgical clinic in Tübingen.

All of Perthes' works were of the highest standard and outstanding in originality. In his *Habilitation* dissertation (for qualification of professorship) he conceptualized utility of a suction pump to maintain negative intrathoracic pressure for treatment of empyema and pneumothorax.

His work on venous disease is signified by the Perthes' test for detecting obstruction of the communicating and deep veins. He devised operations to treat bony deformities and to reconstruct tendons, for example for paralysis of the radialis muscle. Perthes established the principles of radiation filtration and developed the foundation of deep radiation therapy. His research on juvenile rheumatoid arthritis led to the description of osteochondritis coxae juvenilis – the condition that bears his name, Perthes' disease.

While enjoying the Christmas season in the mountains of Switzerland, he suffered a fatal heart attack. It was an untimely death as he was still a prolific surgeon, an active teacher and a productive scientist.

Subfascial Dissection and Perforating Vein Ablation

14

Mark D. Iafrati and Thomas F. O'Donnell Jr.

Introduction

The indications for and benefits of subfascial ligation of incompetent perforating veins are enumerated in other chapters in this text. While the classic Linton operation or the stocking seam incision to approach perforating veins provides excellent exposure it is plagued by unacceptably high wound complication rates.[1–3] Modifications of the open approaches (Chapter 9) have decreased wound complication rates; however, complete visualization of the subfascial space is difficult with these limited incisions. In recent years endoscopic approaches to perforator ligation have been developed both in Europe and in the United States. These minimally invasive techniques provide exposure to the entire subfascial space allowing complete perforator ablation, while minimizing trauma to the skin and underlying tissues. The operation is comprised of three conceptually simple steps; incision, subfascial dissection, and disruption of perforators. Although simple in design, proficient performance of subfascial endoscopic perforator surgery (SEPS) requires a familiarity with laparoscopic instrumentation (Chapter 10), surgical anatomy (Chapter 2), and experience with videoscopic surgery.

Treatment of patients with chronic venous insufficiency (CVI) requires an understanding of many facets of this disease. Treatment of superficial reflux is usually indicated as the initial intervention. When incompetent perforating veins (ICPVs) are noted, the operative treatment of superficial reflux and ICPVs can be combined as an out-patient proce-

dure. While treatment of the superficial and perforating systems has been shown to improve mild deep venous reflux[4] and result in reliable ulcer healing, ulcer recurrence rates may approach 100% in long term studies when severe untreated DVI is present.[5]

When our group introduced endoscopic subfascial ligation of perforators in the US in 1991, we were employing saline instillation for dissection and maintenance of the the subfascial plane.[6] Most instruments required 10-mm ports and there were no specifically designed dissection aids for this procedure. During the last 5 years considerable attention has been focused on the instrumentation and techniques involved in SEPS. Despite the advances in instrumention, a universally accepted approach has not yet emerged. While all techniques share the principle of locating incisions cephalad to the area of most severe skin changes, the means of creating and maintaining the subfascial working space as well as the methods of perforator interruption vary widely. This chapter will review some of the contemporary approaches to subfascial dissection and perforator division.

Technique

A minimally invasive approach to the ligation of incompetent perforating veins requires careful planning and appropriate instrumentation. We have found preoperative marking of ICPVs using duplex ultrasound to be an important adjunct in this procedure

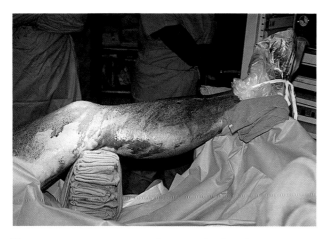

Fig. 14.1. SEPS preparation. Photograph of a left leg prepared with betadyne and positioned for subfascial endoscopic ligation of perforators. The lower leg is elevated and is parallel to the table. A stack of towels at the knee and a padded stand at the ankle maintains this position. Elevation allows for instrument movements which are unencumbered by either the contralateral leg or ipsilateral thigh and knee.

(Chapter 7). Although in ideal cases the entire subfascial space is explored it is useful to define the location of the largest perforators to ensure their division. Either general or regional anesthesia are acceptable and perioperative antibiotics and deep vein thrombosis prophylaxis are advised. Once the leg is prepared with betadyne, positioning is important. Elevating the lower leg parallel to the table provides maximum freedom for instrument movement (Fig. 14.1). The primary considerations relevant to incision placement are outined in Table 14.1.

Since the primary impetus for the development of SEPS is the reduction of wound complications, minimizing trauma to the compromised tissues in the lower leg is imperative. The constaints on instrument mobility can be addressed by allowing adequate space between port sites and the bony encumbrances of the knee and tibia. Finally a dualing instrument phenomenon is encountered when the scope and instrument shaft vie for the same space in a small tunnel. Separating the instru-

ments provides a triangulation effect, improving visualization and mobility. Using these guidelines our usual approach is demonstrated in Fig. 14.2. The first incision accommodates a 10-mm port and is located at least 10 cm distal to the tibial tuberosity and 2 cm lateral to the edge of the tibia. A 5-mm port is then placed under direct vision after creating and insufflating the subfascial tunnel. This port is located 5 cm posterior and distal to the first. Both incisions may be placed more distally on the leg if healthy skin is available. These incisions may also be used for avulsion of branch varicosities or to strip the greater saphenous vein.

Creation and maintenance of the subfascial working space is crucial. After the first incision is made, a finger can be used to create the initial space.

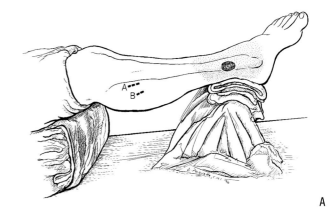

A

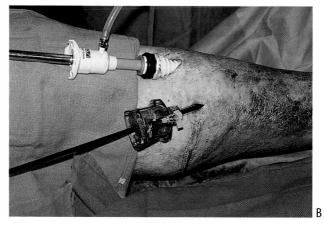

B

Fig. 14.2. Incision placement in SEPS. **A** Sketch demonstrating the incision sites for port placement in SEPS. Incisions are proximal to the area of lipodermatosclerosis (violet) and ulceration. Incision (A) accommodates a 10-mm port and is located at least 10 cm distal to the tibial tuberosity and 2 cm lateral to the edge of the tibia. Incision (B) accommodates a 5-mm port and is located 5 cm posterior and distal to the first incision. **B** Photo demonstrating the usual configuration of an anteriorly placed 10-mm port accommodating the scope with a 5-mm port placed posterior and caudal for the operating instruments.4

Table 14.1. Considerations for incision placement

1. Incisions should be placed in the relatively normal skin of the upper calf
2. Ports placed too close to the knee or tibia limit instrument movement
3. Ports placed too close to each other result in a "dualing instrument" phenomenon

At this point a number of options exist. For very limited dissections, manual retraction with conventional right angle retractors provides exposure for up to 10 cm from the incision. Video optics are useful even when this limited approach is used; however, conventional scissors and dissectors may be used. While the use of video imaging does extend the range of dissection in this limited incision approach complete subfascial exploration is not achieved. We therefore stongly advocate approaches which provide access to the entire subfascial space.

The subfascial space is a potential space, which separates the soleus and gastrocnemius muscles from the overlying fascia. This potential space within the superficial posterior compartment is normally bridged by fatty connective tissue but where chronic venous disease is present may have dense fibrotic changes, especially if ulceration is present. Creation and maintenance of an actual working space in this plane is the first unique aspect of the SEPS approach. Fig. 14.3 demonstrates the location of this surgically expanded plane.

The initial dissection of this subfascial plane may be accomplished with or without specific dissection aids (Chapter 13). We have found that use of a balloon dissector quickly creates a subfascial space which can then be maintained with CO_2 insufflation or mechanical retraction. Two types of devices are currently available. The first type utilizes an extrusion balloon which is packaged on a stiff trocar and covered with a peel-away sheath (General Surgical Innovations, Cupertino, CA). This device is inserted through the initial incision and is distended with 200–300 ml of saline (Fig. 14.4). As the balloon deploys along the length of the leg it can be guided by applying external pressure. This device provides a consistent working space (Fig. 14.5), with most perforators pushed toward the tibia. The balloon is usually deflected around dense fibrosis from ulceration or previous surgery. While this limits the utility of the dissection it lessens the potential for injury. An alternative device utilizes direct visualization and incremental balloon distension to create a working space (Guident, Mendlo Park, CA) (Fig. 14.6). Both devices provide a reliable working space. Direct visualization in the Guident system provides a theoretical safety advantage, but repetitive inflation of the dissecting balloon is cumbersome.

Although we have found that balloon dissection provides a convenient starting point for perforator dissection which we believe expedites the operation, this step is not mandatory (Chapter 12). The laparoscope may itself be used as a blunt dissector, although this necessitates frequent cleaning of the lens. Scope covers or recessed optics may lessen this problem. Alternatively, any number of conventional laparoscopic instruments may facilitate the initial dissection (Fig. 14.7).

Special Considerations in Perforator Dissection

While the initial subfascial dissection and the exposure of mid-calf perforating veins is typically straightforward there are a number of circumstances which deserve comment. Although the mid-calf subfascial working space is often generous (2 × 2 cm in cross-section), as shown in Fig. 14.3 this space quickly narrows as the operation is carried toward the ankle (Fig. 14.8). This small space, combined with the noncompliant skin and fibrotic subcuta-

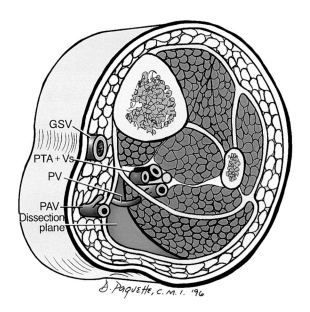

Fig. 14.3. Cross-sectional anatomy. The sketch shows a cross-section of the lower leg demonstrating the working space (Cyan) for SEPS which is created in a subfascial plane within the superficial posterior compartment. The fascia is pink, a perforating vein (PV) is shown crossing the subfascial space connecting the posterior tibial (PTV) and posterior arch veins (PAV). The peroneal and anterior tibial neurovascular bundles are omitted. The greater saphenous vein (GSV) is identified.

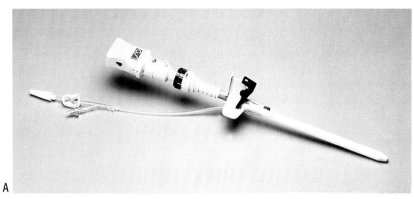

A

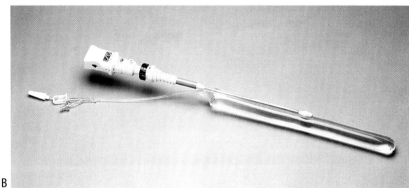

B

Fig. 14.4. Space maker balloon dissector (GSI, Upertino CA). **A** This balloon is inserted on a stiff trocar with a covering sheath. **B** The sheath is removed and the balloon is distended with saline. The balloon distends longitudinally creating the subfascial plane. The balloon and trocar are then removed leaving a 10-mm port in place.

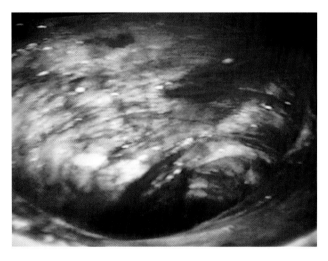

Fig. 14.5. Subfascial tunnel. Subfascial working space obtained by the use of balloon dissection and CO_2 insufflation. The tibia and most perforating veins will be located along the left side of this picture.

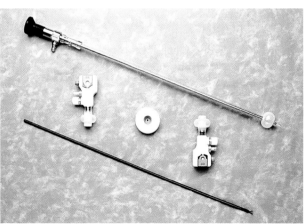

Fig. 14.6. Vaso view balloon dissection system (Guident, Menlo Park, CA). This through viewing balloon dissection device uses incremental balloon distention under direct visualization to create a subfascial or subcutaneous space.

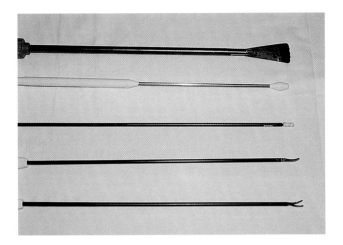

Fig. 14.7. Laparoscopic instrumentation. A wide variety of laparoscopic instruments may be utilized for subfascial dissection. Pictured here from top to bottom are a fan refractor, blunt dissector, Kitner, curved dissector, curved scissor.

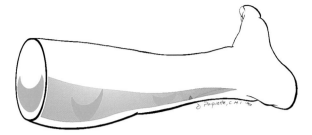

Fig. 14.9. Fasciotomy of the superficial posterior compartment. Distal longitudinal division of the superficial fascia of the superficial posterior compartment allows radial expansion of the narrow confines near the ankle. Both increased working space and depth of vision are obtained and represented by the magenta-colored area in this figure.

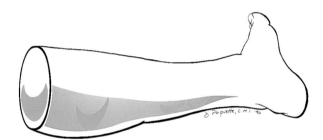

Fig. 14.8. Superficial posterior compartment. This sketch highlights the fascial enclosure of the superficial posterior compartment of the lower leg (cyan). Note the marked tapering of this space near the ankle. The narrow confines in the distal reaches of this compartment pose significant technical challenges to SEPS.

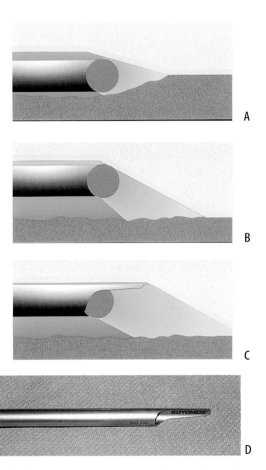

Fig. 14.10. Mechanical retraction combined with insufflation. Exposure in the lower leg may be limited even with the use of CO_2 insufflation and a fasciotomy, as in **A**. In **B** the working space (cyan) is enhanced by applying an upward force on the scope. Since the fascia (pink) is reflected over the end of the scope, the visual field is further augmented by use of a 30° lens. Significantly greater depth of field is obtained by adding a retracting hood, **C**. This hood extends the point of retraction without narrowing the field of view. **D** photo: retracting hood for a 10-mm endoscope (Smith & Nephews Endoscopy, Andover, MA).

neous tissues associated with CVI, results in an extremely tight working space. Reaching these supramalleor perforators represents the greatest limitation of our current technology. However several maneuvers may be employed in this situation. Division of the investing fascia may significantly increase the available space (Fig. 14.9). Upward retraction using the scope is a useful maneuver which may be further enhanced by the use of a 30° lens and a retracting hood (Fig. 14.10). Excessive force should be avoided as tissue injury at the trocar site is possible, as is injury to the saphenous nerve. These interventions provide some improvement in visualization but the working space remains confined. Using 5-mm rather than 10-mm instruments reduces the area needed to manipulate the instruments in this long tunnel. Finally, in

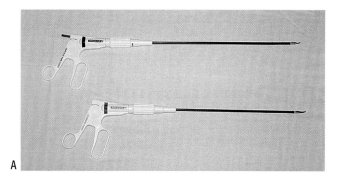

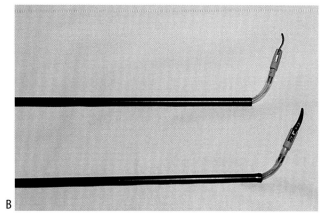

Fig. 14.11. Roticulating instruments. Dissectors and scissors with roticulating movement (US Surgical Corp., Norwalk, CT) facilitate dissection when operating in long narrow planes during SEPS. The roticulating end allows the instrument shaft to run parallel with the scope while the working end crosses the field of view past the end of the scope. **A** demonstrates the scissors and dissectors in the straight configuration. **B** close-up view of the scissor (top) and dissector (bottom) in the extended (bent) configuration.

selected cases the use of roticulating dissectors and scissors (US Surgical Corp, Norwalk, CT) helps to avoid the dualing shaft problem (Fig. 14.11). Providing downward pressure with the instrument shaft further enhances distal exposure.

Dissection beneath active ulcers represents the major limitation of balloon dissection. These dense connective tissues are resistant to most blunt dissection but can be dissected sharply with scissors. Fortunately, we have not found reoperative cases to be a major problem. In our experience with 5 patients with prior open subfascial ligation of perforators the planes dissected without difficulty. While ICPVs are frequently found in the vicinity of ulcers, Hanrahan et al. found that only 26% of ulcers covered perforating veins.[7] Furthermore, although sharp dissection beneath ulcers can be tedious we have found the perforating veins to generally be located at the periphery of the ulcers. Therefore,

although complete dissection is ideal we concentrate our efforts at the sites of preoperatively identified ICPVs and may accept incomplete dissection if the known perforators have been addressed.

To this point we have limited our discussion to exploration of the superficial posterior compartment. However, detailed anatomic studies (Chapter 2) have shown that while muscular perforating veins reliably cross this plane, only a minority of direct ICPVs (Cockett and paratibial perforators) can be accessed in the superficial posterior compartment. These direct perforators originate from the greater saphenous vein or its tributaries and join the posterior tibial veins. These perforators can be accessed by dividing the deep fascia (Fig. 14.12). The fasciotomy is performed with a laparoscopic scissor and dissection is carried out bluntly. In the lower leg this dissection exposes the deep posterior compartment and the Cockett perforators. The posterior tibial neurovascular bundle may be encountered during this dissection and care should be exercised to avoid injury to these structures. Division of the fascia more superficially allows extrafascial exposure of perforating veins. In the mid to upper calf, the fasciotomy exposes paratibial perforators which are immediately adjacent to the tibia or within a duplicated fascial layer. The paratibial perforators may be disrupted without risk to adjacent structures.

Perforator Disruption

The goal of SEPS is to stop the pathologic flow of blood from the deep venous system through incompetent perforating veins to the superficial venous system. Since rehabilitative and reconstructive options for perforator incompetence are not practical we are forced to pursue ablative surgical techniques. The various methods of subfascial dissection outlined previously are all designed to facilitate exposure (Fig. 14.13) and disruption of incompetent perforating veins.

The approaches to perforator disruption vary widely and include simple division with external compression, electrocoagulation, ultrasonic coagulation, and clips. The choice of technique should be guided by several principles, as outlined in Table 14.2. Since no device is ideal in all circumstances we will review the merits of each.

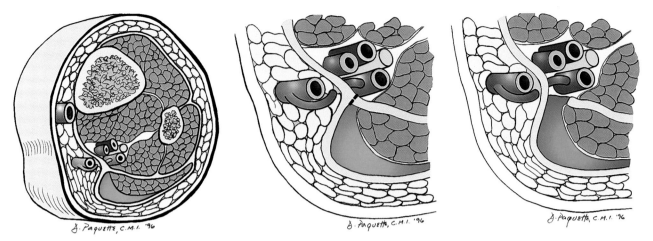

Fig.14.12. Fasciotomy for access to direct perforating veins. **A** A perforating vein originating from a subcutaneous axial vein such as the saphenous or posterior arch vein traverses to the posterior tibial vein in the deep posterior compartment without entering the initial dissection plane in the superficial posterior compartment. **B** A magnified view of a direct perforating vein, outside the initial dissection plane. The dashed line indicated the site of fascial division for access to the deep posterior compartment. **C** An incision in the fascia allows extension of the dissection plane into the deep posterior compartment for control of these direct perforating veins.

Uncontrolled disruption of ICPVs provides a rapid and permanent solution. This method has been used in a blind fashion (Fig. 14.14) with control of hemorrhage by external compression.[8] This technique does not allow direct visualization of perforators and its use is limited to the superficial posterior compartment, potentially missing important perforators. When videoscopic techniques are employed, simple division of perforators is still an option but it mandates exsanguination and use of a tourniquet to maintain a blood-free operative field. Although we occasionally use simple perforator division to disrupt the most distal perforator when space limitations preclude other techniques we advocate use of more hemostatic methods when possible.

Electrocautery devices quickly divide even the largest perforating veins, especially when emptied of blood. While hemostasis is improved compared to

Table 14.2. Principles for perforator disruption

1. The disruption should be permanent
2. Disruption of proximal perforating veins should not impair access to the distal leg
3. Injury to adjacent nerves and blood vessels should be avoided
4. The device should be small to allow its use when space is limited

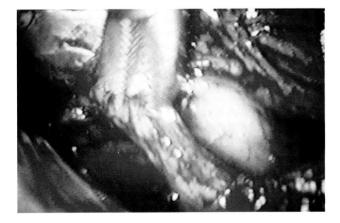

Fig. 14.13. Perforating vein. Endoscopic view of a perforating vein. Dissection is being completed with a curved laparoscopic dissector. Note that the vein is decompressed by the use of exsanguination and a tourniquet.

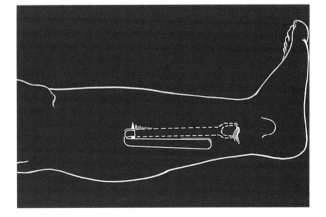

Fig. 14.14. Blind disruption of incompetent perforating veins. The sketch depicts a minimally invasive technique for subfascial perforator disruption. In this shearing technique described by Edwards, perforators are not directly visualized and hemostasis is obtained by external compression.

simple uncontrolled division of perforators, electrocautery is less reliable than other techniques and tissue vaporization necessitates frequent lens cleaning. The greatest problem with cautery is the potential for heat energy to be conducted to adjacent nerves or veins. Injury to the saphenous nerve can result in paresthesias, while injury to the posterior tibial veins may predispose to deep venous thrombosis, and saphenous vein injury could compromise its future use as a conduit for bypass. Collateral damage is minimized by the use of bipolar cautery, however current equipment is cumbersome and energy delivery is not easily regulated.

Ultrasonic coagulation utilizes a high-frequency oscillating arm within pincer jaws to coagulate and divide tissues. This device relies on a combination of pressure and harmonic oscillation to hemostatically divide the veins. The oscillating limb has three surfaces which may be chosen. (Fig. 14.15) By adjusting the contact surface area the amount of tissue coagu-

lated may be varied. In general, larger surface contact provides better coagulation, but takes more time, causes more vaporization and results in grater energy transfer. The ability to dissect, divide, and coagulate tissues without exchanging instruments improves the tempo of the operation. Heat conduction is less than with cautery but the current device is only available in a 10-mm shaft size which makes it impractical for use when working space is limited. When this device is used for perforator disruption, either the medium or large surfaces should be used with firm pressure to ensure hemostasis.

Endoscopic clip appliers have been widely used in laparoscopic cholecystectomy and other laparoscopic procedures. They are relatively secure, easy to use, and do not conduct any heat. Traditional 10-mm devices are difficult to use in the narrow confines of the leg but 5-mm devices are now available (Fig. 14.16). Although the jaws are smaller on the 5-mm Ligaclip Allport (Ethicon Endo-Surgery,

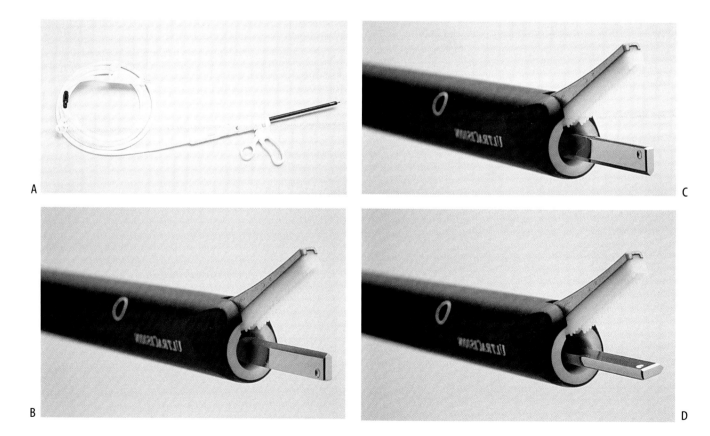

Fig. 14.15. Ultrasonic scalpel. **A** Ultrasonic scalpel (Ultracision, Smithfield, RI) with handset and cable. **B–D** Demonstrate the 10-mm shaft with its adjustable oscillating arm. As the contact surface increases from **B** to **D**, the time and energy required to divide tissues increases as does the security of hemostasis.

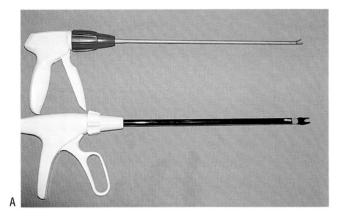

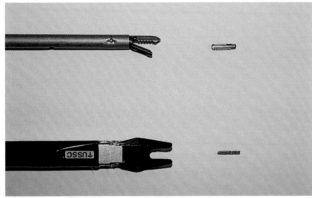

Fig. 14.16. Endoscopic clip appliers. **A** 5-mm (Ethicon Endo-Surgery, Cincinnati, OH) (top) and 10-mm (US Surgical Corp. Norwalk, CT) (bottom) multifire endo clip appliers. **B** Close-up view of the 5- and 10-mm clip appliers and clips. Note that although both clips are 9 mm in length the 5-mm Ethicon device uses a higher profile clip.

Cincinnati, OH) it uses 9-mm clips which are equivalent in length to most 10 mm devices. Perforating veins may be interrupted by placing a single clip across the vessel, however distal dissection is often facilitated by doubly clipping and then dividing the vein. We have not found clip dislodgement to be a problem, and although exchanging instruments may be awkward at times this is our preferred technique for perforator control.

Conclusion

The techniques and instrumentation for SEPS have been greatly refined over the last few years. Using the methods outlined in this and other chapters in this text, most incompetent perforating veins can be disrupted. However dissection and division of ICPVs near the ankle or under ulcers remains a challenge. We believe that even these challenges will be overcome by continued improvements in techniques and technology.

References

1. Burnand K, O'Donnell TF, Thomas ML, Browse NL (1976) Relation between postphlebitic changes in the deep veins and results of surgical treatment of venous ulcers. Lancet 1:936–938
2. Johnson WC, O'Hara ET, Corey C, Widrich WC, Nabseth DC (1985) Venous stasis ulceration; effectiveness of subfascial ligation. Arch Surg 120:797–800
3. Silver D, Cikrit D (1989) Operative management of perforator vein incompetence. In: Rutherford R (ed) Vascular Surgery WB Saunders Co., Philadelphia
4. Padberg FT, Hobson RW, Pappas PJ, Araki CT (1996). Hemodynamic improvement with superficial venous ablation in combined deep and superficial venous insufficiency. American Venous Forum, San Diego, CA J Vasc Surg 24:711–718
5. Burnand KG, O'Donnell TF, Lea TM, Browse NL (1977) The relative importance of incompetent communicating veins in the production of varicose veins and venous ulcers. Surgery 82:9–14
6. O'Donnell TF (1992) Surgical treatment of incompetent communicating veins. In: Bergan JJ, Kistner RL (eds) Atlas of Venous Surgery. WB Saunders, Philadephia, pp 111–124
7. Hanrahan L, Araki C, Rodriguez A, Kechejian G, LaMorte W, Menzoian J (1991) Distribution of valvular incompetence in patients with venous stasis ulceration. J Vasc Surg 13:805–812
8. Edwards JM (1976) Shearing operations for incompetent perforating veins. Br J Surg 63:885–886

Profile

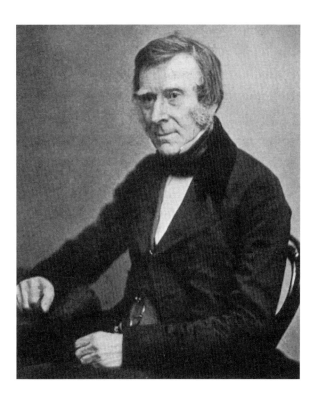

Sir Benjamin Collins Brodie
1783–1862

Benjamin Collins Brodie was the only person ever named president of three distinguished medical societies of England, the Royal Society, the General Medical Council, and the Royal College of Surgeons.

Son of a parish rector, who taught him Greek and Latin, at age 18 Ben Brodie studied anatomy in London under Abernethy at St Bartholomew's Hospital. Later he became pupil and assistant of Sir Everard Home, brother-in-law of John Hunter. In 1808 he was appointed to the surgical staff of St George's Hospital, and soon he was considered to be one of the most dexterous surgeons in London. From 1812 he systematically started compiling a treatise that was to become an authoritative source on varicose veins, on diseases of joints, injuries of the brain, and chronic abscess of bones. This was published in the series of Medico Chirurgical Transactions and is considered his greatest literary contribution to practical surgery. He operated on many patients with varicose veins and designed a test to evaluate venous valve incompetence. He treated varicose veins by severing the vessel above and below the varicosity.

Brodie's interest in the different fields of surgery was remarkable. He described an operation for fistula in ano, recognized the significance of the sentinel pile at the lower end of the fissure, observed the physiological changes in digestion following ligation of the common duct, prepared treatises on urology and the action of local nervous afflictions, and reported on chronic cystic mastitis, Brodie's tumor.

In 1819, at the age of 36, he was appointed professor of comparative anatomy and physiology at the Royal College of Surgeons. Following the retirement of Sir Astley Cooper in 1828, Sir Brodie was considered to be the leading surgeon in England. In 1832 he was appointed Sergeant-Surgeon to the King, William IV.

Comparison of Open Linton Operation with Subfascial Endoscopic Perforator Vein Surgery

15

Cees H. A. Wittens

Robert Linton first recognized the necessity of interrupting incompetent perforating veins to cure varicose ulcers following deep phlebitis. Descriptions of these veins, however, were scanty and incomplete at that time. Since a more accurate knowledge of these veins was necessary for the proper treatment of perforating veins and ulcers, Linton studied and described the anatomy of the perforating veins of the lower extremity.[1] Subsequently, he developed the radical surgical treatment described elsewhere in this volume.[2] His operation had a four-fold purpose: 1. to remove all enlarged superficial veins, 2. to subfascially ligate and divide all perforating veins of the lower leg, 3. to interrupt the superficial femoral veins distal to the profunda vein, and 4, to partially excise the deep fascia of the lower leg in an attempt to restore the lymphatic drainage. His initial technique involved three longitudinal incisions (anterolateral, posterolateral, and medial) for complete ligation of the perforators.

In 1953, Linton began using only a medial incision since most perforators could be reached through this incision[3] (Fig. 15.1). However, this operation still necessitated an incision through unhealthy skin and fat for a direct approach to the incompetent perforating veins. Although Linton preferred to perform this procedure after the ulcerations had been healed completely by bed rest and compression therapy, he himself noticed that his incision did not always heal by primary intention. Although the operation proved to be successful, it was complicated by delayed wound healing, skin necrosis, and wound infection in up to 58% of the cases.[4–7]

However, since Linton's paper, the cornerstone in the treatment of venous ulcers has been based on preventing the abnormal transmission of high ambulatory pressure to the superficial veins. This is done by interruption of the perforating veins.

Multiple modifications of Linton's technique have been advocated to avoid wound complications. Cockett advised not dividing the deep fascia surrounding the soleus muscle because of its role in the calf pump mechanism. He performed an extrafascial ligation of the incompetent perforators in addition to excision of the ulcer.[4] However, the subcutaneous exploration has become obsolete because of many disappointing experiences caused by difficulties in identification of perforating veins. Dodd described a posteromedial subfascial approach to obviate dissection of unhealthy skin.[8]

The Rob procedure achieved posterior subfascial ligation of perforating veins via a long "stocking-seam" incision.[9] A final modified operative approach

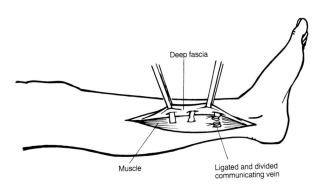

Fig. 15.1. Schematic drawing of a modified Linton procedure.

to the problem of wound healing was described by DePalma in 1974 using multiple small parallel, oblique skin incisions (see Chapter 9) in the natural skin lines along the medial aspect of the lower extremity.[10] He proposed subcutaneous as well as subfascial dissection, depending on the degree of lipodermatosclerosis.

For the most part, however, others abandoned surgery for post-thrombotic vein incompetence and turned to injection sclerotherapy.[11–13] This was instigated not only by the high complication rate of traditional surgical methods but also by a growing controversy about the role of calf perforating veins in the etiology of venous ulceration.[14,15]

A prerequisite for DePalma's method as well as sclerotherapy is accurate location of perforating veins. This is of special interest because recently the dogma of predilection sites of perforating veins has been questioned.[16] Perforator detection by clinical methods,[17] venography,[18] infrared photography,[19] fluorescein injection with ultraviolet scanning,[20] and ultrasonography[21] have all been ried. No single method has been found to identify the site of all incompetent perforating veins accurately. The use of duplex ultrasonography will likely improve perforator detection but the technique is time-consuming and very operator-dependent if reproducible results are to be obtained.[22]

Although some authors still question the benefit of conventional surgical procedures, Negus and Friedgood treated 109 ulcerated legs and showed an 84% healing rate after subfascial ligation of incompetent perforating veins using the Linton and Dodd approach.[23] They suggested that a more optimistic attitude towards surgical treatment of this "crux medicorum" was justified. Good to excellent results after surgical therapy directed at the perforating veins have also been described by others.[6–24]

Between 1961 and 1971, over 1 000 patients were followed up after perforating vein ligation for periods ranging between 5 and 9 years with an overall recurrence rate of 10%.[25] A review of the 10 most recent reports of subfascial ligation of perforators revealed a recurrence rate of 15% in 767 limbs.[26] Complications included deep vein thrombosis, pulmonary embolism, flap necrosis, wound infections, and a wound complication rate of 17%. These recurrence and complication rates were found in patients in whom all types of medical management had failed, thus representing the most severe expressions of venous insufficiency.

Recently, however, minimally invasive procedures have been developed and described for subfascial perforator division in patients with varicose veins and lipodermatosclerosis. The term SEPS (subfascial endoscopic perforator surgery) has been adopted. The use of fiberoptics,[27] rigid endoscopic instruments,[28] or mediastinoscopes[29,30] allows subfascial ligation and sectioning of all perforating veins under direct vision with minimal trauma.

Only a few retrospective studies have been published describing the results of endoscopic dissection. Jugenheimer and Junginger reported acceptable results of endoscopic subfascial sectioning of incompetent perforating veins in 103 legs of 72 patients with primary varicose veins.[31] In this retrospective study, subfascial endoscopy was combined with conventional excision of varices in 94%. Postoperative delayed wound healing was observed in only 2.9%. Two patients (1.9%) complained of dysesthesia in the distribution of the sural nerve. Other complications included extended subcutaneous hematoma in 5.8% and postoperative dysesthesia in the distribution of the saphenous nerve in 9.7%. However, the question remains unanswered as to whether these complications were associated with the endoscopic procedure or with vein stripping. After a mean follow-up of 27 months, newly formed or persistent incompetent perforating veins were detected in 2 patients (1.9%).

Severe subfascial infection necessitating repeat surgical intervention on both legs was described in a patient operated upon bilaterally by Wittens et al.[29] Using a mediastinoscope, 40 recurrent or protracted venous leg ulcers were treated by subfascial endoscopy.[30] After a mean of approximately 3.9 years, only one patient (2.5%) developed a recurrent ulcer. Endoscopic subfascial dissection of incompetent perforating veins is a promising technique as a surgical alternative in the treatment of venous ulceration. This is in line with renewed interest in venous surgery and the modern trend towards minimally invasive surgery.[32–33]

No prospective, randomized studies have been published comparing open and endoscopic perforator surgery. It can be questioned if endoscopic surgery is as effective in eradicating incompetent perforating veins as the open Linton operation. In Rotterdam, in 1994, a prospective study compared these two approaches. Only patients with venous ulceration of the lower leg were treated. There was a special interest in the number and localization of

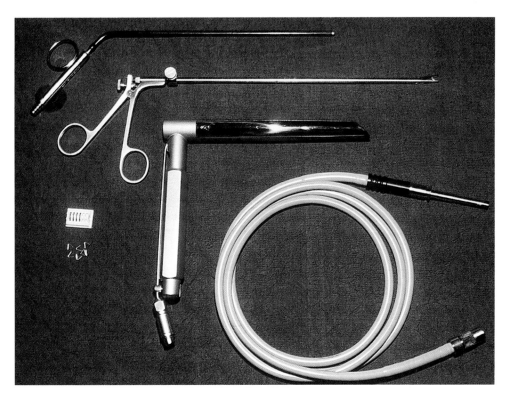

Fig. 15.2. Instruments used for the randomized trial: suction tube, clip applier, mediastinoscope, light cable.

perforating veins on the medial side of the lower leg. We made use of a mediastinoscope and a long clipping instrument and gained subfascial access via a small incision on the medial side of the lower limb (Fig. 15.2).

Patterns of venous insufficiency were determined by color-flow duplex ultrasonography by an experienced vascular technologist before operation at 6 weeks postoperatively. All determinations were made using a linear-array transducer with a 7.5 MHz imaging/5 MHz pulsed-wave Doppler color-flow duplex system (P700, Philips Medical Systems, Eindhoven, The Netherlands) (Fig. 15.3) with the patient in a near upright standing position (Fig. 15.4A, B). Perforating veins were defined as vessels penetrating the fascia and constituting continuously traceable connections between the superficial and deep venous systems. The only criterion for insufficiency was reverse venous flow demonstrated on the Doppler spectral display during the relaxation phase after active dorsiflexion of the ankle and/or manual compression of the foot. Insufficiency was determined to be present if reverse flow persisted for longer than 0.3 sec (Fig. 15.5). A sterile conductivity gel and transparent dressing were used for duplex evaluation of the ulcer bed. The number, localization

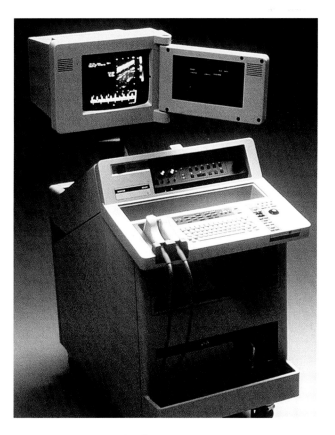

Fig. 15.3. Doppler color-flow duplex system (P700, Philips Medical Systems, Eindhoven, The Netherlands)

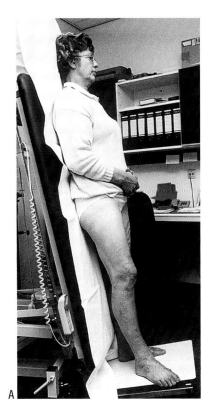
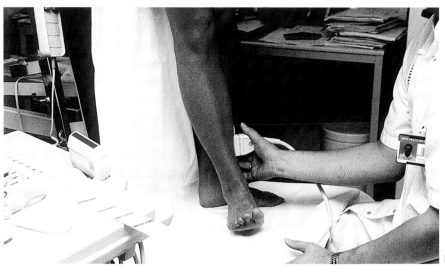

Fig. 15.4. A Patient on a special table to facilitate the color-flow duplex examination of the venous system in an erect position. **B** Easy access for the vascular laboratory technician to perform a thorough venous examination on the medial aspect of the lower leg.

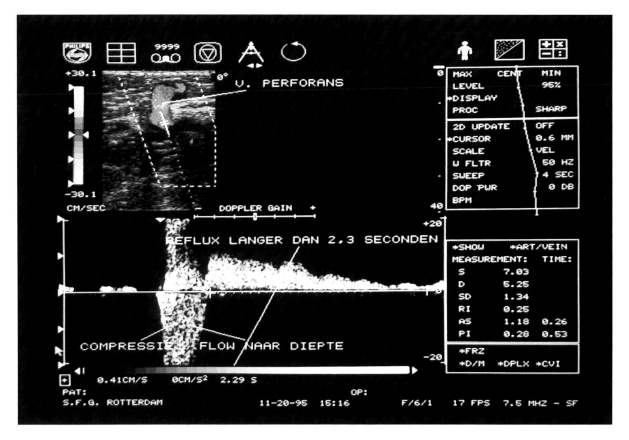

Fig. 15.5. Incompetent perforating vein identified by color-flow duplex examination.

and presence or absence of insufficiency of the perforating veins at the medial and dorsal side of the lower leg were noted. The distance of each perforating vein to the sole of the foot was measured in centimeters.

After 15 months, 39 patients were included and an interim analysis was done. Patient characteristics are shown in Table 15.1. The number and location of competent and incompetent perforating veins detected with duplex ultrasonography and during operation are found in Tables 15.2 and 15.3.

During endoscopic surgery, all perforating veins were clipped as close to the fascia as possible (Fig. 15.6A, B). The perforating veins often divide close to the muscle. This might allow persisting connections between the deep venous system and the superficial system if only one branch is clipped close to the muscle. This is prevented by clipping as close to the fascia as possible (Fig. 15.7A, B). If necessary, perforators were clipped and divided (Fig. 15.8A, B).

Table 15.3. Number and location of incompetent, competent, and false-negative perforating veins on the medial side of the lower leg during preoperative duplex ultrasonography (in cm above foot sole) in patients randomized to endoscopic exploration.

Location	Incompetent PF	Competent PF	False-negative PF
0–5	2	0	0
6–10	4	0	0
11–15	13	2	1
16–20	13	3	2
21–25	8	1	2
26–30	4	0	0
31–35	1	0	0
36–40	1	0	0
Totals	62	6	5

Table 15.1. Patient characteristics.

	Open (n = 19)	Endoscopic (n = 20)
Age (years)	70 (36–89)	64 (33–89)
Sex ratio (M/F)	3/16	9/11
Diabetes mellitus	1	0
Recurrent ulceration	12	13
Duration of present ulcer period (days)	249 (14–1825)	299 (20–3650)
Duplex findings preoperatively		
Superficial incompetence	13	14
Deep incompetence	14	11
Incompetent perforating vein	2.1 (1–5)	2.3 (1–5)

Table 15.2. Number and location of incompetent, competent, and false-negative perforating veins on the medial side of the lower leg during preoperative duplex ultrasonography (in cm above foot sole) in patients randomized to open exploration.

Location	Incompetent PF	Competent PF	False-negative PF
0–5	1	0	2
6–10	3	1	4
11–15	11	2	3
16–20	13	2	1
21–25	7	1	1
26–30	5	2	0
31–35	2	0	0
36–40	0	0	0
Totals	42	8	11

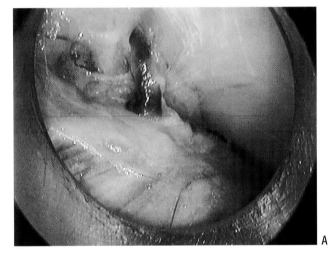

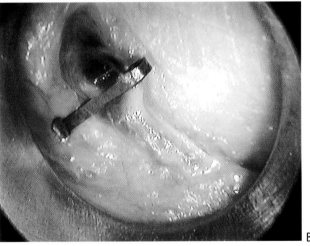

Fig. 15.6. A Perforating vein by endoscopic exploration. **B** Clipped perforating vein.

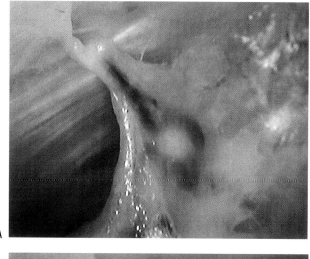

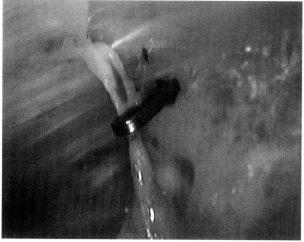

Fig. 15.7. A Perforating vein that branches immediately in the subfascial region. **B** Properly clipped branching perforating vein, namely along the fascia.

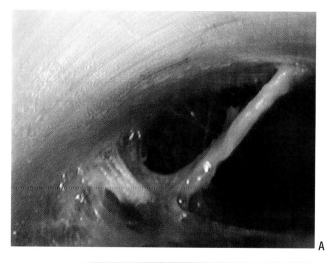

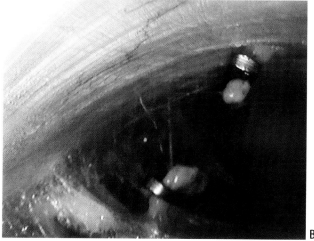

Fig. 15.8. A Perforating vein. **B** Double clipped and dissected perforating vein.

In the open group, no perforating veins were found with duplex ultrasonography 6 weeks after surgery. The complete absence of these perforating veins strongly confirms the thoroughness of the Linton procedure. In the endoscopic surgery group, 6 incompetent perforating veins in 4 patients were found at duplex ultrasonography 6 weeks after surgery. Two patients were the ones in whom 3 preoperatively diagnosed perforating veins could not be confirmed at operation. The localization of the postoperative perforating veins was similar to the preoperative duplex examination. That is, near the anterior margin of the tibia. The ulcers of both patients did not heal.

In one patient, two "new" incompetent perforating veins were detected. This patient had suffered from venous ulceration for more than 45 years.

Multiple recurrences on both legs were caused by combined deep and superficial venous incompetence. The ulcer did not heal post perforator interruption although initial improvement in the size of the ulcer was achieved (Fig. 15.9). Six months postoperatively, a squamous cell carcinoma was found in the ulcer.

In the fourth patient, a perforating vein was detected at the same level as was detected preoperatively. This was confirmed and clipped during endoscopy. This persisting perforating vein could have been caused by a slipped clip or a branched perforating vein. In spite of perforator persistence, the ulcer healed uneventfully within 5 weeks.

In the other 17 patients, no persistent or recurrent perforating veins could be detected at postoperative duplex ultrasonography.

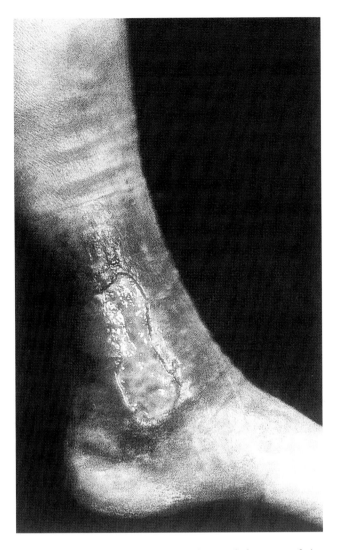

Fig. 15.9. Severe venous ulcer on the medial aspect of the lower leg.

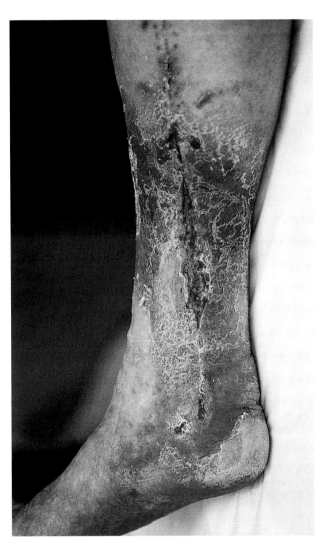

Fig. 15.10. Wound complication following a Linton procedure.

After a follow-up period of 46 weeks, 17 of 19 patients in the open group and 17 of 20 patients in the endoscopic group had healed. Thus, overall results were similar. There were no wound complications in the endoscopic group but there were 10 wound infections in the open group (Fig. 15.10). We concluded that subfascial endoscopic perforator surgery was an effective method by which to identify and occlude the incompetent perforating veins in patients with venous ulceration on the medial side of the lower leg. However, special attention must be paid to the presence of an intermuscular septum near the anterior margin of the tibia (Fig. 15.11) which is present in about 30% of patients. If such a septum is identified, it has to be opened completely

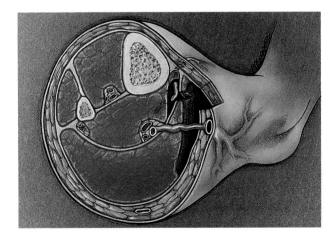

Fig. 15.11. Artist's drawing of incision of the intermuscular septum and entry into the deep posterior compartment.

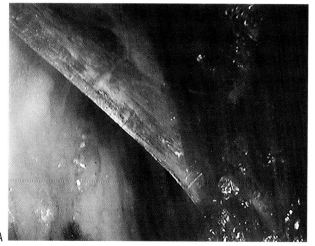

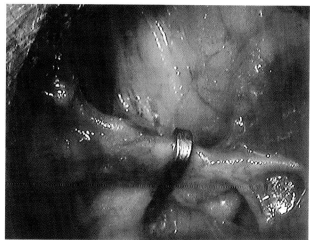

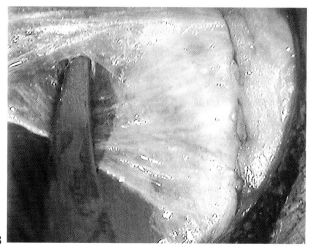

Fig. 15.12. **A** Endoscopic aspect of an intramuscular septum at the anterior margin of the tibia. **B** Dissection of the septum with scissors. **C** Large clipped incompetent perforating vein in the intermuscular septum.

because large perforating veins may be in it or behind it (Fig. 15.12A, B, C). In 2 patients of this series, 3 perforating veins were probably missed due to the fact that the septum intermusculare was not identified.

In order to visualize as much of the fascia as possible, a new endoscope by Olympus has been developed (Fig. 15.13). This has an optical system facing the fascia with a working channel which allows easy clipping and/or cutting as close to the fascia as possible. Due to the combination of a single-port mechanical dissection device and continuous CO_2 insufflation, a good overview ("cave view") (Fig. 15.14) is created during the procedure. This allows perfect quality control at the end of the procedure. We conclude that use of a single-port endoscope permits: 1. identification of nearly all perforating veins in patients with far-advanced stages of chronic venous insufficiency, 2. exploration of the entire

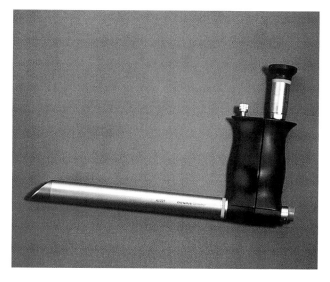

Fig. 15.13. Newly designed Olympus mechanical dissection endoscope with an optical system facing the fascia, a working channel along the fascia, and a CO_2 insufflation system.

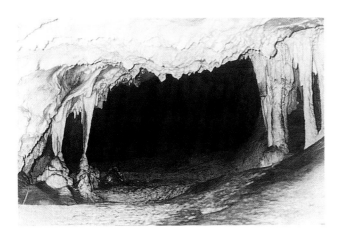

Fig. 15.14. The "cave view."

subfascial area, and 3. splitting of the medial intermuscular septum when present. This is important to prevent the persistence of incompetent perforating veins. These, in our study, related to failure of ulcer healing.

References

1. Homans J (1917) The etiology and treatment of varicose ulcer of the leg. Surg Gynecol Obstet 24:300–311
2. Linton RR (1938) The communicating veins of the lower leg and the operative technique for their ligation. Ann Surg 107:582–593
3. Linton RR (1953) The postthrombotic ulceration of the lower extremity: Its etiology and surgical treatment. Ann Surg 138:415–432
4. Cockett FB (1955) The pathology and treatment of venous ulcers of the leg. Br J Surg 43:260–278
5. Haeger K (1966) Five-year results of radical surgery for superficial varices with or without coexistent perforator insufficiency. Acta Chir Scand 131:38–49
6. Field P, Van Boxel P (1971) The role of the Linton flap procedure in the management of stasis, dermatitis, and ulceration in the lower limb. Surgery 70:920–926
7. Puts JP, Gruwez JA (1993) Surgical treatment of the postthrombotic syndrome: Improvement of the Linton operation by use of piracetam. Br J Surg 80(suppl):115
8. Dodd H (1964) The diagnosis and ligation of incompetent perforating veins. Ann R Coll Surg Engl 34:186–196
9. Healey RJ, Healey EH, Wong R, Schaberg FJ (1979) Surgical management of the chronic venous ulcer: The Rob procedure. Am J Surg 137:556–559
10. DePalma RG (1974) Surgical therapy for venous stasis. Surgery 76:910–917
11. Fegan WG (1963) Continuous compression technique of injecting varicose veins. Lancet 2:109–112
12. Hobbs JT (1968) The treatment of varicose veins: A random trial of injection compression therapy versus surgery. Br J Surg 55:777–780
13. Henry MEF, Fegan WG, Pegum JM (1971) Five-year survey of the treatment of varicose ulcers. Br Med J 2:493–494
14. Recek C (1971) A critical appraisal of the role of ankle perforators for the genesis of venous ulcers in the lower leg. J Cardiovasc Surg 12:45–49
15. Burnand KG, Lea Thomas M, O'Donnell TF, Browse NL (1976) The relationship between postphlebitic changes in the deep veins and results of surgical treatment of venous ulcers. Lancet 1:936–938
16. Fischer R, Fullemann HJ, Adler W (1992) A propos d'un dogme phlebologique sur les localisations des perforantes de Cockett. Phlébologie 45:207–212
17. Editorial (1970) Hidden perforating veins. Br Med J 1:186
18. Townsend J, Jones H, Edmund-Williams J (1967) Detection of incompetent perforating veins by venography at operation. Br Med J 3:583–585
19. Beesley WH, Fegan WG (1970) An investigation into the localization of incompetent perforating veins. Br J Surg 57:30–32
20. Chilvers AS, Thomas MH (1970) Method for the localization of incompetent ankle perforating veins. Br Med J 2:577–579
21. O'Donnell TF, Burnand KG, Clemenson G, Thomas ML, Browse NL (1977) Doppler examination vs. clinical and phlebographic detection of the location of incompetent perforating veins. Arch Surg 112:31–35
22. Hanrahan LM, Kechjian GJ, Cordts PR et al. (1991) Patterns of venous insufficiency in patients with perforating veins. Arch Surg 126:687–691
23. Negus D, Friedgood A (1983) The effective management of venous ulceration. Br J Surg 70:623–627
24. Wilkinson GE, Maclaren IF (1986) Long-term review of procedures for venous perforator insufficiency. Surg Gyn Obstet 163:117–120
25. Negus D (1985) Prevention and treatment of venous ulceration. Ann R Coll Surg Engl 67:144–148
26. Cikrit DF, Nichols K, Silver D (1988) Surgical management of refractory venous stasis ulceration. J Vasc Surg 7:473–478
27. Fischer R (1989) Surgical treatment of perforating veins: Endoscopic treatment of incompetent Cockett veins. Phlébologie 1040–1041
28. Hauer G (1985) Die endoscopische subfasciale Diszision der Perforansvenenvorlaufige mitteilung. VASA 14:59
29. Wittens CHA, Bollen ECM, Kool DR, van Urk H, Mul T, van Houtte HJKP (1993) Goede resultaten van subfasciale endoscopie als behandeling van insufficiente Vv. perforantes. Ned Tijdschr Geneesk 137:1200–1204
30. Pierik EGJM, Wittens CHA, van Urk H (1995) Subfascial endoscopic ligation in the treatment of incompetent perforating veins. Eur J Vasc Endovasc Surg 2:24–27
31. Jugenheimer M, Junginger Th (1992) Endoscopic subfascial sectioning of incompetent perforating veins in treatment of primary varicosis. World J Surg 16:971–975
32. Fitzpatrick JM, Wickham JEA (1990) Minimally invasive surgery. Br J Surg 77:721–722
33. Kitslaar PJEHM, Rutgers PH (1993) Varicose veins and the vascular surgery: From nuisance to challenge. Eur J Vasc Surg 7:109–112

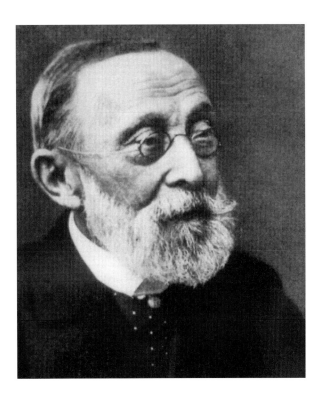

Rudolf Ludwig Karl Virchow
1821–1902

Virchow was born in Pomerania and died in Berlin. At the age of 22, he received his medical degree from the University of Berlin and immediately was appointed to the Charité and within 2 years was a prosector in anatomy and assistant in the clinic. At the age of 25, he began his life work in pathology and quickly rose to the position of Professor of Pathology at Würzburg, and finally Professor of Pathology at the University of Berlin.

Among his contributions was the first true description of the cellular pathology of leukemia. He described the progressive leukocytosis and the anemia which followed. At autopsy, he noted the enormous enlargement of lymph glands and spleen and studied, by microscopy, the anatomy of the leukemic cells. His volume on cellular pathology, first published in 1859, was reprinted as recently as 1971.

In his work in pathology, Virchow served as an experimental pathologist introducing the scientific method into investigations. It was said by William Henry Welch that, "Between the years 1846 and 1856, Virchow constructed the whole doctrine of [thrombo]embolism upon the basis of anatomical, experimental, and clinical investigation which, for its completeness, accuracy, and just discernment of the truth, must always remain a model for scientific research in medicine." Although he made many contributions to the pathology of arteriosclerosis, he is best known for his prescient observations on the triad which leads to thromboembolic disease.

His scientific contributions ensure his place in history but it is less well known that he served in the Reichstag for 13 years. He was the leader of a radical party which openly opposed Bismarck. In his earliest schooling, he displayed two life-long characteristics: academic brilliance and rebellion against established rules. In the clinics, he was appalled by the poverty and starvation of peasants and became committed to overthrow of the bureaurocratic futile government. He was a sympathetic but minor participant in the German revolution of 1848. In 1861, he was elected to the Prussian Diet.

It was Virchow's careful, even meticulous work and observations which allowed the overturning of the doctrine proposed by John Hunter that venous thrombosis followed the inflammation of the wall of a vein. In his monumental, 514-page book *Thrombosis and embolism* published in 1856, Virchow established the foundation upon which all present knowledge of thromboembolic disease is based.

By the turn of the century, his tremendous medical contributions had been recognized and brought to him international acclaim and many honors. He was labeled a Renaissance man and his brilliance extended widely. At age 81, he suffered a fractured femur and his health declined rapidly. He died in 1902.

Deep Venous Thrombosis Prophylaxis   16

Graham F. Pineo and Russell D. Hull

Introduction

Pulmonary embolism is responsible for approximately 150 000 to 200 000 deaths per year in the United States.[1,2] Despite significant advances in the prevention and treatment of venous thromboembolism (venous thrombosis and pulmonary embolism), pulmonary embolism remains the most common preventable cause of hospital death.[3] Venous thromboembolism usually occurs as a complication in patients who are sick and hospitalized, but it may also affect ambulant and otherwise healthy individuals. It is, therefore, vital that efforts continue to find means of managing venous thromboembolism that are safer and more effective. Many patients who die from pulmonary embolism succumb suddenly or within 2 h after the acute event, i.e., before therapy can be initiated or take effect.[4] Effective and safe prophylactic measures against venous thromboembolism are now available for most high-risk patients.[5-8] Prophylaxis is more cost-effective for preventing death and morbidity from venous thromboembolism than is the treatment of established disease. This review highlights practical approaches to the prevention of venous thromboembolism. In the absence of data from randomized clinical trials, recommendations for prophylaxis of deep vein thrombosis following perforator vein surgery can be made based on estimates of risk from comparable surgical procedures.

Pathogenesis of Venous Thromboembolism

Deep vein thrombosis most commonly arises in the deep veins of the calf muscles or, less commonly, in the proximal deep veins of the leg. Deep venous thrombosis confined to the calf veins is associated with a low risk of clinically important pulmonary embolism.[9-12] However, without treatment, approximately 20% of calf vein thrombi extend into the proximal venous system[13,14] where they may pose a serious and potentially life-threatening disorder. Untreated proximal venous thrombosis is associated with a 10% risk of fatal pulmonary embolism and at least a 50% risk of non-fatal pulmonary embolism or recurrent venous thrombosis.[11,12,15] Furthermore, the postphlebitic extremity is afflicted with extensive proximal venous damage and carries its own high risk for recurrent thrombosis (Fig. 16.1).

It is now well established that clinically important pulmonary emboli arise from thrombi in the proximal deep veins of the legs.[16-20] Other less common sources of pulmonary embolism include the deep pelvic veins, renal veins, the inferior vena cava, the right heart, and occasionally axillary veins. the clinical significance of pulmonary embolism depends on the size of the embolus and the cardiorespiratory reserve of the patient.

It is widely accepted that venous thromboembolism is a single disorder[21-23] and, therefore, the

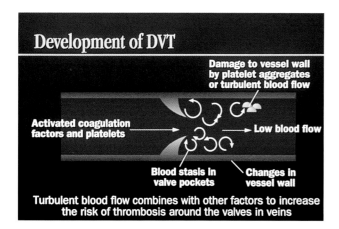

Fig. 16.1. This figure describes the elements which lead to deep venous thrombosis. In patients undergoing the SEPS procedure, a coagulopathy may be present and there may be a higher incidence of activated coagulation factors and platelets to interact and damage the venous wall.

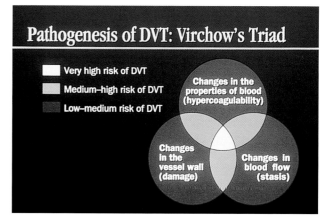

Fig. 16.2. In this figure, the three elements of genesis of venous thrombosis are shown to be interactive. Some patients requiring the SEPS procedure may carry a diagnosed or undiagnosed coagulopathy. The procedure may be associated with inadvertent damage to the femoral vein at the time of saphenectomy, and the patient may be subjected to unusual couch rest or even bed rest.

treatment of venous thrombosis or pulmonary embolism is similar. The diagnostic approach may start with the legs or the lungs, beginning with the least invasive test and proceeding to the more invasive tests.

Prevention of Venous Thromboembolism

Without prophylaxis, the frequency of fatal pulmonary embolism ranges from 0.1% to 0.8% in patients undergoing elective general surgery,[24–26] 2% to 3% in patients undergoing elective hip replacement,[27] and 4% to 7% in patients undergoing surgery for a fractured hip.[28] Factors increasing the risk of postoperative venous thrombosis include advanced age, malignancy, previous venous thromboembolism, obesity, heart failure, or paralysis (Fig. 16.2). It is surprising that physicians and surgeons still do not comply with the recommendations for prophylaxis of venous thromboembolism despite the fact that there is convincing evidence for the efficacy and safety of a number of agents.[5–8,28,29] In a recent retrospective audit of hospitals in Massachusetts, it was shown that prophylaxis of venous thromboembolism even in high-risk patients was grossly under-

utilized, particularly in non-teaching hospitals.[30] In orthopedic surgery, as shown in surveys conducted in England and Sweden, some form of prophylaxis, usually in the form of drugs, is used in the majority of cases.[31,32]

There are two approaches to the prevention of fatal pulmonary embolism: (a) secondary prevention involves the early detection and treatment of subclinical venous thrombosis by screening postoperative patients with objective tests that are sensitive for venous thrombosis; and (b) primary prophylaxis is carried out using either drugs or physical methods that are effective for preventing deep vein thrombosis. The latter approach, primary prophylaxis, is preferred in most clinical circumstances. Furthermore, prevention of deep venous thrombosis and pulmonary embolism is more cost-effective than treatment of the complications when they occur.[33–37] Secondary prevention by case-finding studies should never replace primary prophylaxis. It should be reserved for patients in whom primary prophylaxis is either contra-indicated or relatively ineffective.

The ideal primary prophylactic method is described in Table 16.1. The prophylactic measures most commonly used are low-dose or adjusted-dose unfractionated heparin, low-molecular-weight heparin, oral anticoagulants (International Normalized Ratio, explained below under Laboratory Monitoring and Therapeutic Range, of 2.0–3.0), and intermittent

Table 16.1. Features of an ideal prophylactic method for venous thromboembolism

Effective compared with placebo or active approaches
Safe
Good compliance with patient, nurses and physicians
Ease of administration
No need for laboratory monitoring
Cost-effective

pneumatic leg compression. More recently, dose-finding studies on the prevention of venous thrombosis following orthopedic surgery have been performed with specific antithrombin agents, i.e., hirudin[38] and hirulog.[39] Other less common measures include the use of aspirin and intravenous dextran.

Ideally, prophylaxis should be started before surgery and continued until the patient is fully ambulant. In North America, prophylaxis for high-risk procedures such as total joint replacement has been started postoperatively because of concern for perioperative bleeding. Clinical trials are currently underway to compare the efficacy and safety of pre-operative prophylaxis with postoperative commencement of prophylaxis. No data are available to allow specific recommendations for continued prophylaxis in patients discharged from hospital; this topic is also being studied in clinical trials.

Patterns of clinical practice with respect to the prevention of venous thromboembolism and the appropriate use of anticoagulants for the treatment of thrombotic disease have been influenced very strongly by recent consensus conferences. The American College of Chest Physicians has held 4 consensus conferences on antithrombotic therapy. Recommendations from the fourth American College of Chest Physicians Consensus Conference on Antithrombotic Therapy have recently been published.[40] Rules of evidence for assessing the literature were applied to all recommendations regarding prevention and treatment of thrombotic disease, thereby indicating which recommendations were based on solid clinical evidence, which were based on extrapolation of evidence from related clinical disorders, and which were based only on non-randomized clinical trials or case series.[41] Data from the European Consensus Conference on the Prevention of Venous Thromboembolism were published in International Angiology in 1992.[8] In that report a number of unanswered questions relating to the prevention of venous thrombosis were identified:

Continuing risk of venous thromboembolism following discharge for total hip replacement, including economic analysis of benefit

Compare pre vs. postoperative commencement of prophylaxis

Cost-effectiveness of low-molecular-weight heparin vs. standard therapy in the prevention and treatment of deep vein thrombosis

Safety and efficacy of low-molecular-weight heparin vs. adjusted dose heparin in the treatment of deep vein thrombosis in pregnancy

Comparison of low dose heparin on low-molecular-weight heparin on total mortality and fatal pulmonary embolism in moderate risk surgery

Comparison of low-molecular-weight heparin and foot impulse technology in high and moderate risk patients

Risk of deep vein thrombosis in minimally invasive abdominal or orthopedic surgery

Prospective registry of spinal/epidural anaesthesia-induced hemorrhage, with preoperative prophylaxis

Potential hemorrhagic interaction between anti-coagulants and nonsteroidal anti-inflammatory drugs

Role of long-term low-molecular-weight heparin in the treatment of deep vein thrombosis

Effectiveness and safety of low-molecular-weight heparin in the treatment of pulmonary embolism

Improved efficacy of ultrasonography over IPG in the diagnosis of asymptomatic deep vein thrombosis

Do intermittent pneumatic compression or graduated compression stockings enhance pharmacologic agents?

These unanswered questions were readdressed at the recent International Consensus Conference on Prevention of Venous Thrombosis, and many remain unanswered. Endoscopic perforator vein surgery fits into the category of minimal to moderate risk surgery, for which no prospective studies have as yet been reported. However, some patients with proven previous DVT may be in the high risk category (Fig. 16.3).

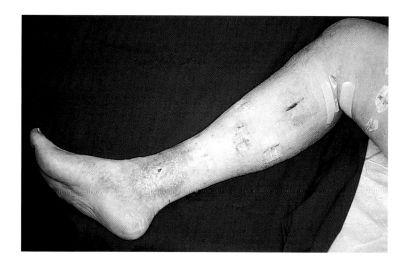

Fig. 16.3. Some patients requiring the SEPS procedure may have a history of previous deep venous thrombosis, corroborated by either phlebography or duplex imaging.

Diagnosis of Postoperative Venous Thromboembolism

The clinical diagnosis of deep vein thrombosis and pulmonary embolism (venous thromboembolism) is imprecise, as many clinical conditions can produce the same signs and symptoms. Furthermore, postoperative venous thrombosis is frequently asymptomatic. Therefore, objective studies, preferably imaging examinations, are required to establish the diagnosis of venous thromboembolism or a screening test to detect venous thrombosis that occurs in spite of prophylaxis. In clinical trials, objectively demonstrated postoperative venous thrombosis is the usual outcome event of interest.

The objective studies which have been assessed for the detection of postoperative venous thrombosis include the I[125] fibrinogen uptake test, ascending venography, and ultrasonography. The fibrinogen uptake test has been useful in the detection of venous thrombosis following thoracoabdominal surgery,[42] but it has been less useful in operative procedures involving the lower leg, such as total hip or total knee replacement.[43,44] It is unlikely that it would be useful following endoscopic perforator vein surgery. Furthermore, the test is dependent on the use of human blood products for the extraction of fibrinogen, and for that reason it is not available in most countries.

B-mode ultrasound with compression, color flow Doppler ultrasound and duplex ultrasonography have all been assessed for the detection of asymptomatic venous thrombosis following high risk

surgery.[45–47] These tests have a high sensitivity and specificity for the diagnosis of symptomatic venous thrombosis, and single reports have reported a high sensitivity for the diagnosis of venous thrombosis in asymptomatic patients. However, a recent meta-analysis which critically assessed all of the available reports indicated that the sensitivity of all of these ultrasound studies is inadequate for the accurate diagnosis of postoperative venous thrombosis.[48] Meta-analyses may be flawed and duplex scans are in common use.

Ascending bilateral phlebography has been the gold standard in the past for the diagnosis of postoperative venous thrombosis, but it remains so today only in highly complex patients.[49,50] Ascending phlebography would be the diagnostic test of choice, for the detection of venous thrombosis following endoscopic venous surgical procedures if duplex scans were unsatisfactory.[49,50]

Specific Prophylactic Measures

Low-dose Heparin

The effectiveness of low-dose heparin for preventing deep vein thrombosis has been established by multiple randomized clinical trials. Low-dose subcutaneous heparin is usually given in a dose of 5000 units 2 h preoperatively, and then postoperatively every 8 or 12 h. Most of the patients in these trials underwent abdominal or thoracic operations particularly for gastrointestinal disease, but patients having gynecological and urological operations as well as mastectomies or vascular procedures were also included. Pooled data from meta-analyses confirm that low-dose heparin reduces the incidence of all deep-vein thromboses, proximal deep-vein thromboses, and all pulmonary emboli including fatal pulmonary emboli.[5–8] The International Multicenter Trial also established the effectiveness of low-dose heparin for preventing fatal pulmonary embolism, a clinically striking reduction from 0.7% to 0.1%.[26]

The incidence of major bleeding complications is not increased by low-dose heparin, but there is an increase in minor would hematomas. The platelet count should be monitored regularly in all patients on low-dose heparin to detect the rare but significant development of heparin-induced thrombocytopenia. Low-dose heparin has the advantage that it is relatively inexpensive, is easily administered, and does not require anticoagulant monitoring.

Adjusted-dose Heparin

The use of adjusted-dose subcutaneous heparin was shown to be an effective approach for prophylaxis compared with low-dose heparin in patients undergoing total hip replacement.[51] Adjusted-dose heparin therapy decreased the incidence of deep-vein thrombosis significantly (13% vs. 39%) without any increase in the frequency of bleeding complications. In a more recent study by the same group, adjusted-dose heparin was compared with low-molecular-weight heparin.[52] The decrease in the incidence of deep-vein thrombosis was not as striking (16% vs. 12%) and there was a surprisingly high incidence of proximal vein thrombosis (13%) in the adjusted heparin group. Adjusted-dose heparin has not become popular because of the time and expense required for laboratory monitoring.

Low-molecular-weight Heparin

A number of low-molecular-weight heparin fractions have been evaluated by randomized clinical trials in moderate-risk general surgical patients.[53–59] In randomized clinical trials comparing low-molecular-weight heparin with unfractionated heparin, the low-molecular-weight heparins given once or twice daily have been shown to be as effective or more effective in preventing thrombosis.[53–59] In most of the trials, similarly low frequencies of bleeding for low-molecular-weight heparin and low-dose unfractionated heparin were documented, although the incidence of bleeding was somewhat higher with unfractionated heparin when various bleeding endpoints were combined.[53]

A number of randomized control trials have been performed with low-molecular-weight heparin comparing it with either placebo, intravenous dextran, unfractionated heparin, or warfarin for the prevention of venous thrombosis following total hip replacement[60–69] (Table 16.2). The drugs under investigation and their dosage schedules vary from one clinical trial to another, making comparisons

Table 16.2. Randomized controlled trials of low molecular weight heparin prophylaxis for deep vein thrombosis following hip replacement surgery: total deep vein thrombosis and bleeding

Reference	Treatment	No. of patients	Total deep vein thrombosis (%)	Total bleeding (%)
Turpie et al.[60]	Enoxaparin	40	10.0	4.0
	Placebo	40	60.6	4.0
Torholm et al.[61]	Dalteparin	58	16.0	NA[a]
	Placebo	54	35.0	NA[a]
Lassen et al.[62]	Tinzaparin	93	31.0	9.5
	Placebo	97	45.0	12.6
Danish Enoxaparin Study Grup.[63]	Enoxaparin	108	6.5	13.9
	Dextran 70	111	21.6	23.4
Levine et al.[64]	Enoxaparin	258	19.4	5.1
	Unfractionated heparin	263	23.2	9.3
Leyvraz et al.[52]	Nadroparin	198	12.6	0.5
	Unfractionated heparin	199	16.0	1.5
Eriksson et al.[65]	Dalteparin	67	30.2	1.5
	Unfractionated heparin	68	42.4	7.4
Planes et al.[66]	Enoxaparin	120	12.5	2.4
	Heparin	108	25.0	1.8
Colwell et al.[67]	Enoxaparin	136	21.0	10.0
	Enoxaparin	136	6.0	12.0
	Heparin	142	15.0	12.0
Hull et al.[68]	Tinzaparin	332	21.0	4.1
	Warfarin	340	23.0	3.8
Hamulyak et al.[69]	Nadroparin	195	13.8	1.2[b]
	Acenocoumaral	196	13.8	2.6

[a] NA = not available
[b] refers to clinically important bleeding

across trials difficult. Furthermore, it has been shown that even within the same clinical trial there can be considerable inter-center variability.[68] Low-molecular-weight heparin was usually started preoperatively in the European trials, in contrast to North American trials where it was started 12–24 h postoperatively. This may account for the lower total deep vein thrombosis rates seen in most of the European trials. Total bleeding rates varied quite widely across trials as well, making comparisons difficult.

Although the number of patients undergoing total knee replacement now equals those undergoing total hip replacements, there have been fewer trials in this patient population.[68–72] The reported clinical trials are shown in Table 16.3. Although the rates of deep vein thrombosis with low-molecular-weight heparin are significantly lower than those with warfarin, the rates continue to be high.

Recent meta-analyses have shown low-molecular-weight heparin to be more effective than unfractionated heparin in the prevention of venous thrombosis, but the risk of bleeding is slightly higher.[73] It should be noted, however, that the findings of meta-analyses evaluating the low-molecular-weight heparins should be interpreted with caution, because all the low-molecular-weight heparins differ. The low-molecular-weight heparins have the advantage that they can be given once a day at a constant dose with-out any laboratory monitoring.[74] A decision analysis compared low-molecular-weight heparin with warfarin but, because of limited data, the cost-effectiveness estimates were uncertain.[75] An economic analysis based on a prospective clinical trial[68] using actual costs in

Canada and the United States demonstrated that low molecular weight heparin was less costly than warfarin in Canada but more costly than warfarin in the United States for the prevention of venous thrombosis following total joint replacement.[75] In out-patient SEPS procedures fractionated heparin prophylaxis is inexpensive compared to other choices.

The low-molecular-weight heparinoid, Danaproid (Organon) has been evaluated in patients undergoing surgery for cancer,[76] hip fractures,[77,78] and total hip replacement.[79] The thrombosis rates were similar with Danaproid and unfractionated heparin in patients undergoing cancer surgery.[76] Compared with placebo, the rates of deep vein thrombosis following total hip replacement were significantly lower (15.5% vs. 56.6%). In patients undergoing surgery for hip fracture, the deep-vein thrombosis rates were significantly lower compared with intravenous dextran[78] (13% vs. 35%) and with low intensity warfarin (7% vs. 21%).[79] More blood transfusions were required in the dextran group. Danaproid has been reported in case series to be an effective alternative for anticoagulation in patients with heparin-induced thrombocytopenia. Unfortunately, it has been found that heparinoid may cross-react in patients with heparin-induced thrombocytopenia, making its use less attractive (Fig. 16.4).

Oral Anticoagulants

For prophylaxis, oral anticoagulants can be commenced preoperatively, at the time of surgery, or in the early postoperative period. Oral anticoagulants commenced at the time of surgery or in the early postoperative period may not prevent small venous thrombi from forming during surgery, or soon after

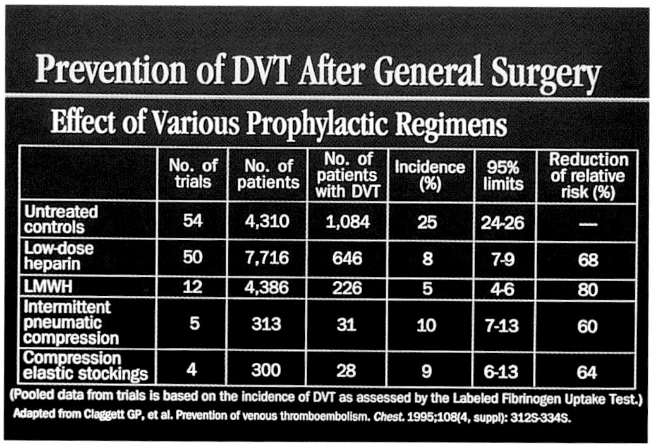

Table 16.3. Randomized control trials of low molecular weight heparin prophylaxis for deep vein thrombosis following total knee replacement: total deep vein thrombosis and bleeding

Reference	Treatment	No. of patients	Total deep vein thrombosis (%)	Total bleeding (%)
Leclerc et al.[70]	Enoxaparin	41	20.0	6.1
	Placebo	54	65.0	6.2
Hull et al.[68]	Tinzaparin	317	45.0	4.4
	Warfarin	324	54.0	2.4
Leclerc et al.[71]	Enoxaparin	206	37.0	33.0
	Warfarin	211	52.0	30.2
Heit et al.[72]	Ardeparin	230	25.0[a]	9.0
	Warfarin	222	36.0[a]	5.0
Hamulyak et al.[69]	Nadroparin	65	24.6	2.6[b]
	Acenocoumaral	61	37.7	1.3

[a] Venogram on operated leg only
[b] refers to clinically important bleeding

Prevention of DVT After General Surgery
Effect of Various Prophylactic Regimens

	No. of trials	No. of patients	No. of patients with DVT	Incidence (%)	95% limits	Reduction of relative risk (%)
Untreated controls	54	4,310	1,084	25	24-26	—
Low-dose heparin	50	7,716	646	8	7-9	68
LMWH	12	4,386	226	5	4-6	80
Intermittent pneumatic compression	5	313	31	10	7-13	60
Compression elastic stockings	4	300	28	9	6-13	64

(Pooled data from trials is based on the incidence of DVT as assessed by the Labeled Fibrinogen Uptake Test.) Adapted from Claggett GP, et al. Prevention of venous thromboembolism. *Chest*. 1995;108(4, suppl): 312S-334S.

Fig. 16.4. As illustrated in this chart, the effectiveness of thromboprophylaxis has been established conclusively.

surgery, because the anticoagulant effect is not achieved until the third or fourth postoperative day. However, oral anticoagulants are effective in inhibiting the extension of these thrombi, thereby preventing clinically important venous thromboembolism.

The postoperative use of warfarin has been compared with low-molecular-weight heparin[68,71] or intermittent pneumatic compression with little or no difference in the incidence of postoperative venous thrombosis or bleeding.[80-82] When warfarin was initiated in small doses 7–10 days preoperatively to prolong the prothrombin time (PT) 1.5–3.0 sec and then less intense warfarin was started the night of surgery, the results were similar to those when warfarin was started postoperatively.[80,83]

Compared with placebo, very low doses of oral anticoagulants (warfarin 1 mg per day) decreased the postoperative thrombosis rate in patients undergoing gynecologic surgery or major general surgery[84] and decreased the thrombosis rate in indwelling central line catheters.[85] There was no increase in bleeding rates. Very low dose warfarin, however, did not provide protection against deep-vein thrombosis following hip or knee replacement.[86]

Intermittent Leg Compression

The use of intermittent pneumatic leg compression prevents venous thrombosis by enhancing blood flow in the deep veins of the legs, thereby preventing venous stasis. It also increases blood fibrinolytic activity, which may contribute to its antithrombotic properties. Intermittent pneumatic leg compression is effective for preventing venous thrombosis in moderate-risk general surgical patients[87] and in patients undergoing neurosurgery.[88-90] In patients undergoing hip surgery, intermittent pneumatic compression of the calf is effective for preventing calf vein thrombosis, but it is relatively ineffective against proximal vein thrombosis.[91]

Intermittent pneumatic compression of the calf decreased distal venous thrombosis following knee replacement, but proximal thrombosis rates remained high.[92] Studies with calf and thigh compression significantly decreased the incidence of both distal and proximal thrombosis rates.[93]

Intermittent pneumatic compression is virtually free of clinically important side effects and offers a valuable alternative in patients who have a high risk of bleeding. It may produce discomfort in the occasional patient, and should not be used in patients with overt evidence of leg ischemia caused by peripheral vascular disease. A variety of well-accepted, comfortable, and effective intermittent pneumatic devices are currently available which may be applied preoperatively, at the time of operation, or in the early postoperative period. These devices should be used for the entire period until the patient is fully ambulatory with only temporary removal for nursing care or physiotherapy.

Graduated Compression Stockings

The use of graduated compression stockings reduces venous stasis in the limb by applying a graded degree of compression to the ankle and the calf, with greater pressure being applied more distally in the limb. Clinical trials have demonstrated graduated compression stockings to be effective for preventing postoperative venous thrombosis in low-risk general surgical patients[94-96] and in selected moderate-risk patients (neurosurgical).[90] A recent meta-analysis confirmed that the use of graduated compression stockings reduced venous thrombosis following moderate-risk surgery.[97] However, there was inadequate information to verify whether the use of graduated compression stockings in combination with other forms of prophylaxis resulted in any further risk reduction.[97] Furthermore, the use of graduated compression stockings along with other prophylactic measures in patients undergoing high-risk surgery has not been adequately studied.

Specific Recommendations

The recommended primary prophylactic approach depends on the patient's risk category and the type of surgery.

In assessing the literature relating to the prevention of venous thromboembolism, the rules of evidence as defined by Cook et al. have been used.[41] They are summarized as follows:

Level I – Randomized trials with low false-positive (a) and low false-negative (b) errors

Level II – Randomized trials with high false-positive (a) and high false-negative (b) errors

Level III – Non-randomized concurrent cohort studies

Level IV – Non-randomized historical cohort studies

Level V – Case series

Unless indicated, all recommendations in the following section are based on Level I evidence.

Low-risk Patients

Apart from early ambulation, specific prophylaxis is usually not recommended. However, prophylaxis for low-risk patients is recommended in certain circumstances. It is the clinical custom in some countries to use graduated compression stockings but this is not based on evidence from clinical trials. Many patients having SEPS arrive at surgery wearing some form of support.

Moderate-Risk Patients

General Abdominal, Thoracic, or Gynecologic Surgery

In moderate-risk patients the use of subcutaneous low-dose heparin (5000 units every 8 or 12 h) or subcutaneous low-molecular-weight heparin is recommended.[5,8,40] Subcutaneous low-molecular-weight heparin is as effective as subcutaneous heparin prophylaxis, and has the advantage of a once-daily injection. An alternative recommendation is the use of intermittent pneumatic compression until the patient is ambulatory. This method is indicated in patients at high risk for bleeding. Pharmacological methods may be combined with graduated compression stockings in selected patients.

Neurosurgery

These patients should receive intermittent pneumatic compression. This approach may be used in conjunction with graduated compression stockings.[8,40] Low-dose heparin is an acceptable alternative.

Endoscopic Perforator Vein Surgery

The incidence of venous thrombosis following endoscopic perforator vein surgery is unknown. However many of the patients have had spontaneous DVT previously. In estimating the incidence of venous thrombosis following surgical procedures in which case-finding studies have not been carried out, an estimation can be made based on the incidence of venous thrombosis following surgical procedures of comparable risk. Such an extrapolation may not be valid for operative procedures on veins, although the risk of DVT following vein stripping is low. The duration of the procedure, length of anaesthetic and tissue trauma represents a mild risk for thrombosis, the fact that the procedure is carried out in a low flow system under tourniquet and entails endothelial cell damage might increase the likelihood of postoperative thrombosis. Therefore, prophylaxis against deep vein thrombosis for these procedures in the high risk patient is warranted. The recommended prophylaxis would be low-dose heparin or low-molecular-weight heparin with our without the use of graduated compression stockings or the non elastic trreatment of existing leg ulcer.

High-risk Patients

Elective Hip Replacement

Several approaches are effective. Subcutaneous low-molecular-weight heparin given once or twice daily is effective and safe. Several such agents are approved for use in Europe and North America. At present in North America, these agents are approved for postoperative use only. Prophylaxis with oral anticoagulants adjusted to maintain an INR of 2.0 to 3.0 is effective and is associated with a low risk of bleeding.[8,40] Other effective approaches include adjusted-dose subcutaneous heparin and intermittent pneumatic compression. However, rates of proximal venous thrombosis are higher with intermittent pneumatic compression than with the other approaches.

Elective Knee Replacement

Although intermittent pneumatic compression was shown in earlier studies to be effective and to be a still-useful alternative, the current prophylaxis of choice is low-molecular-weight heparin given once or twice daily postoperatively.[68–70] Oral anticoagulants are less effective than low-molecular-weight heparin and cannot be recommended.

Hip Fractures

Two approaches to prophylaxis are available: oral

anticoagulation[83] (INR = 2.0 to 3.0) or fixed-dose subcutaneous low-molecular-weight heparin started preoperatively.[40] The combined use of intermittent pneumatic compression with low-molecular-weight heparin or warfarin may provide additional benefit in certain patients (not Level 1).

Multiple Trauma

Multiple trauma represents a high risk for thrombosis.[40] At present there are no recommendations based on Level I evidence. Intermittent pneumatic compression has been recommended, where feasible, because it eliminates any risk for bleeding. Other alternatives include low-molecular-weight heparin, low-dose heparin, and warfarin based on extrapolation from other high-risk situations such as hip fracture and hip replacement surgery. Insertion of an inferior vena cava filter has been recommended for very high-risk situations where anticoagulants may be contraindicated, but this recommendation is based on Level III and Level IV data.

Acute Spinal Cord Injury Associated with Paralysis

Low-molecular-weight heparin is the most effective prophylaxis.[40] Adjusted-dose heparin has also been shown to be effective. Low-dose heparin and intermittent pneumatic compression are less effective. Combining intermittent pneumatic compression with low-molecular-weight heparin or adjusted-dose heparin may provide additional benefit, but this is not supported by data.

Conclusion

For prophylaxis of DVT in SEPS patients much can be learned from experience with other surgical procedures. Effective prophylaxis is available for patients undergoing general surgery, although it is disappointing that such measures are not applied more uniformly. Low-dose subcutaneous unfractionated heparin and low-molecular-weight heparin are used most extensively, with sequential intermittent compression recommended in selected cases. For orthopedic surgery the options include low-molecular-weight heparin, warfarin or IPC. For endoscopic venous surgery, low-dose heparin or low-molecular-weight heparin are recommended, with graduated compression stockings especially in the high risk patient with DVT. Future studies will examine the use of combined modalities and the use of newer antithrombotic agents. The ultimate goal for clinicians is to minimize the incidence of fatal pulmonary embolism in all patients undergoing these special surgical procedures.

References

1. Dismuke SE, Wagner EH (1986). Pulmonary embolism as a cause of death. The changing mortality in hospitalized patients. JAMA 255:2039–2042
2. Dalen JE, Alpert JS (1975) Natural history of pulmonary embolism. Prog Card Dis 17:257–270
3. Anderson FA, Wheeler HB, Goldberg RJ et al. (1991) A population-based perspective of the hospital incidence and case-fatality rates of deep vein thrombosis and pulmonary embolism. Arch Int Med 151:933–938
4. Donaldson GA, Williams C, Scanell J et al. (1963) A re-appraisal of the application of the Trendelenburg operation to massive fatal embolism. N Engl J Med 268:171–174
5. Clagett GP, Reisch JS (1988) Prevention of venous thromboembolism in general surgical patients. Results of meta-analysis. Ann Surg 208:227–240
6. Collins R, Scrimgeour A, Yusef S et al. (1988) Reduction in fatal pulmonary embolism and venous thrombosis by peri-operative administration of subcutaneous heparin. N Engl J Med 318:1162–1173
7. Colditz GA, Tuden RL, Oster G (1986) Rates of venous thrombosis after general surgery: combined results of randomized clinical trials. Lancet 19:143–146
8. Nicolaides AN, Arcelus J, Belcaro G et al. (1992) Prevention of venous thromboembolism. Int Ang 11:151–158
9. Hull RD, Hirsh J, Carter CJ et al. (1985) Diagnostic efficacy of impedance plethysmography for clinically suspected deep-vein thrombosis: a randomized trial. Ann Int Med 102:21–28
10. Huisman MV, Buller HE, ten Cate JW et al. (1986) Serial impedance plethysmography for suspected deep venous thrombosis in outpatients. The Amsterdam General Practitioner Study. N Engl J Med 314:823–828
11. Moser KM, Le Moine JR (1981) Is embolic risk conditioned by location of deep venous thrombosis? Ann Int Med 94:439–444
12. Huisman MV, Buller HR, ten Cate JW et al. (1989) Management of clinically suspected acute venous thrombosis in outpatients with serial impedance plethysmography in a community hospital setting. Arch Int Med 149:511–513
13. Kakkar VV, Flanc C, Howe CT et al. (1969) Natural history of post-operative deep-vein thrombosis. Lancet 2:230–233
14. Lagerstedt CI, Fagher BO, Olsson CG et al. (1985) Need for long-term anticoagulant treatment in symptomatic calf-vein thrombosis. Lancet 2:515–518

15. Hull RD, Delmore T, Genton E et al. (1979) Warfarin sodium versus low-dose heparin in the long-term treatment of venous thrombosis. N Engl J Med 301:855–858

16. Huisman MV, Buller HR, ten Cate JW et al. (1989) Unexpected high prevalence of silent pulmonary embolism in patients with deep venous thrombosis. Chest 95:498–502

17. Sevitt S, Gallagher N (1961) Venous thrombosis and pulmonary embolism. A clinico-pathological study in injured and burned patients. Br J Surg 48:475–489

18. Mavor GE, Galloway JMD (1967) The iliofemoral venous segment as a source of pulmonary emboli. Lancet 1:871–874

19. Hull RD, Hirsh J, Carter CJ et al. (1985) Diagnostic value of ventilation-perfusion lung scanning in patients with suspected pulmonary embolism. Chest 88:819–828

20. A collaborative study by the PIOPED Investigators (1990) Value of the ventilation/perfusion scan in acute pulmonary embolism: results of the Prospective Investigation of Pulmonary Embolism Diagnosis (PIOPED). JAMA 263:2753–2769

21. Bone RC (1990) Ventilation/perfusion scan in pulmonary embolism. "The emperor is incompletely attired." JAMA 263:2794–2795

22. Secker-Walker RH (1983) On purple emperors, pulmonary embolism, and venous thrombosis. Ann Int Med 98:1006–1008

23. Stein PD, Hull RD, Saltzman HA et al. (1993) Strategy for diagnosis of patients with suspected acute pulmonary embolism. Chest 103:1553–1559

24. Skinner DB, Salzman EW (1967) Anticoagulant prophylaxis in surgical patients. Surg Gynecol Obstet 125:741–746

25. Shephard RM, White HA, Shirkey AL (1966) Anticoagulant prophylaxis of thromboembolism in post-surgical patients. Am J Surg 112:698–702

26. International Multicentre Trial (1975) Prevention of fatal postoperative pulmonary embolism by low doses of heparin. Lancet 2:45–64

27. Coventry MB, Nolan DR, Beckenbaugh RD (1973) "Delayed" prophylactic anticoagulation: a study of results and complications in 2,012 total hip arthroplasties. J Bone Joint Surg [Am] 55:1487–1492

28. Eskeland G, Solheim K, Skhorten F (1986) Anticoagulant prophylaxis, thromboembolism and morality in elderly patients with hip fracture: a controlled clinical trial. Acta Chir Scand 131:16–29

29. Kakkar V, Stamatakis JD, Bentley PG et al. (1979) Prophylaxis for post-operative deep-vein thrombosis. JAMA 241:39–42

30. Anderson FA, Wheeler HB, Goldberg RJ et al. (1991) Physician practices in the prevention of venous thromboembolism. Ann Int Med 115:581–595

31. Bergqvist D (1980) Prevention of postoperative deep vein thrombosis in Sweden: results of a survey. World J Surg 4:489–495

32. Laverick MD, Croak SA, Mollan RA (1991) Orthopedic surgeons and thromboprophylaxis. Br Med J 303:549–550

33. Salzman EW, Davies GC (1980) Prophylaxis of venous thromboembolism. Analysis of cost-effectiveness. Ann Surg 191:207–218

34. Hull R, Hirsh J, Sackett DL et al. (1982) Cost-effectiveness of primary and secondary prevention of fatal pulmonary embolism in high-risk surgical patients. Can Med Assoc J 127:990–995

35. Oster G, Tuden RL, Colditz GA (1987) A cost-effectiveness analysis of prophylaxis against deep vein thrombosis in major orthopedic surgery. JAMA 257:203–208

36. Bergqvist D, Matzsch T, Jendteg S et al. (1990) The cost-effectiveness of prevention of post-operative thromboembolism. Acta Chir Scand Suppl 556:36–41

37. Hauch O, Kyattar SC, Jorensen LN (1991) Cost-benefit analysis of prophylaxis against deep vein thrombosis in surgery. Semin Thromb Hemost 17 Suppl 3:280–283

38. Eriksson BI, Kalebo P, Ekman S et al. (1996) Prevention of deep vein thrombosis after total hip replacement: direct thrombin inhibition with recombinant hirudin CGP 39393. Lancet 347:635–639

39. Ginsberg JS, Nurmohamed MT, Gent M et al. (1994) Use of hirulog in the prevention of venous thrombosis after major hip or knee surgery. Circulation 90:2385–2389

40. Clagett GP, Anderson A, Heit J et al. (1995) Prevention of venous thromboembolism. Chest 108:312S–334S

41. Cook DJ, Guyatt GH, Lalupacis A et al. (1995) Rules of evidence and clinical recommendations on the use of antithrombotic agents. Chest 108:227S–230S

42. Kakkar VV, Nicolaides AN, Renney JT et al. (1972) ^{125}I-labelled fibrinogen test adapted for routine screening for deep vein thrombosis. Lancet 1:540–544

43. Harris WH, Salzman EW, Athanasoulis C et al. (1975) Comparison of ^{125}I-fibrinogen count scanning with phlebography for detection of venous thrombi after elective hip surgery. N Engl J Med 292:665–671

44. Kakkar VV (1977) Fibrinogen uptake test for detection of deep vein thrombosis. A review of current practice. Semin Nucl Med 7:229–244

45. Cronan JJ, Dorfman GS, Scola FH et al. (1987) Deep venous thrombosis: US assessment using vein compressibility. Radiology 162:191–194

46. Lensing AWA, Prandoni P, Brandjes DPM et al. (1989) Accurate detection of deep-vein thrombosis by real-time B-mode ultrasonography. N Engl J Med 320:342–345

47. Lensing AWA, Levi MM, Buller HR et al. (1990) Diagnosis of deep-vein thrombosis using an objective Doppler method. Ann Intern Med 113:9–13

48. Wells PS, Lensing AW, Davidson BL, Prins MH, Hirsh J (1995) Accuracy of ultrasound for the diagnosis of deep venous thrombosis in asymptomatic patients after orthopedic surgery: a meta-analysis. Ann Intern Med 122:47–53

49. Rabinov K, Paulin S (1972) Roentgen diagnosis of venous thrombosis in the leg. Arch Surg 104:134–144

50. Lensing AWA, Buller HR, Prandoni P et al. (1992) Contrast venography, the gold standard for the diagnosis of deep vein thrombosis: improvement in observer agreement. Thromb Hemost 67:8–12

51. Leyvraz PF, Richard J, Bachmann F et al. (1983) Adjusted versus fixed dose subcutaneous heparin in the prevention of deep-vein thrombosis after total hip replacement. N Engl J Med 309:954–958

52. Leyvraz PF, Bachmann F, Hoek J et al. (1991) Prevention of deep vein thrombosis after hip replacement: randomised comparison between unfractionated heparin and low molecular weight heparin. Br Med J 303:543–548

53. Kakkar VV, Cohen AT, Edmonson RA et al. (1993) Low molecular weight versus standard heparin for prevention of venous thromboembolism after major abdominal surgery. Lancet 341:259–265

54. Kakkar VV, Murray WJG (1985) Efficacy and safety of low-molecular-weight heparin (CY216) in preventing postoperative venous thromboembolism: a co-operative study. Br J Surg 72:786–791

55. Bergqvist D, Matzsch T, Brumark U et al. (1988) Low-molecular-weight heparin given the evening before surgery compared with conventional low-dose heparin in preven-

tion of thrombosis. Br J Surg 75:888–891

56. Samama M, Bernard P, Bonnardot JP et al. (1988) Low-molecular-weight heparin compared with unfractionated heparin in prevention of postoperative thrombosis. Br J Surg 75:128–131

57. The European Fraxiparin Study Group (1988) Comparison of a low-molecular-weight heparin and unfractionated heparin for the prevention of deep vein thrombosis in patients undergoing abdominal surgery. Br J Surg 75:1058–1063

58. Caen JP (1988) A randomized double-blind study between a low-molecular-weight heparin Kabi 2165 and standard heparin in the prevention of deep-vein thrombosis in general surgery. A French multicentre trial. Thromb Haemost 59:216–220

59. Leizorovicz A, Picolet H, Peyrieux JC et al. (1991) Prevention of perioperative deep vein thrombosis in general surgery: a multicentre double-blind study comparing two doses of logiparin and standard heparin. Br J Surg 78:412–416

60. Turpie AGG, Levine MN, Hirsh J et al. (1986) A randomized controlled trial of low-molecular-weight heparin (enoxaparin) to prevent deep-vein thrombosis in patients undergoing elective hip surgery. N Engl J Med. 315:925–929

61. Tørholm C, Broeng L, Jørgensen PS et al. (1991) Thromboprophylaxis by low-molecular-weight heparin in elective hip surgery: a placebo controlled study. J Bone Joint Surg [Br] 73B:434–438

62. Lassen MR, Borris LC, Christiansen HM et al. (1991) Prevention of thromboembolism in 190 hip arthroplasties. Acta Orthop Scand 62:33–38

63. The Danish Enoxaparin Study Group (1991) Low-molecular weight heparin (Enoxaparin) vs Dextran 70. Arch Int Med 151:1621–1624

64. Levine MN, Hirsh J, Gent M et al. (1991) Prevention of deep vein thrombosis after elective hip surgery: a randomized trial comparing low molecular weight heparin with standard unfractionated heparin. Ann Int Med 114:545–551

65. Eriksson BI, Kälebo P, Anthmyr BA et al. (1991) Prevention of deep vein thrombosis and pulmonary embolism after total hip replacement. J Bone Joint Surg [Am] 73A:484–493

66. Planes A, Vochelle N, Fagola M et al. (1991) Prevention of deep vein thrombosis after total hip replacement: the effect of low-molecular-weight heparin with spinal and general anesthesia. J Bone Joint Surg [Br] 73B:418–423

67. Colwell CW, Spiro TE, Trowbridge AA et al. (1994) Use of Enoxaparin, a Low-Molecular-Weight Heparin, and Unfractionated Heparin for the Prevention of Deep Venous Thrombosis after Elective Hip Replacement. J Bone Joint Surg 76A:3–14

68. Hull RD, Raskob GE, Pineo GF et al. (1993) A comparison of subcutaneous low-molecular-weight heparin with warfarin sodium for prophylaxis against deep-vein thrombosis after hip or knee implantation. N Engl J Med 329:1370–1376

69. Hamulyak K, Lensing AWA, van der Meer J, Smid WM, van Ooy A, Hoek JA, for the Fraxiparine Oral Anticoagulant Study Group (1995) Subcutaneous low-molecular-weight heparin or oral anticoagulants for the prevention of deep-vein thrombosis in elective hip and knee replacement? Thromb Haemost 74:1428–1431

70. Leclerc JR, Geerts WH, Desjardins L et al. (1992) Prevention of deep vein thrombosis after major knee surgery – a randomized, double-blind trial comparing a low-molecular-weight heparin fragment (Enoxaparin) to placebo. Thromb Haemost 67:417–423

71. Leclerc JR, Geerts WH, Desjardins L et al. (1996) Prevention of venous thromboembolism after knee arthroplasty – a randomized, double-blind trial comparing a low molecular weight heparin fragment (Enoxaparin) to Warfarin. Ann Intern Med 124:619–626

72. Heit J, Berkowitz S, Bona R et al. (1995) Efficacy and safety of Normiflow (a LMWH) compared to warfarin for prevention of venous thromboembolism following total knee replacement: a double-blind, dose-ranging study. Thromb Haemost 73:A739. [abstract]

73. Nurmohamed MT, Rosendaal FR, Büller HR et al. (1992) Low molecular weight heparin in the prophylaxis of venous thrombosis: a meta-analysis. Lancet 340:152–156

74. O'Brien BJ, Anderson DR, Goeree, R (1994) Cost-effectiveness of enoxparin versus warfarin prophylaxis against deep-vein thrombosis after total hip replacement. Can Med Assoc J 150:1083–1089

75. Hull RD, Raskob GE, Pineo GF, et al. (1997) subcutaneous low-molecular weight heparin vs. warfarin for prophylaxis of deep vein thrombosis after hip or knee implantation. arch. Interm. Med; 157:298–303

76. Gallus A, Cade J, Ockelford P et al. (1993) Orgaran (Org 10172) or heparin for preventing venous thromboembolism after elective surgery for malignant disease? A double-blind, randomized mutlicentre comparison. Thromb Haemost 70:562–567

77. Bergqvist D, Kettunen K, Fredin H et al. (1991) Thromboprophylaxis in hip fracture patients – a prospective randomized comparative study between ORG 10172 and dextran. Surgery 109:617–622

78. Gerhart TN, Yett HS, Robertson LK et al. (1991) Low-molecular-weight heparinoid compared with warfarin for prophylaxis of deep vein thrombosis in patients who are operated on for fracture of the hip. A prospective, randomized trial. J Bone Joint Surg 73A:494–502

79. Hoek J, Nurmohamed MT, ten Cate H et al. (1989) Prevention of deep vein thrombosis following total hip replacement by a low-molecular-weight heparinoid. Thromb Haemost Suppl 62:1637

80. Francis CW, Pellegrini VD, Marder VJ et al. (1992) Comparison of warfarin and external pneumatic compression in prevention of venous thrombosis after total hip replacement. JAMA 267:2911–2915

81. Paiement F, Wessinger SJ, Waltman WC et al. (1987) Low-dose warfarin versus external pneumatic compression for prophylaxis against venous thromboembolism following total hip replacement. J Arth 2:23–26

82. Kaempffe FA, Lifeso RM, Meinking C (1991) Intermittent pneumatic compression versus Coumadin: prevention of deep vein thrombosis in lower-extremity total joint arthroplasty. Clin Orthop 269:89–97

83. Powers PJ, Gent M, Jay R et al. (1989) A randomized trial of less intense postoperative warfarin or aspirin therapy in the prevention of venous thromboembolism after surgery for fractured hip. Arch Int Med 149:771–774

84. Poller L, McKernan A, Thomson JM et al. (1987) Fixed minidose warfarin: a new approach to prophylaxis against venous thrombosis after major surgery. Br Med J 285:1309–1312

85. Bern MM, Lokich JJ, Wallach SR et al. (1990) Very low doses of warfarin can prevent thrombosis in central venous catheters. Ann Int Med 112:423–428

86. Dale C, Gallus A, Wycherley A et al. (1991) Prevention of venous thrombosis with minidose warfarin after joint replacement. Br Med J 303:224

87. Roberts VC, Sabri S, Beely AH et al. (1972) The effect of

intermittently applied external pressure on the hemodynamics of the lower limb in man. Br J Surg 59:233–236

88. Turpie AGG, Gallus A, Beattie WS et al. (1977) Prevention of venous thrombosis in patients with intracranial disease by intermittent pneumatic compression of the calf. Neurology 27:435–438

89. Turpie AG, Delmore T, Hirsh J et al. (1979) Prevention of venous thrombosis by intermittent sequential calf compression in patients with intracranial disease. Thromb Res 16:611–616

90. Skillman JJ, Collins RR, Coe NP et al. (1978) Prevention of deep vein thrombosis in neurosurgical patients: a controlled, randomized trial of external pneumatic compression boots. Surgery 83:354–358

91. Hull RD, Raskob G, Gent M et al. (1990) Effectiveness of intermittent pneumatic leg compression for preventing deep vein thrombosis after total hip replacement. JAMA 263:2313–2317

92. Hull RD, Delmore TJ, Hirsh J et al. (1979) Effectiveness of intermittent pulsatile elastic stockings for the prevention of calf and thigh vein thrombosis in patients undergoing elective knee surgery. Thromb Res 16:37–45

93. Mckenna R, Galante J, Bachmann F et al. (1980) Prevention of venous thromboembolism after total knee replacement by high-dose aspirin or intermittent calf and thigh compression. Br Med J 1:514–517

94. Turner GM, Cole SE, Brooks JH (1984) The efficacy of graduated compression stockings in the prevention of deep vein thrombosis after major gynaecological surgery. Br J Obstet Gynaecol 91:588–591

95. Ishak MA, Moreley KD (1981) Deep venous thrombosis after total hip arthroplasty: a prospective controlled study to determine the prophylactic effect of graded pressure stockings. Br J Surg 68:429–432

96. Allan A, Williams JT, Bolton JP et al. (1983) The use of graduated compression stockings in the prevention of postoperative deep vein thrombosis. Br J Surg 70:172–174

97. Wells PS, Lensing AWA, Hirsh J (1994) Graduated compression stockings in the prevention of postoperative venous thromboembolism. Arch Int Med 154:67–72

SECTION 4
Supportive Therapy

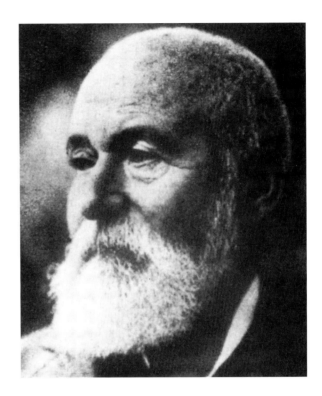

Paul Gerson Unna
1850–1929

The father of dermatohistopathology, Paul Gerson Unna, was born in Hamburg, Germany, in a family full of artists and physicians. He received his medical degree in Strassburg where he studied under von Recklinghausen, Kussmaul and Waldeyer. Dermatology captured his interest early, and he wrote his doctoral thesis on the development and anatomy of the skin.

In the late 1800s, when dermatology was mostly a descriptive science, Unna soon distinguished himself as the best-known dermatologist in the world, despite his lack of affiliation with an academic institution. His private clinic, which opened in 1888, became a world-famous center for dermatology. He was a Renaissance man reincarnated into the nineteenth century. He excelled in the development of dermatologic microscopy, staining technics, bacteriology, mycology and the study of leprosy. However, first and foremost he was an excellent practical therapist who introduced a vast armamentarium of salves, plasters and ointments for the treatment of skin diseases. The "Unna boot," the glycerine-gelatine mixture used for compression dressings to treat varicose ulcers and pruritic dermatitis is one of many of his practical discoveries.

Unna's academic productivity was exceptional. He authored over 500 publications and a monumental book of 1225 pages, *Histopathology of skin diseases*. In 1927 he became Honorary Professor of the University of Bonn. His peers characterized him as an honest man in medical research not for the purpose of monetary gain. His love of music persisted throughout his life and he was an accomplished cellist.

Compression Therapy for Treatment of Lower Extremity Chronic Venous Insufficiency and Venous Stasis Ulcers

Alexander D. Nicoloff, Mark R. Nehler, Gregory L. Moneta and John M. Porter

Introduction

Although surgical solutions for the treatment of lower extremity chronic venous insufficiency (CVI) and venous ulceration continue to be explored and implemented, non-operative management remains the primary approach to treatment world-wide. It has long been known that strict bed rest and leg elevation are effective modes of treatment. However, the impracticality of this has led to ambulatory therapy with the goals of controlling symptoms, promoting the healing of ulcers, and preventing ulcer recurrence.

Theories Behind Compression Therapy

Compression therapy remains the current "gold standard" treatment for CVI with or without ulceration. Although the mechanism of benefit of compression therapy remains unknown, three theories have received the most attention. Multiple studies have examined the effects of compression therapy on deep venous dynamics. Some reports describe improvement in ambulatory venous pressures and venous recovery times.[1] Christopoulos et al. (1987) studied 22 patients with superficial venous insuf-

ficiency and 9 patients with deep venous disease. Dorsal foot veins were cannulated and both ambulatory venous pressure (AVP) and venous recovery times (VRT) were measured. Ten tiptoe movements were performed by each patient with and without elastic compression stockings. The patients with superficial venous insuffiency were tested with thigh-high stockings and showed a 48% decrease in AVP and a 114% increase in VRT ($P<0.01$ compared to similar testing without stockings). In patients with deep venous disease, knee-high stockings resulted in an 18% decrease in AVP ($P<0.01$) and a 58% increase in VRT (not significant). Other researchers, however, have not found any significant changes in AVP or VRT with elastic stockings.[2] We measured AVP and VRT in 9 healthy patients and 16 patients with deep venous disease. Ten tiptoe exercises were performed. Four varieties of elastic compression stockings including 30–40 torr and 40–50 torr above- and below-knee stockings were evaluated in each patient. In patients with deep venous disease, no differences were found in AVP or VRT measured with or without the stockings.

Compression therapy may lead to improvements in skin and subcutaneous tissue microcirculatory hemodynamics. Using laser Doppler flowmetry, an impairment in venoarteriolar reflex resulting in a dependency-induced resting cutaneous hyperemia can be demonstrated in patients with CVI. A similar hyperemic response is not seen in controls without venous disease. Christopoulos et al. (1991) demonstrated improvement of the venoarteriolar reflex with 40 mmHg compression (measured at the ankle) stockings, but not with 20 mmHg compression stockings.[3]

Compression therapy may also result in a direct effect on subcutaneous pressures. Increased subcutaneous pressures resulting from external compression may act to counteract transcapillary hydrostatic forces that otherwise result in capillary leakage, edema formation and subsequent poor cutaneous diffusion of oxygen and other nutrients. In the laboratory, supine perimalleolar subcutaneous pressures are increased with elastic compression in lower extremities with CVI.[4] Increased skin capillary density with edema resolution can also be demonstrated with videomicroscopy. In addition, skin tcPO$_2$ may also increase following edema resolution.[5]

Elastic Compression Stockings

Since their development by Conrad Jobst in the 1950s, elastic compression stockings have become

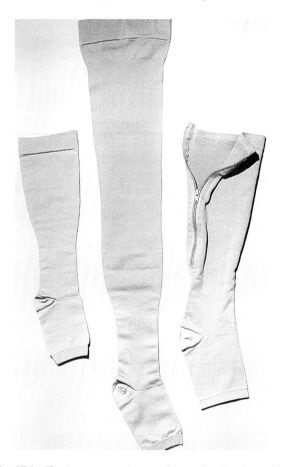

Fig. 17.1. Elastic compression stockings showing knee-high, thigh-high, and zippered knee-high versions.

the most widely accepted treatment for CVI and venous ulceration. It is said Jobst noted partial resolution of his own symptoms of CVI while standing in a swimming pool. His design of the first ambulatory, gradient, compression stocking is thought to have been an attempt to reproduce the hydrostatic pressure gradient of a column of water.

Currently, elastic compression stockings are manufactured by various companies in an assortment of lengths, compositions, and strengths (Fig. 17.1). Multiple clinical reports have documented the benefit of elastic compression stockings for treatment of CVI. Elastic compression decreases limb edema and provides symptomatic relief of the pain or discomfort in patients with CVI. Often the sense of limb heaviness and fatigue frequently experienced with CVI is relieved as well.

Compression therapy is also the standard initial treatment of venous ulceration associated with CVI. At our institution, the treatment of venous ulceration in virtually all cases is local wound care combined with ambulatory compression therapy using primarily elastic compression stockings (Table 17.1).[6,7] At the time of the initial assessment, patients with severe edema may be placed at bed rest for 5–7 days and those with obvious cellulitis treated with a broad spectrum antibiotic such as ciprofloxacin. Severe stasis dermatitis is treated with hydrocortisone cream (1%) applied twice daily to involved areas surrounding the ulcer. No topical agents are used directly on the ulcer. Local wound care consists only of mild soap and water scrubbing followed by dry cotton gauze dressing changes twice daily (Fig. 17.2). After the resolution of severe edema and cellulitis, patients are fitted with 30–40 mmHg elastic compression stockings. They are instructed to wear them daily while ambulatory and to remove them at

Table 17.1. The Oregon protocol for treatment of venous stasis ulceration[7]

1. Initial period of bed rest with limb elevation either at home or in the hospital
2. Systemic antibiotics (IV or oral) to treat any associated cellulitis
3. Elastic compression stockings are then fitted following adequate edema reduction
4. Daily ulcer cleansing and dry gauze dressing changes
5. Corticoid ointment to areas of stasis dermatitis surrounding the ulcer, as needed
6. Continued use of elastic compression stockings for life following ulcer healing

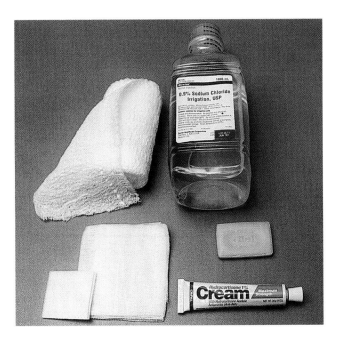

Fig. 17.2. Basic local wound care supplies used in the Oregon protocol including a mild antiseptic soap, cotton gauze dressings, normal saline solution, and hydrocortisone cream (1%) for areas of stasis dermatitis.

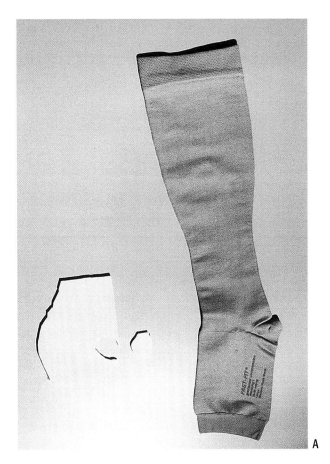

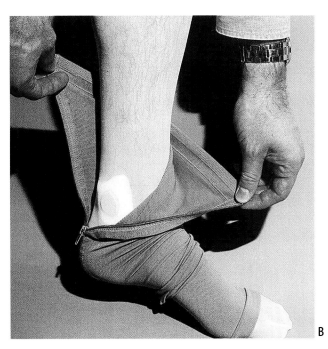

Fig. 17.3.A Sponge wedge cut for placement over a ulcer where ankle topography requires added compression. A knee-high elastic stocking is also shown. **B** A sponge wedge in place over a gauze dressing and beneath a silk stocking liner. A zippered elastic stocking is being applied. A simple nylon stocking can be substituted for the silk liner.

night prior to bed. The stockings cover and hold the dry gauze dressing in place. Sponge wedges are placed over the ulcer and gauze dressing for added compression on limb areas where uniform compression is difficult or increased compression is desirable (Fig. 17.3). Daily ambulatory compression therapy is continued for life. Stockings are replaced every 3–6 months to maintain compression strength.

We analyzed our results with elastic compression therapy for venous stasis ulcers in 113 patients over a 15-year period.[8] Complete ulcer healing was achieved in 99 of 102 (97%) patients who were compliant with stocking use. Only 6 of 11 (55%) patients who were non-compliant with the use of elastic compression stockings healed their ulcer. Mean time to ulcer healing was 5.3 months. Seventy-three patients were available for long term follow-up. At a mean follow-up of 30 months there was a 16% incidence of ulcer recurrence in patients who remained compliant with elastic compression therapy. One hundred percent of ulcers recurred in patients who where non-compliant with the recommendation for long-term elastic compression stocking therapy.

The ability to ensure compliance with elastic stockings is a significant problem for patients and physicians. Patients may complain of discomfort

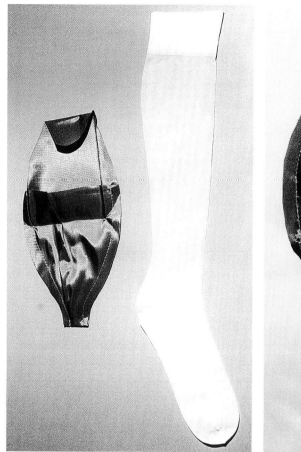
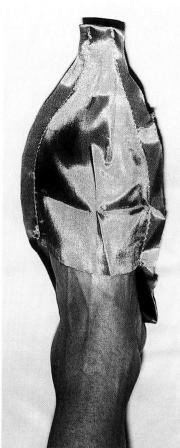
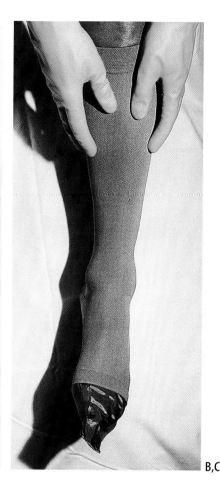

A   B,C

Fig. 17.4.A Nylon toe liner and silk stocking liner for easier application. **B** The toe liner in place. This is easily removed after the stocking is applied by pulling on the exposed portion. **C** Knee-high elastic compression stocking placed over the liners using latex gloves.

and/or difficulty in applying the stockings. We have found patient intolerance of compression can be greatly ameliorated by initially wearing the stockings for short periods, 10–15 minutes, and subsequently gradually increasing this time until they can be worn continuously during ambulation. Another approach is to start with a lower compression strength stocking, such as 20–30 mmHg, allowing the patient to gradually adjust to the compression before moving to a higher strength stocking.

Stocking application can also be aided by various commercially available devices. These include silk stocking and toe liners, zippered compression stockings, and latex gloves (Fig. 17.4). The latter we have found to provide a better grip and easier application of the stockings. Mechanical devices such as metal frames upon which stockings can be loaded to aid application are also available (Fig. 17.5). Infrequently, however, some patients are still unable to

apply or tolerate the elastic compression stockings. In such cases alternative forms of compression are utilized.

Paste Gauze Boots

The paste gauze compression dressing is another common form of compression therapy. Originally developed by the German dermatologist Unna in 1896, this dressing now exists in many variations referred to popularly as an "Unna boot". Most consist of a gauze wrap covered with a zinc-oxide-based paste containing various other ingredients thought to aid in wound care. A typical Unna boot consists of a 2–3 layer dressing usually requiring

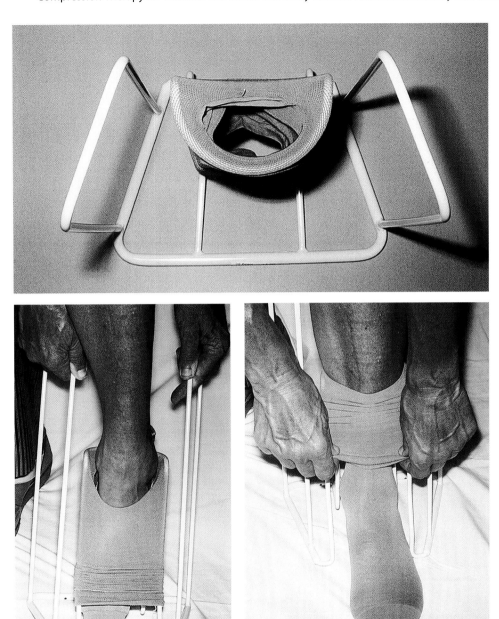

Fig. 17.5. Application of an elastic compression stocking using the Butler® device which holds the stocking open allowing the patient to step into it. The handles can then be used to pull the stocking over the leg.

application by trained personnel. When we utilize Unna boots, we apply a 2-layer dressing consisting first of the Unna-Flex® stretchable gauze dressing with a zinc oxide, acacia, glycerin, castor oil, and white petroleum paste. This is followed by a Co-Flex® elastic dressing. Both layers are applied with graded compression (Fig. 17.6). The Unna-Flex is a non-hardening dressing which, unlike earlier ver-

sions of the Unna boot, does not become stiff after application. Bandages are changed weekly or as needed for increased amounts of drainage.

Although Unna boots do not require patient education and participation in application, they do require follow-up at least weekly. This, as well as the fact that many patients find them uncomfortable to wear, often adversely affects compliance. Another

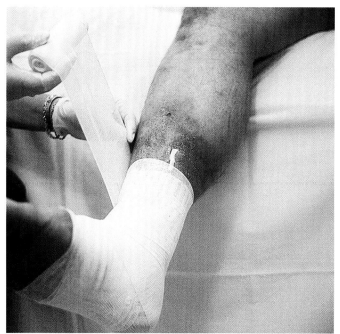 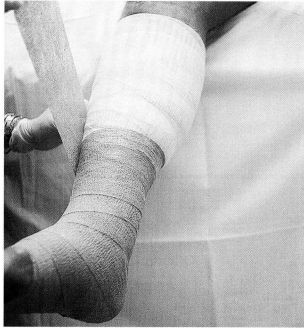

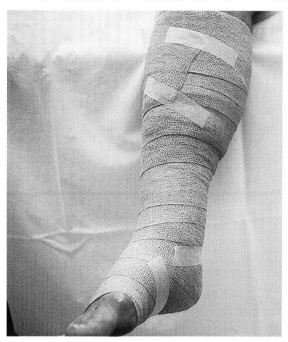

Fig. 17.6. Sequential views of an Unna boot application. The Unna-Flex® rolled gauze dressing with a zinc oxide based paste is first applied with graded compression from the forefoot to below the knee. An elastic cohesive (Co-Flex®) dressing is then applied over this also using graded compression.

been compared to other forms of compression therapy. A randomized prospective trial of 21 patients[10] with venous ulcers compared Unna boots to light-strength compression stockings (24 mmHg at the ankle). Both groups healed their ulcers with average healing times of 7.3 weeks for the Unna boot group compared to 18.4 weeks (11.8 weeks excluding the 78 weeks required for healing for 1 patient with multiple calf ulcers) for the compression stockings group.

Another randomized 12-month study compared Unna boot therapy to polyurethane foam dressings with elastic compression wraps in 26 patients with CVI and venous ulcers. The Unna boot group was found to have a faster healing rate and greater overall wound healing.

The Unna boot has also been compared to hydrocolloid dressings (DuoDERM®) in a 6-month study of 87 venous ulcers in 84 patients. Seventy percent of ulcers healed with Unna boot therapy compared to only 38% of ulcers treated with hydrocolloid dressings alone.[11] A separate study comparing Unna boots to hydrocolloid dressings and elastic compression bandages revealed no significant difference in healing rates after 12 weeks.[12]

potential disadvantage is that the ulcer cannot be monitored except between applications of the boot. The technique is also expensive and compression strength is operator-dependent and, therefore, can be inconsistent. Occasionally, contact dermatitis may necessitate discontinuation of Unna boot therapy.

In a recent 15-year review of 998 patients, Unna boot bandage treatment healed 73% of venous ulcers in a mean time of 9 weeks.[9] The Unna boot has also

Other Forms of Elastic Compression

Most studies suggest inferior results when alternative forms of bandaging are compared to elastic stockings or Unna boot therapy. However, if effective compression can be achieved and maintained, excellent results in initial ulcer healing are possible.[10,11] One study evaluated a 4-layer dressing composed of orthopedic wool, crepe bandages, and elastic cohesive wraps in treatment of 126 patients previously refractory to simple elastic bandages.[13]

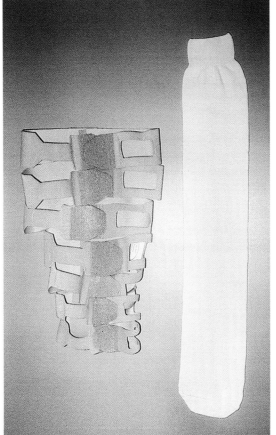
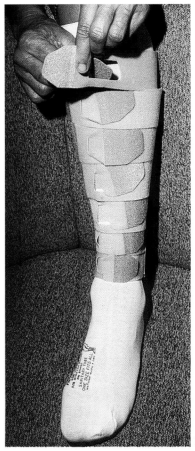
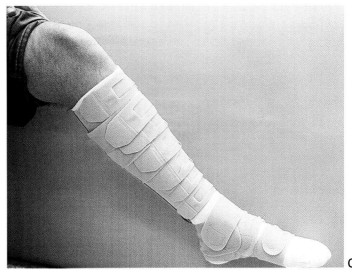

Fig. 17.7. **A** The CircAid® device with inner sock demonstrating the multiple nonelastic Velcro® straps. **B** Application of the rigid device with the top strap being adjusted. Note the interdigitation of the Velcro® straps. **C** The device in place with the foot extension strap.

Measurement of compression at the ankle showed a decline of only 10% after one week. After 12 weeks of treatment 74% of ulcers healed.

The legging compression orthosis (CircAid®) is an excellent alternative to bandaging or elastic stocking treatment of CVI. It can be applied by the patient or care-giver without special training and is easily adjusted to tailor for individual fit, accommodating changes in leg size as edema resolves (Fig. 17.7). It is particularly useful for obese patients with very large or unusually shaped legs and for patients who lack the hand strength to apply elastic stockings. The device consists of multiple, pliable, adjustable, compression bands that are secured with Velcro® around the leg from the ankle to the knee. A sock is provided to place under the orthosis and over dressings. The CircAid® has been evaluated in a trial of 15 venous ulcers in 13 patients who were unable to wear elastic stockings. Fifty-three percent

of ulcers were healed at 12 months.[14] Although these results are modest, our anecdotal experience with the CircAid® in a small group of patients has been favorable in both edema reduction and ulcer healing. We use this device as our first alternative choice in patients who are unable or unwilling to wear elastic compression stockings.

Adjunctive Compression Devices

Many adjunctive compression devices exist. External pneumatic compression devices providing sequential, graded, intermittent, pneumatic compression have received the most attention (Fig. 17.8). Used widely in hospitalized patients for prophylaxis of deep venous thrombosis, intermittent pneumatic

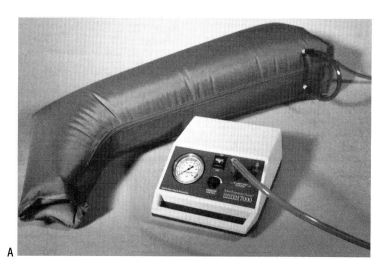

A

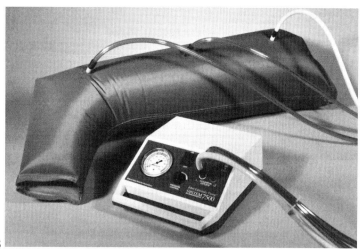

B

Fig. 17.8. Two variants of intermittent pneumatic compression devices. **A** The Jobst Extremity Pump intermittent pneumatic sleeve which is single chambered; and **B** the sequential pneumatic sleeve which is multi-chambered allowing gradient compression (Courtesy of Jobst, a Beiersdorf Company).

compression (IPC) devices have been evaluated for treatment of venous stasis and venous ulceration in several recent reports. In one trial, 8 patients with CVI (documented by phlebography) and venous ulcers present for 1–60 months were treated with IPC for 45 minutes, 5 days a week for 2 weeks.[15] IPC was then continued twice a week until healing of the ulcer was achieved. The lower extremities were wrapped with elastic compression bandages and the ulcers dressed with saline gauze between IPC treatments. All ulcers healed within a mean time of 5 weeks. In comparing this to a mean healing time of 13 weeks in an earlier set of patients treated with elastic compression stockings alone, the authors concluded that the addition of IPC therapy led to faster ulcer healing. A second, randomized study compared IPC and 30–40 mmHg compression stockings to the stockings alone for 3 months in patients with CVI and venous ulceration.[16] Ulcer healing occurred in 10 of 21 (48%) patients in the IPC group compared to only 1 of 24 patients in the stocking alone group. While the use of IPCs has not gained widespread acceptance, the results of these studies indicate a possible adjunctive role for these devices in the treatment of venous ulcers refractory to ambulatory compression stockings alone. Currently, however, routine use of IPC in the treatment of patients with venous ulcers is not recommended.

Summary

Compression therapy remains the primary mode of treatment for chronic venous insufficiency worldwide. For the treatment of venous ulcers it offers the best combination of simplicity, efficacy, and cost-effectiveness. Ambulatory elastic compression stockings are the best all-around mode of compression therapy and continue to be the "gold standard" of treatment for chronic venous insufficiency and venous ulceration. Paste gauze boots and the legging orthosis are reasonable alternatives if elastic compression is not tolerated, while pneumatic compression devices can be used as adjuncts in treating ulcers refractory to compression bandages alone.

References

1. Christopoulos DG, Nicolaides AN, Szendro G et al. (1987) Air plethysmography and the effect of elastic compression on venous hemodynamics of the leg. J Vasc Surg 5:148–159
2. Mayberry JC, Moneta GL, DeFrang RD, Porter JM (1991) The influence of elastic compression stockings on deep venous hemodynamics. J Vasc Surg 13:91–100
3. Christopoulos DG, Nicolaides AN, Belcaro, Kalodiki E (1991) Venous hypertensive microangiopathy in relation to clinical severity and effect of elastic compression. J Dermat Surg Oncol 17:809–813
4. Nehler MR, Moneta GL, Woodard DM et al. (1993) Perimalleolar subcutaneous pressure effects of elastic compression stockings (Abstract). J Vasc Surg 17:431
5. Kolari PJ, Pekanmaki K (1987) Effects of intermittent compression treatment on skin perfusion and oxygenation in lower legs with venous ulcers. VASA 15:312–317
6. Nehler MR, Moneta GL (1995) Nonoperative therapy for patients with chronic venous insufficiency. In Callow AD, Ernst CB (eds) Textbook of Vascular Surgery Appleton and Lange
7. Nehler MR, Moneta GL (1996) Nonoperative management of chronic venous insufficiency of the lower extremities. In: Gloviczki P, Yao JST (eds) Handbook of Venous Disorders Chapman and Hall London 416–433
8. Mayberry JC, Moneta GL, Taylor LT, Porter JM (1991) Fifteen year results of ambulatory compression therapy for chronic venous ulcers. Surgery 109:575–581
9. Lippman HI, Fishman LM, Farrar RH et al. (1994) Edema control in the management of disabling chronic venous insufficiency. Arch Phys Med Rehabil 75:436–441
10. Hendricks WM, Swallow RT (1985) Management of stasis leg ulcers with Unna's boots versus elastic support stockings. J Am Acad Dermatol 12:90–98
11. Kitka MJ, Schuler JJ, Meyer JP et al. (1988) A prospective, randomized trial of Unna's boot versus Hydroactive dressing in the treatment of venous stasis ulcers. J Vasc Surg 7:478–486
12. Cordts PR, Hanrahan LM, Rodriguez AA et al. (1992) A prospective, randomized trial of Unna's boots versus Duoderm CGF hydroactive dressing plus compression in the management of venous leg ulcers. J Vasc Surg 15:480–486
13. Blair SD, Wright DD, Backhouse LM et al. (1988) Sustained compression and healing of chronic venous ulcers. Br Med J 297:1159–1161
14. Spence RK, Hardesty WH, Brown AS et al. (1992) Experience with the Circaid garment in the treatment of the non-healing venous stasis ulcers. Presented at the 16th Annual World Congress of the International Union of Angiology, Paris
15. Pekanmaki K, Kolari PJ, Kiistala U (1987) Intermittent pneumatic compression treatment for the post-thrombotic leg ulcers. Clin Exp Dermatol 12:350–353
16. Coleridge Smith P, Sarin S, Hasty J, Scurr JH (1990) Sequential gradient pneumatic compression enhances venous ulcer healing: A randomized trial. Surgery 108:871–875

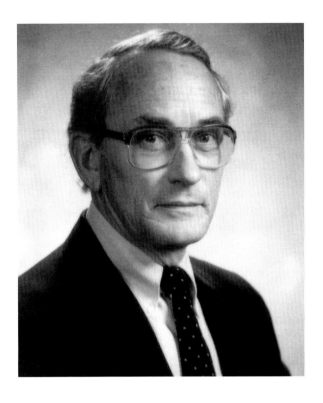

Robert L. Kistner

b. 1927

Although experimental venous valve surgery began in the 1950s coincident with the development of arterial reconstruction, clinical venous reconstruction really began only after the monumental contributions of Robert Kistner of Honolulu. It is difficult to overestimate the contributions of Kistner to venous reconstruction. It was only after his description of reflux correction that surgeons were provided with a battery of operations which could correct the abnormalities of venous pathophysiology. As a direct result of Kistner's contributions, present-day options in direct venous reconstruction are numerous.

Kistner was born into a medical family in St. Louis. The family's education had always been tied to St Louis University where Kistner attended high school, medical school, and a full surgical internship and residency. In the latter part of his medical training, he came under the influence of C. Rollins Hanlon, a thoroughly respected pioneer of cardiac surgery who was later to become Director of the American College of Surgeons.

After a sojourn in the Air Force and a two-year practice in Santa Barbara, California, Kistner traveled to the Cleveland Clinic to become a vascular fellow under Dr Al Humphries. The art of specialty medicine was finally honed at the Cleveland Clinic so it was natural for Kistner to accept an invitation from the Straub Clinic in Honolulu to travel there and bring the new field of peripheral vascular surgery at a very high level to the islands. Interest in developing a very personal type of vascular surgery with ability to do clinical research was stimulated both by Hanlon and Humphries who were "indescribably different types of individuals who shared the common attributes of high intelligence and extreme devotion to medicine and surgery."

On reaching the islands, Kistner was told that it was unlikely that he would ever find enough arterial patients to build a practice. Therefore, he chose early on to see as many venous patients as possible. It is remarkable to contemplate the situation which existed as Kistner developed the first venous valve repair. Working in isolation, he was unaware of the development of descending phlebography in Scandinavia but literally reinvented and used the method in his clinic. It was in the late 1960s that Kistner did the descending phlebography which uncovered massive reflux in a patient whose post-thrombotic changes were limited to the popliteal and distal veins. The proximal superficial femoral valve was well outlined but totally incompetent and so Kistner proceeded with exploration and repair of that valve. The report of this case in the Straub Clinic Proceedings was obscure but led to a series of repairs which were subsequently reported and followed for the next 15 years.

At present, Kistner thinks that ignorance about venous disease is monumental but will begin to change with the new generation of surgeons in training. As he said in his Presidential address to the American Venous Forum, "chronic venous disease is complex and important, and as such, requires definitive diagnoses based on objective criteria." He believes that in the future there will be major changes in management of acute and chronic venous problems and most of this change will be based upon accurate diagnosis.

The Medical Management of Venous Ulcers   18

Thom W. Rooke and Cindy Felty

The medical management of venous ulcers consists of four steps, some of which have been discussed previously. These are (1) confirm the venous nature of the ulcer; (2) eliminate or minimize the underlying cause; (3) create the proper local environment for healing, and (4) use aggressive ancillary measures when necessary.

Step One: Confirm the Venous Nature of the Ulcer

Efforts to treat venous ulcers may be unsuccessful because of misdiagnosis and/or failure to recognize significant comorbid conditions.[1,2] The diagnosis of a venous ulcer can generally be made by history and examination alone, but occasionally confusion as to the etiology of the ulcer may arise. Certain non-venous lesions may mimic venous ulcers (Fig. 18.1A–D), and some patients with venous insufficiency may have ulcers with a non-venous component (i.e., multifactorial ulcers). Non-invasive vascular testing can be helpful when the presence or severity of venous diseases is uncertain[3] (See Chapter 6). Invasive tests, including biopsy, may occasionally be necessary to diagnose an atypical ulcer.

Step Two: Eliminate or Minimize the Venous Insufficiency

Surgical measures to eliminate venous *incompetence* include saphenous vein stripping, avulsion of incompetent varicosities, valve repair, valve auto-transplantation, and perforator ligation; these topics have been dealt with elsewhere. Treatment for venous *obstruction*, including bypass procedures and, in some cases, lytic therapy or venous angioplasty (with or without stenting) may be possible.

For the majority of cases in which a definitive surgical treatment for venous insufficiency is not available, the practitioner must rely upon adequate elastic or non-elastic compression to offset the detrimental effects of venous stasis and ambulatory venous hypertension. (Fig. 18.2) (See-).

Step Three: Create the Proper Local Environment for Healing

Once the underlying problem (i.e. venous insufficiency) has been identified and addressed through surgery or compression, the next step in

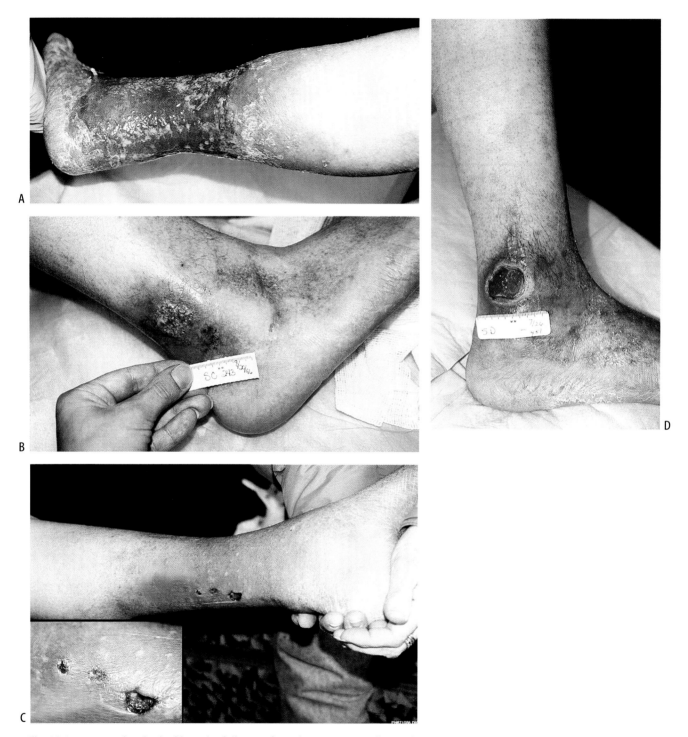

Fig. 18.1. Venous ulcer look-alikes. The following four ulcers were initially misdiagnosed as "venous ulceration". In all cases, subsequent non-invasive testing (plethysmography and/or duplex scanning) failed to show any evidence of venous dysfunction. Alternative diagnoses were eventually established for each of these lesions. **A** *Polycythemia with hydroxyurea therapy.* This 83-year-old female developed erythema and desquamation of the ankle and lower leg following the initiation of hydroxyurea therapy for her polycythemia. The ulcerations and breakdown resolved after hydroxyurea was discontinued. **B** *Vasculitis* This 18-year-old male developed lateral and medial ankle ulcers which failed to heal despite aggressive elastic compression therapy. Biopsy eventually revealed "vasculitis" with microvascular thromboses. **C** *Hypertensive ulcer.* This 73-year-old male had severe, chronic hypertension which was poorly controlled. The ulcers on the medial portion of the ankle were present for at least two years and were extremely painful. They healed following successful treatment of his hypertension. **D** *Cryoglobulinemia.* This 41-year-old female had an ulcer present for six weeks on the lateral posterior ankle region. Subsequent work-up revealed chronic hepatitis C associated with cryoglobulinemia.

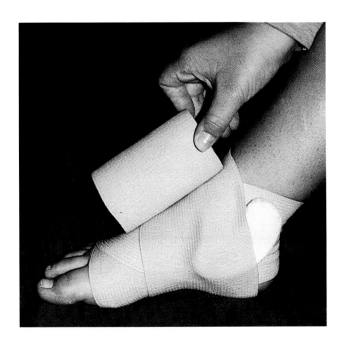

Fig. 18.2. Elastic compression – foam pads. Elastic (or non-elastic) compression can be made more effective in the region of ulcerations by providing compressible foam pads. These pads, which are placed directly over the ulcer, ensure that the compressive forces are adequate at and around the region of the skin breakdown.

wound care is to create the proper local environment for healing. Factors to consider include:

Debride/Clean. Although a few practitioners still advocate the view that eschar is "nature's bandage", most wound care experts now prefer to remove dead tissue from a non-healing ulcer whenever possible.[4] Debridement reduces infection, improves drainage, and enables the care-giver to inspect the wound for otherwise occult tracts, areas of necrosis, etc. (Fig. 18.3A, B). It also permits the environment of the wound surface to be more precisely controlled with regard to factors such as moisture level and air exposure. Several techniques are available for debriding and cleaning wounds. *Sharp* debridement, utilizing scalpels or scissors, is frequently used when large, densely adherent areas of necrotic tissue are present. *Wet-to-dry* dressings are another form of manual debridement. These are usually applied in the form of saline-soaked gauze, which is placed on the wound and allowed to dry. When the dry gauze is physically removed it carries away adherent pieces of eschar. By repeating this two or three times a day for several days, most eschars can be removed. Immersion therapy using a *whirlpool bath* is another way of debriding certain ulcers; the water loosens the eschar while the swirling motion mechanically removes it. Some topical debriding agents contain *enzymes* which break down and soften the eschar. These need to be used with caution to avoid destruction of healthy tissue. An extreme, if somewhat unesthetic, version of mechanical debridement involves the use of *maggots* which can be placed onto a wound and which will selectively consume the eschar.[5,6,7]

Control infection. Bacterial infection can be a contributing factor in many cutaneous ulcerations, especially those produced by diabetes, but its importance in venous ulcers is often controversial. *Infection* (as opposed to *colonization*) includes the occurrence of greater than 10 000 organisms per gram of biopsied tissue,[5] but it is usually impractical to biopsy an ulcer in order to make a diagnosis of infection. *Clinical criteria* for infection include the findings of cellulitis surrounding the ulcer, frank purulence, foul odor, excessive drainage, etc. (Fig. 18.4). The usual causative microbial agents include *Streptococcus* and *Staphylococcus*, although gram-negative bacteria (including *Pseudomonas*) and even fungi may occasionally be implicated. When infection is present oral or intravenous antibiotics are indicated. The value of topical antibiotics in treating an established infection is debatable, although they are widely used by many practitioners as a means of preventing infection in chronic ulcerations.[8]

Maintain an optimum moisture level in the wound. The development, growth, and spread of granulation and epithelial tissues require an appropriate level of moisture within the wound. If the local environment is too dry healing will be inhibited, while too much moisture causes maceration of the surrounding skin. Specific dressings should be chosen primarily to maintain wound moisture at the optimal level (Table 18.1). Dry wounds can be kept moist with occlusive dressings,[9] gels, or other moistening agents, while the secretions from excessively wet wounds can be controlled by absorbent dressings such as calcium alginates or co-polymer starches.

Other factors. Some factors affect the body systemically, and in doing so alter the local environment in ways that affect wound healing. These factors include nutritional status (proteins, vitamins, etc.), the presence of other comorbid conditions, tobacco use,[10] and others.

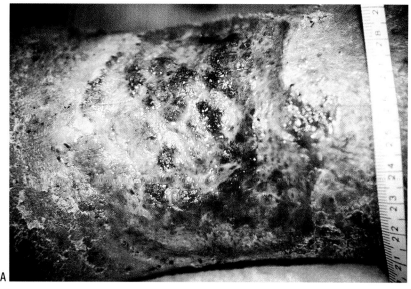

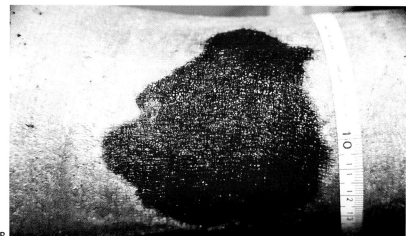

Fig. 18.3. Debridement. Venous ulcer before (**A**) and after (**B**) aggressive debridement therapy. In this case, debridement was accomplished over several visits using sharp instruments wet-to-dry dressings, and whirlpool therapy.

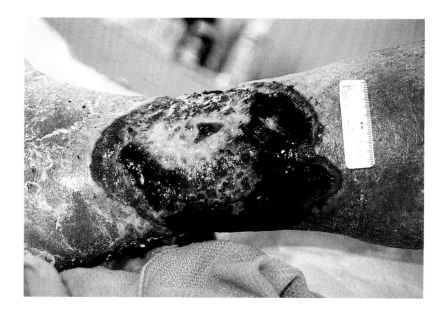

Fig. 18.4. Infection. Typical clinical appearance of an "infected" venous ulcer. Debridement of necrotic material and use of antibiotics lead to rapid improvement in the appearance of this wound.

Table 18.1. Dressings used for the treatment of venous ulcers

Indication Wound Types	Category/Action	Frequency of Change
Dry	Transparent Im	When seal is broken
	Wound gels	Twice a day
	Hydrogel sheets	Once a day
	Telfa	Once a day
Moist	Hydrocolloids	Every 2–5 days
	Gauze dressings	Twice to four times daily
	Iodosorb gel	Every 1–3 days
	Alginates	1–3 times daily
	Co-polymer starches	1–2 times daily
Wet	Foam dressings	1–2 times daily

Step Four: Use of Adjuvant Measures to Promote Healing

A venous ulcer will usually heal with nothing more than elastic compression, good hygiene, and proper control of wound moisture. When these steps fail, additional measures to promote healing may become necessary. For example:

Skin grafting. Various grafts including split thickness, pinch grafts, and flaps are common methods of treating stubborn venous ulcers (see Chapter 19).

Amputation. This may be necessary in debilitating or life-threatening situations, although limb removal should be an extraordinarily rare occurrence in patients with venous disease.

Drugs. Venotrophic agents are not approved for use in the United States. *Systemic antibiotics* have already been mentioned and are probably used in a significant number of patients – whether they are truly needed or not! *Anticoagulants* have utility in some settings, especially when the underlying venous insufficiency is due to recurrent venous thrombosis, but the value of anticoagulation in most settings is unclear. The same is true for antiplatelet agents (including aspirin and the newer platelet inhibitors). *Pentoxifylline* is another agent which may be of theoretical value in venous disease, since a decrease in blood viscosity (caused, in part, by pentoxifylline's ability to increase red blood cell flexibility) might help to promote microvascular flow in certain settings.[11]

Pumps

Controlling limb edema is an important component in the management of venous ulcers.[12] Edema control can be divided, somewhat arbitrarily, into two phases: a)*Edema reduction and* b)*Maintenance of the edema-free state.* As previously discussed in Chapter 17, the religious use of elastic (or non-elastic) compression (i.e., wraps or graduated elastic compression stockings) provides the primary means for keeping edema out of the limb once the swelling has been reduced. It is essential that the limb be fully reduced prior to measurement and fitting for elastic stockings; if the stocking size is determined when the limb is swollen, edema management will be difficult and therapeutic benefit is likely to be small.

How is limb edema reduced? In patients with mild edema, simple leg elevation (sometimes little more than the overnight elevation of the legs on pillows) may be sufficient to remove the swelling. Elastic wraps can accelerate the process. In patients with more severe edema, and especially in those with some associated swelling due to lymphedema, the reduction process is more difficult. *Foam wedges* or even *slings* may enhance rapid reduction by allowing the effects of gravity to be amplified by extreme leg elevation (Fig. 18.5A, B). *Diuretics* may also help to enhance fluid mobilization in some settings.

When these measures fail to reduce edema fully, or to reduce it in a timely fashion, or when edema reaccumulates aggressively despite the patient's use of elastic compression, it may be useful to treat the limb with a *pneumatic compression pump.* For purposes of discussion, pumps can be classified into four major categories.

1. *Single-chamber, sustained pressure.* This was the first type of pump to enjoy widespread usage and is still one of the most common designs. A single pneumatic sleeve encases the involved limb; this sleeve is intermittently inflated to pressures of 80 mmHg or more by an air pump (Figure 18.6).[13] The pressure is typically held for 30–90 seconds, during which time the high pressure encasing the limb acts to mobilize edema fluid. Following a predetermined (and often adjustable) time period, the cuff deflates allowing a temporary restoration of normal limb blood flow, after which the cuff is reinflated and a new cycle begins. The advantage of this type of pump is that it is relatively inexpensive and easy to use. Although it may not be as effective

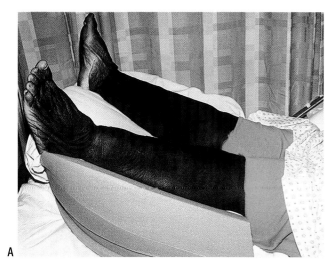

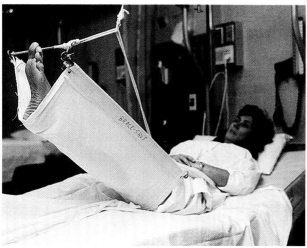

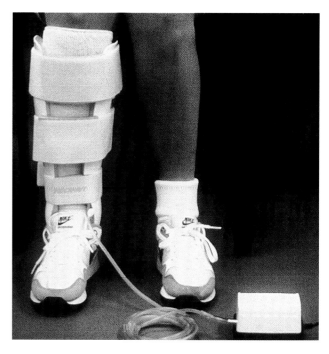

Fig. 18.6. Single chamber pneumatic pump. The pump shown here (EdemaFlo® by the AIRCAST Co.) represents one of the latest advances in pump therapy. This small unit can be used at home or in an ambulatory setting. It provides a comprehensive pressure of up to 90 mmHg, which is delivered for 30 seconds at a time. The pump can be powered by a cigarette lighter (in a automobile) or may be used with a battery pack (which is attached to the waist), thus enabling ambulation.

Fig. 18.5. Controlling edema by leg elevation. Wedges made out of foam (**A**) can be replaced at the foot of the patient's bed to elevate their limb(s) and promote edema reduction. In severe cases, a patient may be hospitalized and treated with sling (**B**) to elevate the leg at 45° or more.

as other pumps, the single-chamber sustained compression model provides an adequate adjunct for many patients.

2. *Multi-chamber sequential sustained pump.* These pumps are similar to the single-chamber types, but employ cuffs with multiple chambers, each of which can be inflated individually and/or sequentially.[14] The goal is to encourage fluid movement and edema reduction by applying a "milking" action to the swollen limb. As with single-chamber pumps, pressures of 60–80 mmHg or more may be used. For some patients the sequential pumps may be more effective than single-chamber pumps (especially when an associated element of lymphedema is present) but not all limbs require the more complex (and usually more expensive) multichamber pumps to obtain adequate edema control.

Some of the newest pumps utilize cuffs with a large number of chambers (up to 10 or more) which can be programmed to simulate various forms of massage (Fig. 18.7). These pumps may require lower cuff pressures to mobilize edema than do the others, making them potentially more comfortable and better tolerated than the higher pressure models; however, the effectiveness of this approach relative to other pumping modalities remains unproven.

3. *Impulse pumps.* In recent years *impulse* pumps have become available (Fig. 18.8). These pumps employ pneumatic cuffs that can be wrapped around the foot or lower leg. At regular intervals (typically every 20 seconds or so) the cuffs are rapidly inflated to a pressure of 100 mmHg or more. After an inflation period lasting 1–3 seconds, the pressure is released. The sudden, forceful application of pressure to the lower end of the extremity drives edema out of the foot and ankle, and improves venous

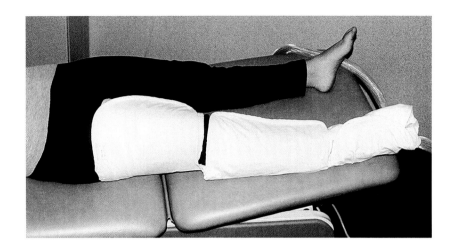

Fig. 18.7. Multi-chamber sequential pump. This prototype, made by Osborn Medical Corp., uses programmed, sequential inflation of multiple chambers in the sleeve to stimulate massage therapy. The pressures produced by this pump are less than those used with most single or multi-chamber pumps.

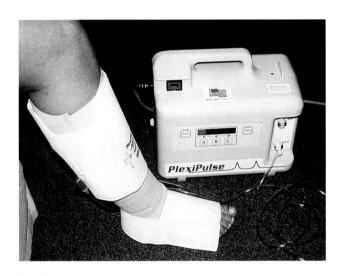

Fig. 18.8. Impulse pump. Impulse pumps (see the PlexiPulse® made by the New Tech Corp.) use short (1–3 second) inflation periods delivered to or three times per minute.

return. Originally employed as a method for preventing deep venous thrombosis in hospitalized patients, these pumps may help to control the edema of venous disease and facilitate ulcer healing.

4. *Cardiac-gated pumps.* Cardiac-gated pumps provide another alternative to high-pressure pumps.[15] The most commonly used pumps are single-chamber models in which the pneumatic cuff covers either the foot and ankle or the entire leg. The inflation occurs rapidly and is triggered by an electrocardiogram, much like an intra-aortic balloon pump. The cuff inflates briefly to 40–60 mmHg in synchrony with the cardiac cycle (Fig. 18.9). Advocates of this approach believe that the cardio-synchronous nature of the pumping provides superior enhancement of both arterial and venous circulation relative to other types of pumps. Unfortunately, there are only limited data on efficacy in the setting of venous ulceration.

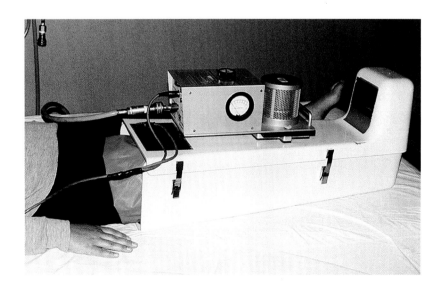

Fig. 18.9. Cardiac-gaited pump. This pump, made by the Circulator Boot Corp., delivers single-chamber limb compression in synchrony with the cardiac cycle.

Platelet-derived Growth Factor

Platelet-derived growth factor is a relatively new and somewhat controversial agent for promoting wound closure.[16,17] The "factor" (or, more likely, a collection of factors) is obtained by disrupting platelets; the platelets may be obtained from the patient or from pooled donors. After processing, the platelet-derived growth factors are applied topically to the wound, usually once or twice daily. The application may be in liquid form (for example, gauze soaked in the factor may be placed on the wound) or, more commonly, it is mixed with collagen to form a paste which is placed in a thin layer on the wound bed. The various platelet-derived factors theoretically work by stimulating the growth, division, and chemotaxis of various cell types.

Most of the available data on the efficacy of platelet-derived growth factor have been derived from work with diabetic (neurotrophic) or ischemic ulcers. Studies involving venous ulcers have been limited.[18] However, it seems logical that the same factors which contribute to poor healing in diabetic or ischemic ulcers might also be important in venous ulcers, and growth factor might therefore be of value in certain settings.

Hyperbaric Oxygen

The role of hyperbaric oxygen as an adjunct to the healing of venous ulcers is poorly defined, but there may be selected cases in which it is of value.[19,20,21] Ulcers which *might* be candidates for treatment with hyperbaric oxygen include those which are infected or associated with ischemia.

Education

As in many other aspects of medicine, educating the patient about the disease process is an important part of any therapeutic program. Patients who understand why ulcers occur and can appreciate the subtleties of dressing changes, good hygiene, and the need for compliance are far more likely to demonstrate successful healing than those who are uneducated. Allied health professionals such as nurses and therapists may complement the physician's role by spending the extra time necessary to ensure that the proper instruction is provided.

References

1. Weingarten MS (1993) The history and diagnosis of venous ulceration. Wounds 5:84–88
2. Hansson C (1994) Optimal treatment of venous (stasis) ulcers in elderly patients. Drugs and Aging 5:323–334
3. Christopherson D, Nicolaides AN, Cook A, Irvine A, Galloway JMD, Wilkinson A (1989) Pathogenesis of venous ulceration in relation to the calf muscle pump function. Surgery 106:829–835
4. Rodeheaver G, Baharesteari MM, Brabec ME, Byrd HJ, Salzberg CA, Scherer P, Vogelpohl TS (1994) Wound healing and wound management: Focus on debridement – An interdisciplinary round table, September 18, 1992, Jackson Hole, WY. Advances in Wound Care 7:22–39
5. Reames MK, Christensen C, Luce E (1988) The uses of maggots in wound debridement. Ann Plast Surg 21:388–391
6. Stoddard SR, Sherman RM, Mason BE, Pelsang DJ (1995) Maggot debridement therapy–an alternative treatment for nonhealing ulcers. J Am Podiat Med Assoc 85:218–221
7. Sherman RA, My-Tien J, Sullivan R (1996) Maggot therapy for venous stasis ulcers. Arch Dermatol 132:254–256
8. Lineaweaver W, Howard R, Soucy D, McMorris S, Freeman J, Crain C, Robertson J, Rumley T (1985) Topical antimicrobial toxicity. Arch Surg 120:213–216
9. Friedman SJ, Su WPD (1984) Management of leg ulcers with hydrocolloid occlusive dressing. Arch Dermatol 120:1329–1336
10. Silverstein P (1992) Smoking and wound healing. Am J Med 93:22S–24S
11. Samlaska CP, Winfeild EA (1994) Pentoxifylline. J Am Acad Dermatol 30:603–621
12. Dickey JW (1991) Stasis ulcers: the role of compliance in healing. So Med J 84:557–561
13. McCulloch JM, Marler KC, Neal MB, Phifer TJ (1994) Intermittent pneumatic compression improves venous ulcer healing. Adv Wound Care 7:22–26
14. Zelikovski A, Zucker G, Eliashiv A, Reiss R, Shalit M (1981) A new sequential pneumatic device for the prevention of deep venous thrombosis. J Neurosurg 54:652–654
15. Dillon RS (1986) Treatment of resistant venous stasis ulcers and dermatitis with the end-diastolic pneumatic compression boot. Angiology 37:47–55
16. Robinson CJ (1993) Growth factors: therapeutic advances in wound healing. Ann Med 25:535–538
17. Ganio C, Tenewitz FE, Wilson RC, Moyles BG (1993) The treatment of chronic nonhealing wounds using autologous platelet-derived growth factors. J Foot Surg 1993;32:263–268
18. Knighton DR, Fiegel VD, Austin LL, Ciresi KF, Butler EL

(1986) Classification and treatment of chronic nonhealing wounds-successful treatment with autologous platelet-derived wound healing factors (PDWHF). Ann Surg 204:322–330

19. Kindwall EP, Gottlieb LJ, Larson DL (1991) Hyperbaric oxygen therapy in plastic surgery: a review article. Am Soc Plast Reconst Surg 88:898–908

20. Kwiecinski MG (1987) Therapeutic value of hyperbaric oxygen in lower extremity ulcerations. J Foot Surg 26:394–396

21. Kindwall EP (1992) Uses of hyperbaric oxygen therapy in the 1990s. Cleveland Clinic J Med 59:517–528

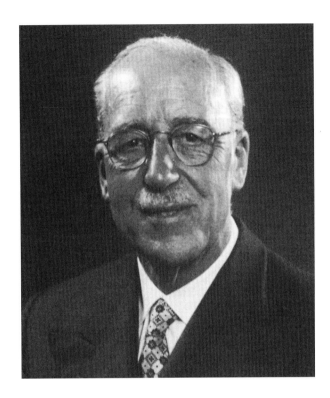

Harold Dodd
1899–1987

Harold Dodd was an unusual man. Born just before the turn of the century, he combined the best attributes of the nineteenth century with the advanced scientific achievements of the twentieth.

While a medical student at the University of Liverpool, he joined the Royal Flying Corps and was a lieutenant pilot from 1918 to 1919. He survived his Royal Air Force career, returned to medicine and graduated in 1922 with distinction in surgery. He continued at Liverpool as house surgeon, registrar, and surgical tutor until 1926. In the next year, he obtained the FRCS (Eng.) and after this, was elected consultant to the King George V Hospital in Illford. He continued as consultant until his retirement in 1964.

Dodd was the first author of the first important textbook dealing with venous insufficiency. His volume, *The pathology and surgery of the veins of the lower limb*, co-authored by Frank B. Cockett, contained a foreword by Robert Linton who remarked there about patients with venous insufficiency saying, "when properly handled, patients with these distressing conditions who are cured or relieved of them are some of the most grateful of surgical patients." In the authors' foreword to their volume, they said, "no finer training ground for surgery is to be found than in dealing with venous conditions. The diagnosis of the exact venous fault needs clinical skill and thoroughness. The operative procedures, though often considered trivial, are actually a testing exercise in exact dissection and good surgical technique which, when mastered, largely overcomes the difficulties of more extensive procedures." A revision of their volume is anticipated with eagerness.

After a career as an aviator and after many triumphs as a consultant surgeon, he studied for the church and was ordained Curate of All Souls, Langham Place in 1970. This career took him until 1982.

His surgical career was distinguished. He was the first President of the Consultants and Specialists Association and President of the section of surgery in the Royal Society of Medicine. He will always be remembered for his lifelong keen interest in the then unfashionable subject of varicose veins, and after publication of his volume with Frank Crockett in 1956, his enthusiasm for the subject never ceased.

This multifaceted man loved gardening and growing things. His friends were often the recipients of raspberries or blackberries when they were in season, and it was said in his obituary, "...he was a warm and steadfast friend to a whole generation of young surgeons whom he encouraged and helped."

Local Management of Chronic Leg Ulcers   19

Craig H. Johnson

The goal of management of chronic leg ulcers is to secure wound healing and skin coverage. This is to relieve chronic infection and preserve limb function. Implicit in the care is an accurate diagnosis and discovery of contributing factors which perpetuate the ulcer. A treatment plan must correct or modify pathology and contributing factors so that the wound bed, surrounding tissue, and entire extremity are able to accept wound coverage. The majority of ulcers of the lower extremity are secondary to venous insufficiency. However, as many as 33% of lower extremity ulcers have a component of arterial insufficiency.[1] An initial presumptive separation into a venous, arterial, or combined group is useful. This directs the starting point of confirmatory diagnosis and treatment.

Preliminary Information

The patient's history should include any inciting traumatic event as opposed to spontaneous development, duration of wound presence and previous attempts at treatment. We feel that tobacco use in all forms should be discontinued immediately. A preliminary diagnosis with the help of ulcer etiology can be based on appearance of the ulcer and non-invasive laboratory data. The ulcers can be classified according to etiology: arterial, venous, or combined. Each contributing factor must be treated to achieve a healed wound. For example, a patient with signi-

ficant arterial insufficiency will need arterial reconstruction to increase the oxygen delivery to the wound. Patients with venous disorders will need correction of these as described elsewhere in this volume.

Initial Treatment

As the initial treatment is begun and after wound assessment, the treatment plan can be developed. Necrotic or devitalized tissue should be treated appropriately. Either local bed-side debridement or formal surgical debridement in the operating room can be done. Each depends on the amount of tissue that must be removed and the patient's sensitivity with regard to need for anesthetic support. Initial saline wet-to-dry dressing changes should be started. These provide gentle mechanical debridement. Wound cultures may be taken. Because the wound is open, antibiotics are usually not necessary. Frank erythema and cellulitis, however, demand antibiotic treatment. In treatment of cellulitis, elevation and bed rest are needed. Otherwise, the antibiotics have very little penetration into the edematous, swollen leg.

Removal of non-viable eschar should be done. This should reveal chronic bleeding, well-perfused, healthy tissue. Debridement may expose vital structures such as tendon, bone, or neurovascular bundles. After eschar removal, dressing changes are resumed until a pinkish-red granulation bed appears. This indicates a healthy wound bed with an intact wound-healing mechanism. Undesirable, copious yellow drainage may signify venous edema and/or lymphatic obstruction.[2] After debridement of devitalized tissue, hygroscopic dressings may be useful to draw edema and fluid away from the wound bed to allow development of healthy granulation. This serofibrinous drainage must be controlled

prior to any attempt at wound coverage. Accumulation of fluid beneath the new coverage will cause failure of the attempt (Fig. 19.1A).

Whirlpool treatment of the involved extremity is also useful to effect gentle mechanical cleaning and minor debridement. Open wounds can usually be treated in a hydrotherapy tank without fear of spread of infection or exacerbation of the wound. In practice, patients begin with dressing changes three

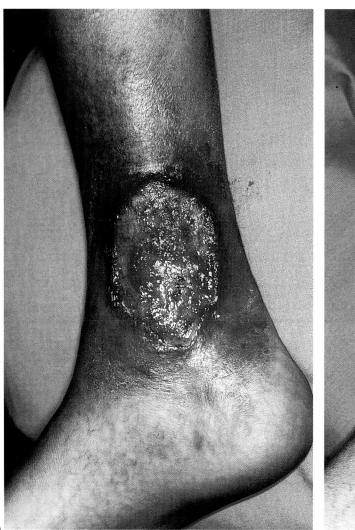 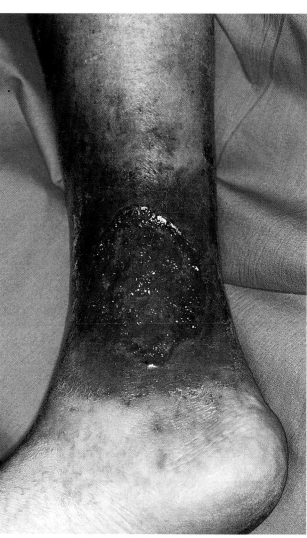

A   B

Fig. 19.1. A Venous stasis ulcer with typical appearance that would not accept split thickness skin grafting. Note the yellowish appearance of the wound bed, the lack of complete granulation issue, and the significant fibrinous exudate denoting moderate serous weepage and drainage. Application of a split thickness skin graft at this juncture would result in near complete loss of the graft. There is not enough well vascularized tissue as evidenced by full granulation, which could support the skin graft by diffusion for the first 48 h that is necessary, prior to capillary inosculatory ingrowth. **B** The same wound after endoscopic subfascial ligation of venous perforators to control the venous hypertension. Note that the granulation tissue now covers the entire bed of the wound. Re-epithelialization of the wound has begun as evidenced by a flattening of the wound crater itself along its outer circumferential edges. New regenerative epithelium is noted at this juncture. There is less drainage, less fibrinous exudate, and the wound bed now has the necessary tissue perfusion such that the skin graft can be supported for the first critical 48–72 h while ingrowth and adherence of the graft occurs to the depths of the wound bed.

times daily, two of which occur immediately after whirlpool treatments in the morning and later in the day (Fig. 19.1B).

Absent paratendon, periosteum, tendon, and bone will not granulate. Further, they will not support a skin graft. These and exposed neurovascular structures require formal coverage procedures.

Tissue Coverage

Nearly all chronic lower extremity ulcers improve with conservative care. However, further wound coverage may be indicated. Two considerations drive this decision. One is the size of the wound. This determines whether it will spontaneously re-epithelialize or whether it is more expedient to accelerate healing with a split-thickness skin graft. Small wounds 2–3 cm in diameter will heal in the same time frame as postoperative immobilization and healing after skin grafting.

A second factor which determines need for further coverage is exposure of vital structures.

The Reconstructive Ladder

The concept of the reconstructive ladder was developed to allow choice of coverage in an orderly and logical fashion. The lower rungs of the ladder are occupied by simpler, more straightforward wound care modalities. As one proceeds up the ladder, the complexity of the coverage process and the overall difficulty of obtaining wound healing is increased. The purpose of the ladder is to promote logical decision making. This then provides the simplest, most reliable, and straightforward method of obtaining the goal of a healed wound (Fig. 19.2).

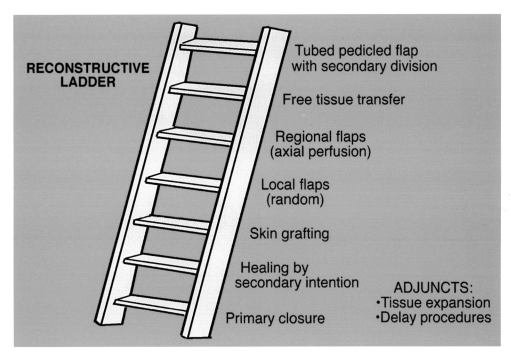

19.2. The concept of the reconstructive ladder allows for logical sequential thinking in order to select the best treatment modality of the patient. The treatment chosen is generally the most simple and straightforward, yet provides the most reliable and reasonable chance for wound healing and return to activities in the most expedient time frame. Wound coverage options generally proceed from a more straightforward to a more complex, technically demanding procedure. Certain adjuncts also facilitate each of the steps on the ladder, including tissue expansion and delay procedures. Delay procedures are preliminary design and partial elevation flaps such that the amount of tissues that can be carried on the planned nutritional supply can be increased. Depending on the size of the wound this is sometimes employed in order to obtain the necessary amount of tissue for coverage of a wound. Tissue expansion can be a useful adjunct as well, however tissue expansion in the lower extremity has a somewhat higher complication rate than its use in other areas of the body. Expander infection is one of the more feared complications, and since most chronic lower extremity ulcers are contaminated or frankly infected, the use of tissue expansion as a treatment modality is somewhat limited.

Venous ulcers are assessed according to adequacy of skin graft coverage. The width of the ulcer and the brawny, woody nature of the surrounding tissues prohibit primary or delayed primary closure. Venous ulcers often have an intact wound-healing mechanism and will display a healthy granulation bed. This is a soft tissue base which will readily accept a split-thickness skin graft (Fig. 19.3). Skin thickness varies throughout the body, but generally split grafts greater than 20/1000 of an inch begin to approach full thickness dermal depth. The advantage of a split thickness skin graft is that the thin graft allows for increased take. This is because the graft must survive for the first 48 h through oxygen diffusion from the underlying bed. Thin grafts allow for a shorter transit barrier to achieve this diffusion. Achievement of this base occurs by following the precepts outlined above. This must accompany controlling or eliminating the underlying cause of the ulcer. For example, elimination of venous hyperten-

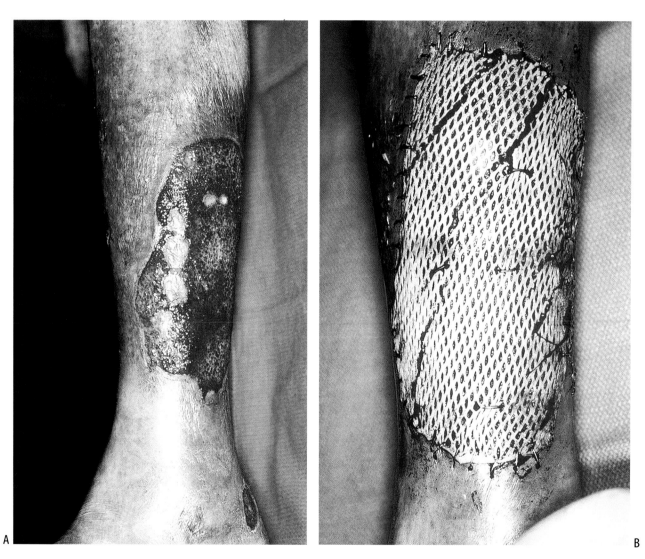

A   B

Fig. 19.3. A A large area of open wound of the left lower extremity secondary to venous stasis. This wound has been previously debrided and treated with wet to dry dressing changes, elevation and hydrotherapy for one week. The bed now displays a healthy granulating wound which is readily able to accept coverage in the form of split thickness skin graft. Note there are no exposed vital structures and the wound shows central islands of regenerating epithelium. **B** A split thickness skin graft which was harvested from the left lateral thigh at 15/1000 of an inch. This thickness is generally referred to in the range of a medium split thickness skin graft. The graft is meshed in a ration of 1.5 to 1. Meshed grafts allow for expansion of the lattice to aid drainage of underlying accumulation of blood and serum. This is significant problem when grafting venous stasis wounds in that serum drainage is often quite perfuse. Anything that lifts the graft off the underlying bed, such as accumulating fluid, be it blood, serum or infectious in origin, will not allow the graft to take. The obvious benefit of the meshed graft is therefore demonstrated in this figure.

sion or reconstitution of arterial perfusion must be accomplished (Figs 19.4a, b, 19.5a–d).

It should be noted that full-thickness skin grafting is rarely, if ever, indicated in the treatment of chronic lower extremity wounds. A split graft has a much greater chance for full take. This is due to its thinness and ability to survive during the first 48 h by oxygen diffusion. Subsequent capillary ingrowth occurs readily in a thin split-thickness graft.

Flap Coverage

The next rung on the ladder involves coverage with local and/or regional flaps. Rarely, small local, randomly based transposition flaps are possible. But an edematous lower extremity or one with compromised arterial perfusion precludes such coverage. Conceptually, the leg below the knee can be divided into thirds. In the proximal third, adequate muscle flap transposition coverage options include use of the medial or lateral heads of the gastrocnemius muscle. These are based on the paired sural arteries from the popliteal artery.[3] These muscles originate from the femoral condyles and insert into the Achilles tendon. The medial head is generally twice the size of the lateral head. Either may be sacrificed without a functional deficit.

Wounds in the middle third of the leg which require flap coverage are generally best treated with transposition of the soleus muscle. This muscle originates from the upper third of the dorsal and medial surfaces of the fibula and mid posterior tibia. It inserts into the Achilles tendon anterior and distal to the insertion of the gastrocnemius muscles. The donor site morbidity and functional impact associated with transposition of the soleus is minimal even in very active individuals. The soleus muscle proximal vasculature arises directly from the popliteal vessels. When these vessels are preserved, the muscle can be transposed with survival of all but the most distal 4–5 cm.

The soleus is predominantly used for mid-tibial defects. It will not consistently reach the lower one-

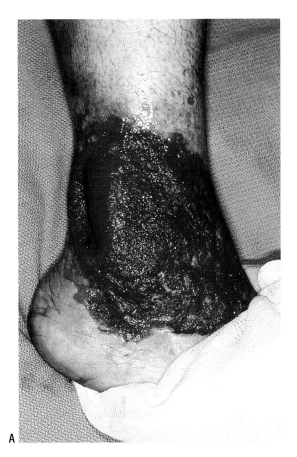

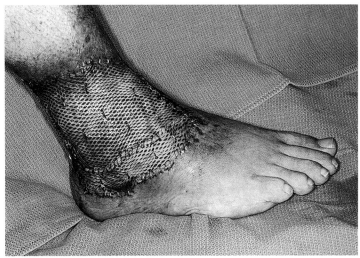

Fig. 19.4.A A large wound secondary to venous stasis which has been treated with debridement, dressing changes and hydrotherapy. With strict elevation the edema has resolved, and the bed is now ready to accept a split thickness skin graft. **B** The same wound after application of a meshed split thickness skin graft of 15/1000 inch. The graft is secured into position with staples, and the patient will then be placed in a bulky, well-padded plaster splint in order to immobilize the ankle joint. Bed rest and immobility will be maintained until the graft is inspected at 5–7 days postoperatively.

A

B

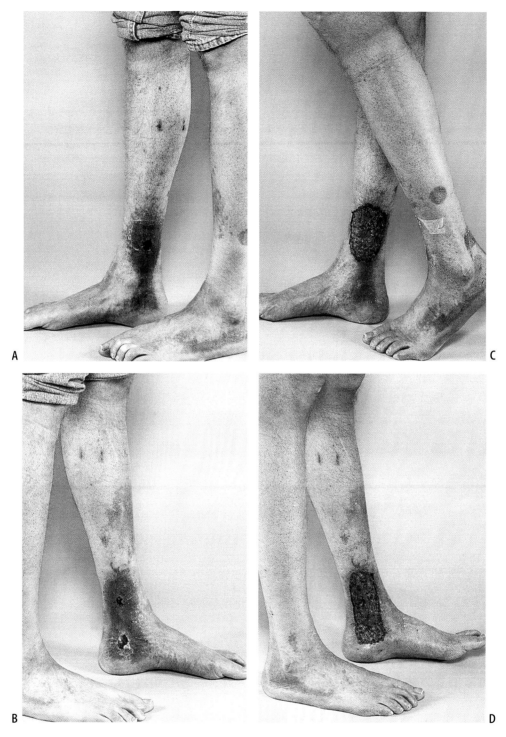

Fig. 19.5.A A 39-year-old white male and bilateral venous stasis skin breakdown. He previously underwent bilateral endoscopic sub-fascial perforator interruption, and his wounds have shown remarkable improvement. He then underwent wide local debridement of his wound back to healthy viable tissue. Because of the excellent underlying bed, local care was instituted. **C, D** The postoperative results after bilateral meshed split thickness skin graft of 15/1000 of an inch harvested from the lateral thigh. Wounds remain healed. The patient is currently ambulatory and participates in distance running events.

third of the lower extremity. The calf can be explored to determine whether the soleus will reach far distally and provide coverage. The soleus has been described for use as a reversed and distally based flap. However, it is seldom used this way because of unreliable survival of such a transfer.

In the lower one-third of the leg, the options for muscle transposition diminish. Yet this is where most chronic venous ulcers are located. The extensor digitorum communis (EDC) muscle has been proposed as an option for a distally based flap to achieve coverage of the distal third of the leg. It will not reach the ankle mortis or the dorsum of the foot. Its vascular anatomy makes it unreliable and it is best to explore the proximally based soleus prior to using the EDC. Free tissue transfer utilizing operating microscope anastomoses should be considered prior to an attempted coverage with the extensor digitorum communis.

Free Flaps

Free tissue transfer becomes an appealing option in large wounds when exposed vital structures and an absent healthy granulation bed are present. Preoperative evaluation includes angiography and assessment of venous drainage. These will be necessary for microvascular anastomoses.[4] In the nontraumatized leg with palpable pulses, it may not be necessary to perform preoperative lower extremity arteriograms. Duplex ultrasound may be adequate. However, a significant number of limbs have mixed arterial and venous deficiencies. Therefore, noninvasive vascular studies and arteriography may be required. Some patients need arterial reconstruction in order to establish adequate inflow to the nonhealing wound. Free tissue transfer can then be performed by using the distal bypass graft, either autogenous or prosthetic, as a source of inflow to the free flap. It is recommended that the venous outflow be established by microvascular anastomosis to the deep system.

Correction of venous reflux, as described elsewhere, is essential to survival of the transferred flap. The free flap actually transplants hundreds of venous valves into the ulcer bed. These valves function to maintain proper venous flow regardless of

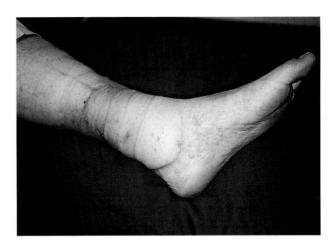

Fig. 19.6. This photograph illustrates a free flap in place 16 years. The tissue transfer was done to treat an intractable, recalcitrant venous ulcer which followed a motorcycle accident, deep venous thrombosis and pulmonary embolization. Note the absence of flap hyperpigmentation or scars. PPG recovery time in the flap was 20 seconds, on the lateral ankle 9 seconds.

the status of the deep venous system. Dunn and colleagues reporting from Worcester described the rationale for free tissue transfer saying, "skin grafting simply covers the wound superficially and the underlying diseased tissue remains prone to ulcer recurrence. Free tissue transfer addresses both the abnormal venous hemodynamics and also provides a healthy tissue bed to achieve long-term healing of refractory ulcers. A radical subfascial ligation is a mandatory part of the procedure and is carried out during the wide excision of the liposclerotic and ulcerated tissues. The transplanted tissue has an additional beneficial effect on the venous hemodynamics because of the presence of the microvenous valves that are present (Fig. 19.6).

Muscle units in these circumstances are almost always transferred without a cutaneous skin island. Once transfer is completed and muscle has been reperfused with the appearance of healthy bleeding tissue, split-thickness skin graft over the muscle is required. In this situation, deep venous valve function has not been improved and ulcer recurrence may follow.

Free Flap Donor Sites

Potential donor sites available for free tissue transfer are numerous. Weinzweig and Schuler have reported

23 consecutive free flaps in which 19 were for venous ulcerations. They have reported a variety of tissue sources, including the rectus muscle, serratus muscle, and omentum. Split-thickness skin graft losses were reported in three of the flaps which used rectus muscle with split-skin covering.[6] The latissimus dorsi muscle is appealing because of minimal donor site morbidity and functional loss. The rectus abdominis muscle is useful with anastomoses performed to the deep inferior epigastric artery and its accompanying venae comitantes. Other muscles which are available include the serratus anterior or the gracilis.

Free tissue transfer to the lower extremity with open injuries and non-healing wounds has progressed to the point where the challenge is not to obtain coverage but to contour and shape the coverage. Now the functional result and esthetic appearance is maximized. With this in mind, the choice of a donor muscle considers donor site morbidity and functional impact and the contour and geometry of the wound. Broad, flat, open wounds are best covered with latissimus muscle with its relatively minimal thickness and expansive shape. In contrast, small, deep, crater-like wounds can be filled with gracilis or rectus abdominis muscles. Both of these are thicker. The gracilis muscle has a rather round, thickened shape which allows it to fill a cavity and obliterate dead space. This is coupled with its minimal donor site morbidity which makes it an especially appealing alternative.

Tube Pedicle Flaps

At the highest rung of the ladder are tube pedicle flaps. Historically, these were a mainstay in plastic surgery. They gave the practitioner a method in which healthy, vascularized tissue could be brought to a wound. The creation of a flap, either random or perfused by a single axial artery, was by elevation from a regional or distant site. This could even be performed using tissue from the opposite extremity. After elevation, the flap was sutured into place and partially inset into the chronic wound. The attachment was allowed to persist for 14–21 days. During this period, vascular ingrowth occurred where the flap was inset in the wound. When enough perfusion

crossed the flap, its original pedicle could be divided and still permit survival. Thus, the flap and donor site could be separated and the remaining portion of the tube pedicle shaped and contoured. Because this required two or three operations and a prolonged waiting period of attachment prior to division, it has been placed in a high position on the ladder and is a less-than-optimal choice. With the advent of microsurgical technique for free flaps and success rates approaching 95% to 98%, the tube pedicle flap is now considered a salvage procedure when flap failure occurs. It remains a choice of last resort should free tissue transfer not be possible.

Ancillary Treatment

Other adjunctive measures that have been used for wound healing coverage include tissue expansion and delay procedures. A delay procedure involves partial elevation of a flap with surgical interruption of a portion of the blood supply to the flap. This is done as a preliminary procedure prior to definitive transfer and coverage. The purpose of the delay procedure is to increase the surviving size and length of a flap. It is most useful in creating larger skin islands which can be carried with muscle flaps for soft tissue coverage. Because of the usual induration in the lower extremity tissues in association with venous ulcers, the delay tactic is not used.

Tissue expansion in the lower extremity has been tried with varying degrees of success.[7,8] In general, the complication rate increases as one moves distally on the lower extremity. Complications include exposure of the tissue expander and infection. Because lower extremity wounds are often colonized and occasionally frankly contaminated and infected, the use of tissue expanders for venous stasis ulcer is not a good choice.

References

1. Colen LB et al. (1987) Limb salvage in the patient with severe peripheral vascular disease: The role of microsurgical free tissue transfer. Plast Reconstr Surg 79:389

2. Marsh JL (ed), Kraemer BA (1993) Leg ulcers: decision making in plastic surgery. Mosby Year Book, Inc., St. Louis, 1993.

3. McCrow J, Arnold PG (eds) (1986) Atlas of muscle and musculocutaneous flaps. Hampton Press Publishing, Inc., Norfolk, Virginia

4. Colen LB et al. (1987) Preoperative assessment of peripheral varicosities diseased patient for free tissue transfer. J Reconstr Microsurgery 4:234–287

5. Dunn RM, Fudem GM, Walton RL, Anderson FA Jr, Malhotra R (1994) Free flap valvular transplantation for refractory venous ulceration. J Vasc Surg 19:525–531

6. Weinzweig N, Schuler J (1997) Effect of free tissue transfer in the treatment of recalcitrant venous stasis ulcerations. Ann Plast Surg (in press).

7. Manders EK, Oaks EK, Au VK et al. (1988) Soft tissue expansion in the lower extremities. Plast & Reconstr Surg 81:208

8. Borges Filho PT, Neves RI, Gemperli R et al. (1991) Soft tissue expansion in lower extremity reconstruction. Clin Plast Surg 18:593

North American Subfascial Endoscopic Perforator Surgery (NASEPS) Registry

Results of the North American Subfascial Endoscopic Perforator Surgery (NASEPS) Registry

20

Sunil S. Menawat, Peter Gloviczki, John J. Bergan and Linda G. Canton

Introduction

Since the mid-1980s, considerable experience has accumulated in Europe with different endoscopic techniques to treat perforator vein incompetence.[1–5] Several groups in the United States and Australia also recognized the advantages of endoscopic procedures and used existing equipment made available by progress in minimally invasive non-vascular surgical technology.[6–10] Recognizing the benefits of perforator interruption and the problems of wound complications and prolonged hospitalization associated with the open procedures, a group of surgeons interested in the care of patients with advanced chronic venous disease decided to evaluate the minimally invasive, endoscopic Linton operation in a multicenter trial. To embark on a series of studies, the registry concept was embraced first to rapidly accumulate useful clinical information. The North American Subfascial Endoscopic Perforator Surgery (NASEPS) Registry was established in 1995 by vascular surgeons from 17 centers in the US and Canada (Table 20.1). The goal of the NASEPS registry was to evaluate the safety and feasibility of endoscopic perforator interruption and simultaneously to collect information on early and late outcomes. The first report of the registry was presented at the 1996 Annual Meeting of the Society for Vascular Surgery, and the data were published recently.[11]

Patients and Methods

The NASEPS registry collected data on patients who underwent subfascial endoscopic vein surgery (SEPS) in 17 institutions in the United States and Canada between 15 June 1993 and 15 February 1996. Each institution submitted completed data sheets on all patients who underwent attempt at SEPS (Fig. 20.1). The method of data collection in most cases was retrospective.

Results

Demographic Data

One hundred and fifty-five SEPS procedures were completed in 148 patients, 81 males and 67 females (Fig. 20.2). The procedure was aborted in 3 additional patients because of technical problems. The mean age of the 148 patients was 56 years. Seven patients had bilateral procedures, but data of only one leg were analyzed for this study.

Table 20.1 Participating centers and surgeons of the NASEPS registry

Emory Clinic	Atlanta, Georgia	Alan Lumsden MD
Jobst Vascular Center	Toledo, Ohio	John P. Pigott MD
		Hugh G. Beebe MD
		Steven M. Dosick MD
		Steven S. Gale MD
		Michael G. Vitti MD
		Ralph C. Whalen MD
Loma Linda Surgery Medical Group	Loma Linda, California	John J. Bergan MD
		Jeffrey L. Ballard MD
Maimonides Medical Center	Brooklyn, New York	Enrico Ascer MD
Mayo Clinic	Rochester, Minnesota	Peter Gloviczki MD
		Sunil S. Menawat MD
Medical College of Wisconsin	Milwaukee, Wisconsin	Robert A. Cambria MD
Mount Sinai Medical Center	New York, New York	Harry Schanzer MD
		Milan Skladany MD
Naval Medical Center	San Diego, California	Jay Murray MD
New England Medical Center	Boston, Massachusetts	Thomas F. O'Donnell MD
		Mark Iafrati MD
Pennsylvania Hospital	Philadelphia, Pennsylvania	Keith D. Calligaro MD
		Matthew J. Dougherty MD
Scripps Memorial Hospital	La Jolla, California	John J. Bergan MD
Straub Clinic & Hospital, Inc.	Honolulu, Hawaii	Robert L. Kistner MD
		Bo G. Eklof MD
		Elna Masuda MD
Toronto General Hospital	Toronto, Ontario, Canada	Peter Kalman MD
		Barry Rubin MD
University of Nevada	Reno, Nevada	Ralph G. DePalma MD
University of Pittsburgh	Pittsburgh, Pennsylvania	Robert Y. Rhee MD
University of Utah	Salt Late City, Utah	Peter F. Lawrence MD
		Spencer W Galt, MD
		Douglas L. Jicka MD
Washington University School of Medicine	St. Louis, Missouri	Brian G. Rubin MD

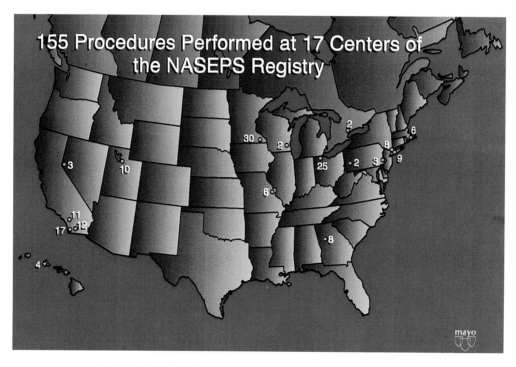

Fig. 20.1. Number of procedures performed in the NASEPS Registry.

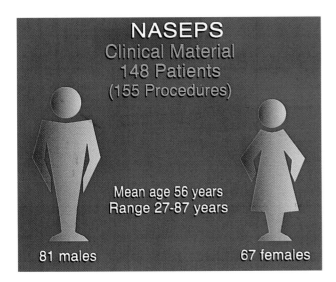

Fig. 20.2. Demographic data.

Risk Factors

At least one risk factor for acute or chronic venous disease was present in 125 (84%) patients. Previous deep venous thrombosis and family history of varicosity were the most frequent risk factors. History of smoking and trauma to the limb were less frequent etiologies (Fig. 20.3).

Clinical Presentation

At presentation skin pigmentation was the most frequent sign of chronic venous disease and pain was the most frequent symptom (Fig. 20.4). Varicose veins were noted in about half the patients. Seventy percent had at least one active ulcer at the time of SEPS and these patients were assigned to clinical Class 6 using the updated CEAP classification of the Joint Societies (Figs 20.5 A, B).[13] Most ulcers were larger than 2 cm in size and had recurred more than once (Figs 20.6 A, B).

Preoperative Evaluation

Preoperative studies included duplex scanning of the leg veins in 110 patients, ascending or descending venographies in 74 patients, and evaluation by impedance, strain gauge, air or photoplethysmography in 50 patients.

Etiology

The etiology of chronic venous disease was primary valvular incompetence in 70% of the patients (Fig. 20.7). Perforator reflux was documented by preoperative studies in 90% of the patients, but SEPS was indicated based on clinical suspicion of perforator incompetence in the remaining 10%. Deep venous reflux with or without occlusive disease was present in 74% of the patients and superficial reflux was seen in 69% (Fig. 20.8 A, B). Combined deep and superficial reflux was present in 51% and only 8 patients (5%) were found to have isolated perforator incompetence.

Preoperative Treatment

Prior to SEPS procedure all patients had received non-operative treatment for venous disease that included compression stockings, elastic wrap or Unna boots (Fig. 20.9). Preoperative patient compliance with non-operative management was estimated to be 75% or better in three-fourth of the patients (Fig. 20.10). Several patients had undergone surgical treatment for their disease before SEPS (Fig. 20.11).

Intraoperative Data

Forty-two patients were treated with SEPS only, 106 patients had concomitant procedures performed for superficial reflux. (Fig. 20.12). Technique for performance of the SEPS procedure varied by surgeons and included those reported earlier in this atlas and published in detail previously.[6-10] A single endoscopic port of various types (Storz endoscope, arthroscope) was used in 66 patients (45%) and two or three laparoscopic ports were used in 82 patients (55%, 2 ports in 79, 3 ports in 3 patients). Carbon-dioxide gas was insufflated into the subfascial space during 78 procedures (53%). In 7 patients a 250 ml balloon expander was used to improve visualization in the subfascial plane. A thigh tourniquet was applied obtain bloodless surgical field in 112 procedures (76%). Tourniquet time averaged 55 min, the number of perforating veins divided averaged 3.8 (Fig. 20.13). Sixty-five percent of the patients were discharged from the hospital the day of surgery or next morning following overnight observation.

Risk Factors for Acute or Chronic Venous Disease in 148 Patients

Risk factors	Patients	
	No.	%
Prevous deep venous thrombosis	45	30
Family history of varicosity	44	30
Smoking	36	24
Limb trauma	31	21
Hypertension*	25	17
Prethrombotic state	23	16
Malignancy	20	14
Obesity	19	12
Cardiac disease**	14	9
Diabetes	10	7
Rheumatoid arthritis	8	5

* Diastolic blood pressure > 90 mm Hg
** Greater than NYHA class 1

mayo
CA-175790d-06

Fig. 20.3. Incidence of risk factor for venous disease.

Signs and Symptoms of Chronic Venous Insufficiency in 148 Patients

Signs and symptoms	Patients	
	No.	%
Pigmentation	136	92
Pain	127	86
Edema	116	78
Ulcer	104	70
Lipodermatosclerosis	103	70
Varicosity	79	53
Venous claudication	21	14

mayo
CA-175790d-07

Fig. 20.4. Clinical presentation.

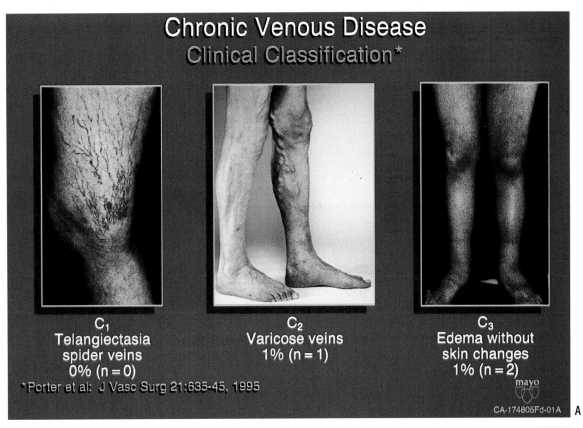

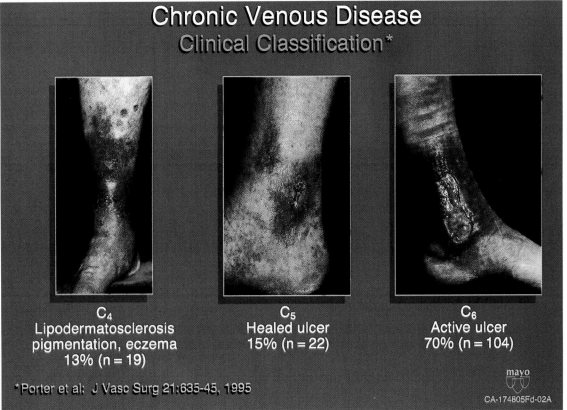

Fig. 20.5A, B. Clinical classification of 148 patients with chronic venous disease.

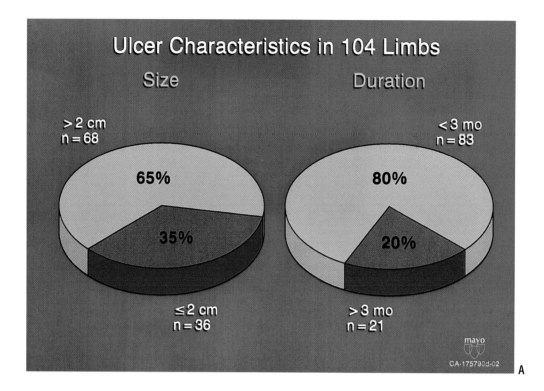

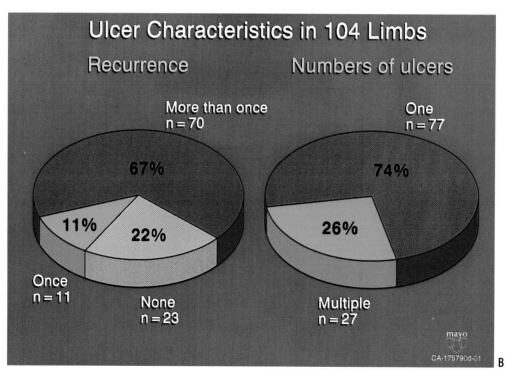

Fig. 20.6A, B. Data on size, duration, number and recurrence of venous ulcers.

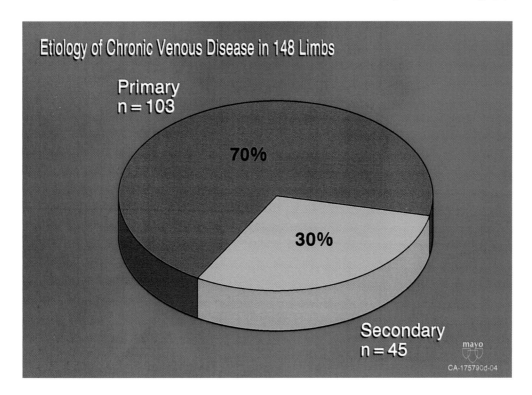

Fig. 20.7. Etiology of chronic venous disease. Note that only 30% of the patients had previous deep vein thrombosis.

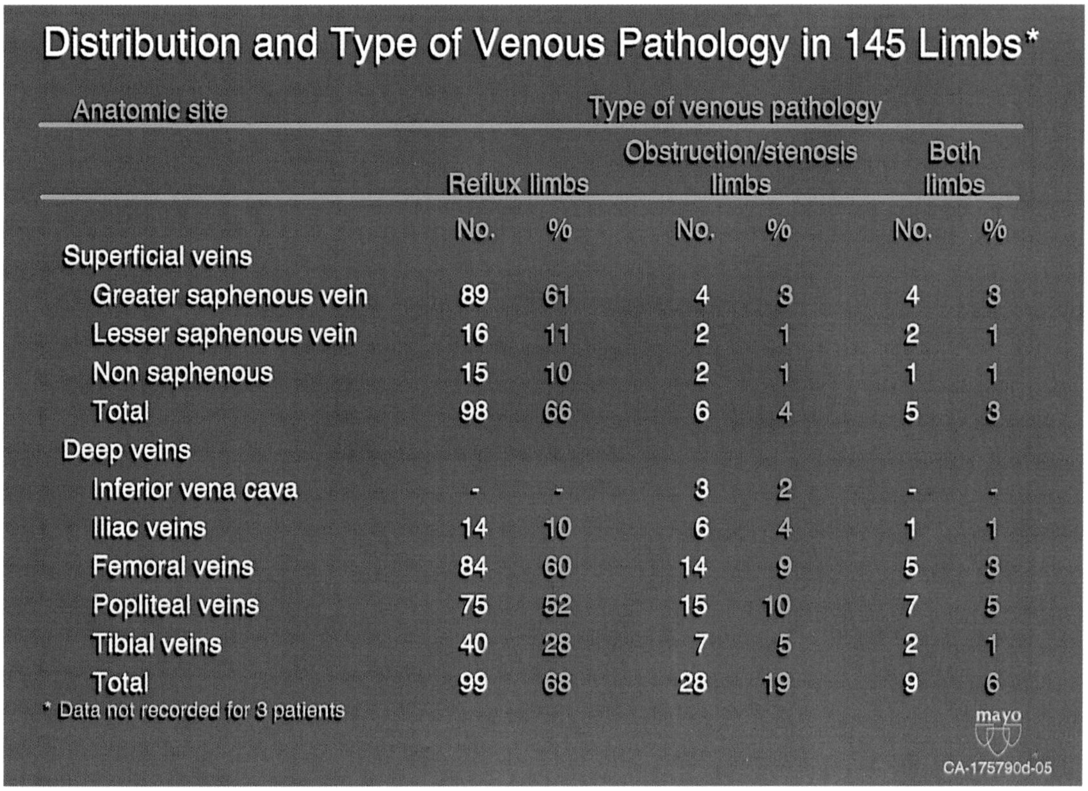

Distribution and Type of Venous Pathology in 145 Limbs*

Anatomic site	Type of venous pathology					
	Reflux limbs		Obstruction/stenosis limbs		Both limbs	
	No.	%	No.	%	No.	%
Superficial veins						
Greater saphenous vein	89	61	4	3	4	3
Lesser saphenous vein	16	11	2	1	2	1
Non saphenous	15	10	2	1	1	1
Total	98	66	6	4	5	3
Deep veins						
Inferior vena cava	-	-	3	2	-	-
Iliac veins	14	10	6	4	1	1
Femoral veins	84	60	14	9	5	3
Popliteal veins	75	52	15	10	7	5
Tibial veins	40	28	7	5	2	1
Total	99	68	28	19	9	6

* Data not recorded for 3 patients

A

Fig. 20.8A, B. Distribution of venous reflux and venous obstruction (part B next page)

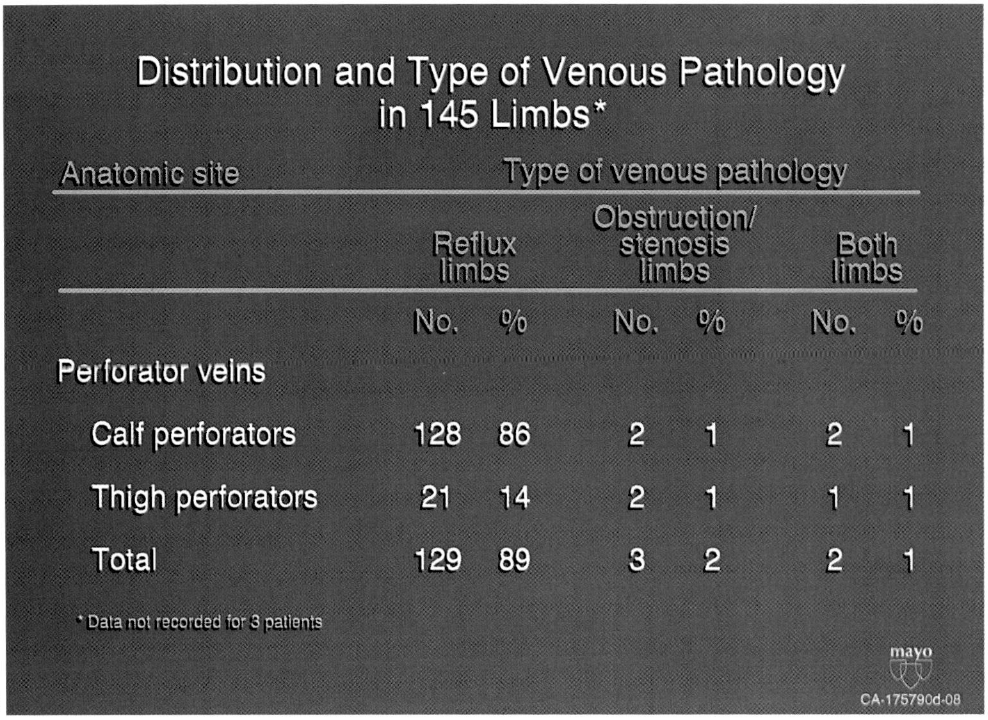

Distribution and Type of Venous Pathology in 145 Limbs*

Anatomic site	Type of venous pathology					
	Reflux limbs		Obstruction/ stenosis limbs		Both limbs	
	No.	%	No.	%	No.	%
Perforator veins						
Calf perforators	128	86	2	1	2	1
Thigh perforators	21	14	2	1	1	1
Total	129	89	3	2	2	1

* Data not recorded for 3 patients

mayo
CA-175790d-08

B

Fig. 20.8B

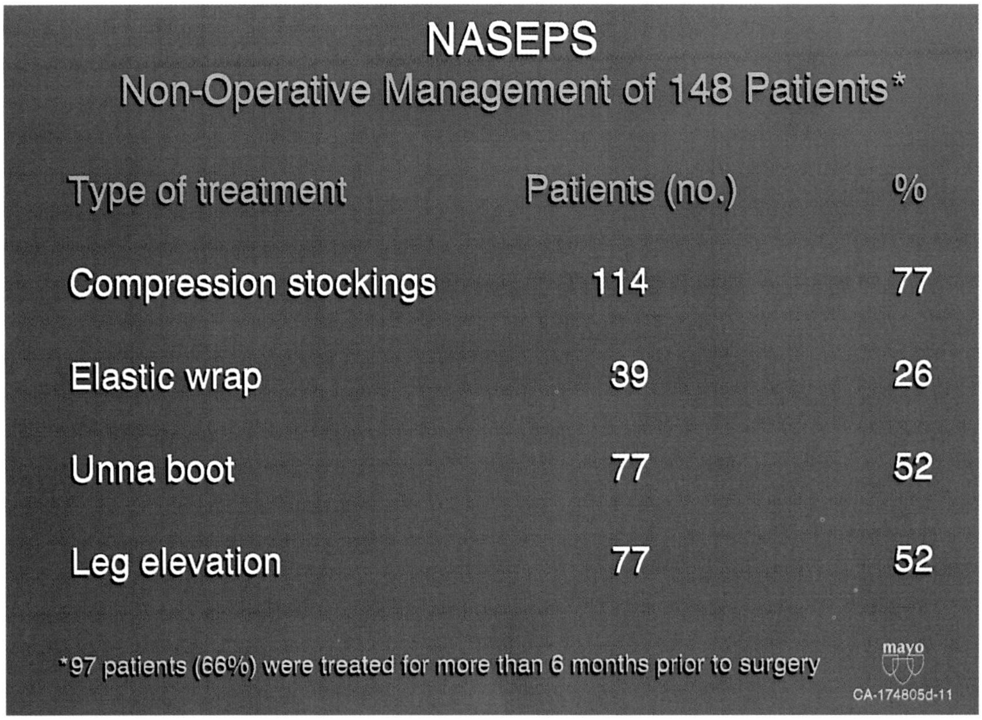

NASEPS
Non-Operative Management of 148 Patients*

Type of treatment	Patients (no.)	%
Compression stockings	114	77
Elastic wrap	39	26
Unna boot	77	52
Leg elevation	77	52

*97 patients (66%) were treated for more than 6 months prior to surgery

mayo
CA-174805d-11

Fig. 20.9. Non-operative management before SEPS procedures.

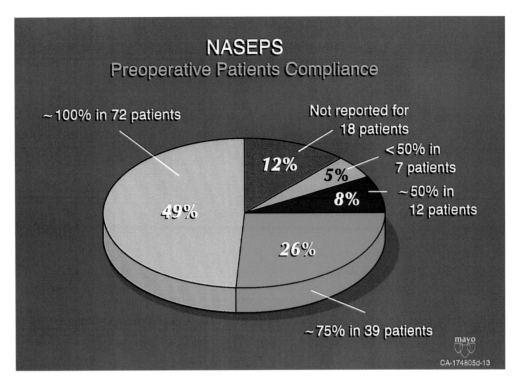

Fig. 20.10. Preoperative patients compliance with non-operative management.

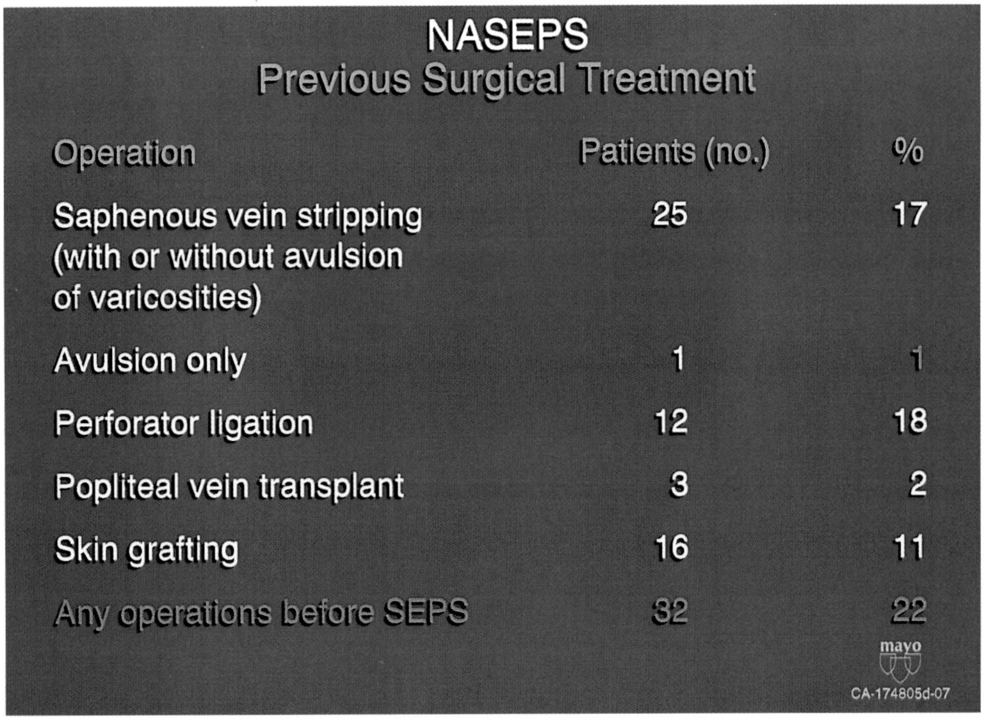

NASEPS
Previous Surgical Treatment

Operation	Patients (no.)	%
Saphenous vein stripping (with or without avulsion of varicosities)	25	17
Avulsion only	1	1
Perforator ligation	12	18
Popliteal vein transplant	3	2
Skin grafting	16	11
Any operations before SEPS	32	22

mayo
CA-174805d-07

Fig. 20.11. Surgical treatment before SEPS procedure.

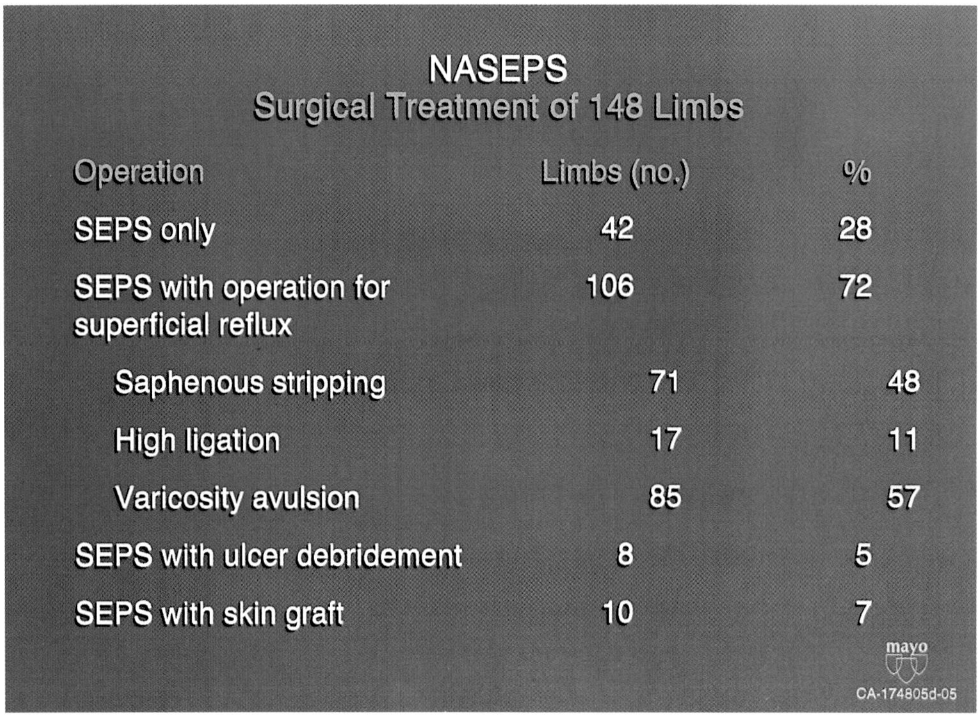

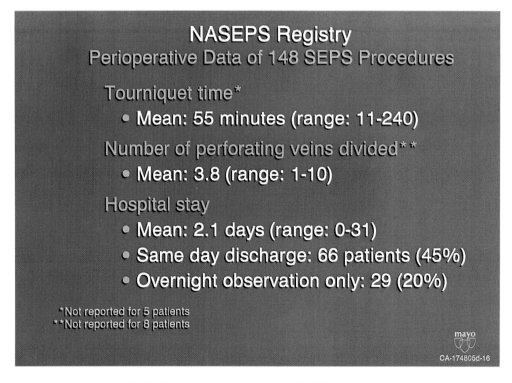

NASEPS
Surgical Treatment of 148 Limbs

Operation	Limbs (no.)	%
SEPS only	42	28
SEPS with operation for superficial reflux	106	72
Saphenous stripping	71	48
High ligation	17	11
Varicosity avulsion	85	57
SEPS with ulcer debridement	8	5
SEPS with skin graft	10	7

Fig. 20.12. SEPS and associated procedures in 148 patients.

NASEPS Registry
Perioperative Data of 148 SEPS Procedures

Tourniquet time*
- Mean: 55 minutes (range: 11-240)

Number of perforating veins divided**
- Mean: 3.8 (range: 1-10)

Hospital stay
- Mean: 2.1 days (range: 0-31)
- Same day discharge: 66 patients (45%)
- Overnight observation only: 29 (20%)

*Not reported for 5 patients
**Not reported for 8 patients

Fig. 20.13. Perioperative data for 148 SEPS procedures.

Complications

No deaths or early clinically evident thromboembolic complications were reported (Fig. 20.14). One patient with protein-C deficiency developed recurrent popliteal vein thrombosis at 2 months, for an incidence of late thrombotic complications of 0.7%. The most frequent complications were infection (6.1%) and saphenous neuralgia (6.7%). One patient developed full thickness skin necrosis from a role-up tourniquet. A statistically significant association between wound infections and the presence of an active ulcer could not be established (Fig. 20.15A). Saphenous neuralgia was significantly more frequent in patients who had avulsion of varicose veins and was also frequent (9.1%) in patients who had concomitant saphenous vein stripping. Differences in surgical technique did not affect the rate of complications (Fig. 20.15 B).

Postoperative Compression Treatment

All patients were advised to continue compression treatment using elastic stockings or elastic wrap. Postoperative estimated patients compliance with this was very similar to preoperative compliance (Fig. 20.16).

Clinical Outcome

Follow-up information to determine ulcer healing was available on 85 of the 104 patients with active ulcers. Healing during early follow-up occurred in 88% of the patients (Fig. 20.17). Average length of follow-up was 5.4 months in those that healed their ulcer and 7.1 months in patients that did not heal the ulcer. The probability of ulcer healing by 3 months after surgery was 67% (95% CI: 55%–76%) (Fig.

NASEPS
Complications

Complications	Early (< 30 days) patients		Late (> 30 days) patients		Total patients	
	no.	%	no.	%	no.	%
Mortality	0	0	0	0	0	0
Thromboembolism	0	0	1	0.7	1	0.7
Wound infection	8	5.4	2	1.3	9*	6.1
Cellulitis	4	2.7	0	0	4	2.7
Superficial thrombophlebitis	3	2.0	2	1.3	5	3.3
Saphenous neuralgia	6	4.0	4	2.7	10	6.7
Skin necrosis	1	0.7	0	0	1	0.7

*1 patient had both early and late wound infection

mayo

CA-174805d-01

Fig. 20.14. Postoperative complications.

Association of Clinical Variables and Early Complications

Clinical variables	Wound infection (%)	P	Saphenous neuralgia (%)	P
Active ulcer	7.6	1.0	3.8	0.34
Saphenous vein stripping	6.1	0.70	9.1	0.08
High ligation	10.0	0.553	0	1.0
Tourniquet time >60 min	4.6	1.0	0	0.182
Avulsion varicosity	7.6	1.0	11.3	0.012
Diabetes	0	1.0	0	1.0

mayo
CA-174805d-04

A

Association of Clinical Variables and Early Complications

Clinical variables	Wound infection (%)	P	Saphenous neuralgia (%)	P
1 endoscope	7.3		7.3	
2 or 3 endoscopes	7.6	1.0	3.9	0.679
CO_2 insufflation	5.8		3.9	
No insufflation	8.9	0.718	7.1	0.680

mayo
CA-174805d-06

B

Fig. 20.15A, B. Association of clinical variables with wound infection and saphenous neuralgia.

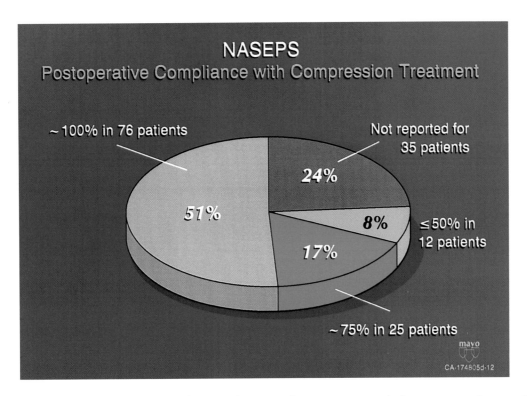

Fig. 20.16. Estimated postoperative compliance with compression treatment was similar to preoperative compliance.

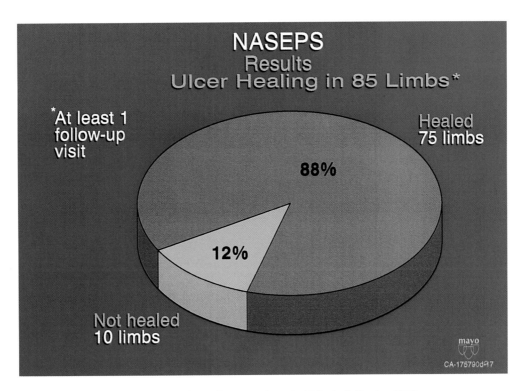

Fig. 20.17. Healing of venous ulcers in 85 limbs following SEPS.

20.18). Mean time to healing in a subset of 31 patients where the exact date of ulcer healing was known was 42 days (median: 38 days, range: 14–144 days) (Fig. 20.19). Ulcer duration, history recurrence, or multiplicity did not significantly influence healing, but small ulcers healed much faster than large ones (Fig. 20.20). To quantitate clinical improvement, preoperative and postoperative clinical scores[13] were calculated in the 114 patients who had at least one follow-up visit after SEPS procedure (Fig. 20.21). A significant improvement was noted from a score of 9.4 preoperatively to 2.9 postoperatively.

Discussion

A review of the data from the NASEPS registry confirmed that the endoscopic Linton operation is safe, with no deaths and no clinically evident thromboembolic complications noted by 30 days after surgery. Thromboembolic complications, however, do rarely occur in the post-thrombotic group and in this study 1 patient developed recurrent deep venous thrombosis 2 months after the operation. Patients with deep venous occlusions and those who have underlying coagulation abnormality are at high risk for this complications. Since the complication of these data the authors are aware of 2 additional patients who developed early deep venous thrombosis following SEPS. Posterior tibial vein thrombosis developed in 1 patient and iliofemoral venous thrombosis in another. Both were managed with full anticoagulation. Pulmonary embolism has never been reported following SEPS procedure. Careful patient selection, avoiding operation in patients with significant underlying deep venous occlusion and, most importantly, perioperative thrombosis prophylaxis, as emphasized in Chapter 16, is recommended in patients prone to develop thrombotic complications.

Wound infection following SEPS is still a problem with an incidence of 6.1% in this series. However, infection appears to occur significantly less frequently than following open procedures,[14–17] supporting data of the randomized study by Wittens et al. as reported in Chapter 15. While a roll-up toumi-

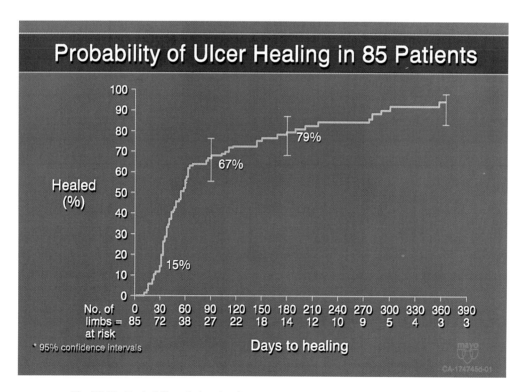

Fig. 20.18. Probability of ulcer healing was 67% at 90 days and 79% at 180 days.

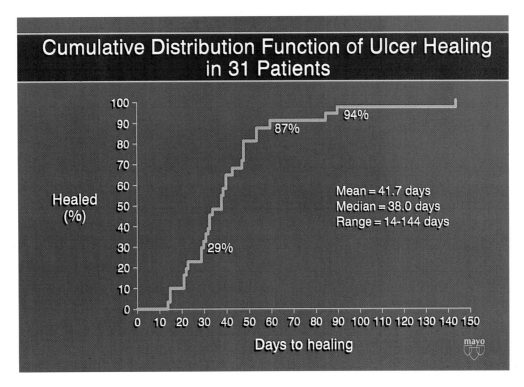

Cumulative Distribution Function of Ulcer Healing in 31 Patients

Mean = 41.7 days
Median = 38.0 days
Range = 14-144 days

Fig. 20.19. Cumulative distribution function of ulcer healing in 31 patients.

Clinical Factors Predicting Healing of Ulcers at 6 Months

Clinical factors	Limbs (no.)	Healed (%)	P
Ulcer duration			
< 3 months	15	7.71	
> 3 months	63	79.6	0.7141
Ulcer size			
< 2 cm	26	93.3	
> 2 cm	52	71.5	0.0039
Ulcer recurrence			
None	17	76.6	
One	9	66.7	
Multiple	55	81.0	0.5396
Ulcer recurrence			
≤ 1	26	73.0	
Multiple	55	81.0	0.6690
Ulcers			
Single	54	71.8	
Multiple	24	72.7	0.2010

CA-174805d-02

Fig. 20.20. Association of clinical factors and ulcer healing at 6 months after SEPS.

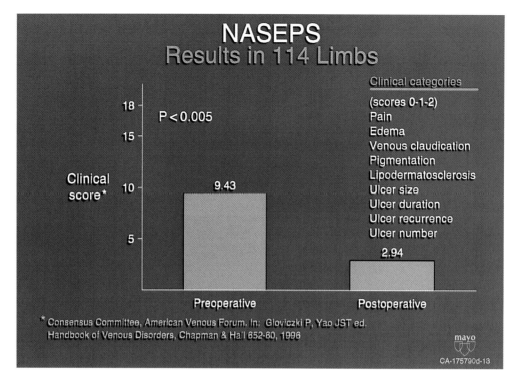

Fig. 20.21. Evaluation of postoperative clinical improvement using clinical scores in 9 categories.

quet resulted in skin necrosis in 1 patients, no complications were noted, when pneumatic tourniquets were used where constant pressure (200–300 mmHg) can be maintained and continuously monitored. Painful subfascial hematoma has been reported in a few patients, emphasizing the need for careful clipping of perforators, or coagulation of smaller vessels during the operation and the need for elastic compression, applied at the end of the operation and used postoperatively.

An important advantage of SEPS over the open Linton operation may lie in a significantly shorter period of hospitalization. Sixty-five percent of the patients entered into the registry were discharged within 24 h and today most centers perform SEPS as an out-patient procedure.

The patients in this series were suffering from severe CVI. Eighty-five percent had active or healed ulcer, all had been treated previously with conservative therapy and 17% had previous operations on superficial veins. Two-thirds of the patients were under treatment for more than 6 months.

The most frequent etiology of venous dysfunction was primary valvular incompetence, confirming findings of other recent studies.[18] The sites of reflux showed significant variability. Sixty-six percent of the patients had superficial, 68% had deep venous reflux and 51% had both. Only 3% had perforator incompetence alone. These findings suggest that patients with CVI should be evaluated to define the sites of valve incompetence and tailor the management accordingly. Patients may benefit from treatment of superficial reflux by superficial venous stripping, avulsion of a cluster of varicose veins, alone or in combination with subfascial perforator interruption.

The early results regarding rapid ulcer healing were evident, with 88% of the patients healing their ulcers in an average of 41 days after surgery. Similar, 90% ulcer healing rate was reported by Mayberry et al. when stringent non-operative measures were used, but mean time to healing was 5.3 months.[19] It is important to note that 66% of the patients entered into the registry underwent non-operative therapy for over 6 months before operation. As reimbursement is limited and length of disability is an important factor in the management of these patients, we may find that surgical treatment including SEPS in combination with compression therapy provides fast ulcer healing with significant cost savings.

Conclusions

Investigators of the NASEPS registry concluded that the minimally invasive, endoscopic Linton operation is a safe procedure, with no postoperative deaths or clinically significant early major thromboembolism reported in 148 procedures performed in 17 centers in the US and Canada. Of the perioperative complications, wound infection with a rate of 6.1% was important. Early results from the registry indicated rapid ulcer healing. Further prospective, randomized trials were recommended to evaluate long-term results, the rate of ulcer recurrence and the final role of SEPS in the treatment of patients with chronic venous disease.

References

1. Hauer G (1985) The endoscopic subfascial division of the perforating veins – preliminary report (in German). VASA 14:59–61
2. Fischer R (1992) Experience with endoscopic perforator interruption (in German). Phlebologie 21:224–229
3. Jugenheimer M, Junginger T (1992) Endoscopic subfascial sectioning of incompetent perforating veins in treatment of primary varicosis. World J Surg 16:971–975
4. Wittens CHA, Pierik RGJ, van Urk H (1995) The surgical treatment of incompetent perforating veins. Eur J Vasc Endovasc Surg 9:19–23
5. Pierik EGJM, Wittens CHA, van Urk H (1995) Subfascial endoscopic ligation in the treatment of incompetent perforating veins. Eur J Vasc Endovasc Surg 9:38–41
6. Sullivan TR, O'Donnell TF (1992) Surgical treatment of incompetent communicating veins. In: Bergan JJ, Kistner RL (eds) Atlas of Venous Surgery. WB Saunders, Philadelphia, pp 111–124
7. Conrad P (1994) Endoscopic exploration of the subfascial space of the lower leg with perforator vein interruption using laparoscopic equipment: a preliminary report. Phlebology 9:154–157
8. Gloviczki P, Cambria RA, Rhee RY, Canton LG, McKusick MA (1996) Surgical technique and preliminary results of endoscopic subfascial division of perforating veins. J Vasc Surg 23:517–523
9. Sullivan TR, O'Donnell TF (1996) Endoscopic division of incompetent perforating veins. In: Gloviczki P, Yao JST (eds) Handbook of Venous Disorders. Chapman and Hall, London pp 482–493
10. Bergan JJ, Murray J, Greason K (1996) Subfascial endoscopic perforator vein surgery (SEPS): a preliminary report. Ann Vasc Surg 10:211–219
11. Gloviczki P, Bergan JJ, Menawat, SS et al. (1997) Safety, feasibility and early efficacy of subfascial endoscopic perforator surgery (SEPS): A preliminary report from the North American registry. J Vasc Surg 25:94–105
12. Porter JM, Moneta GL, International Consensus Committee on Chronic Venous Disease (1995). Reporting standards in venous disease: an update. J Vasc Surg 21:635–645
13. Executive Committee, American Venous Forum (1996) Classification and grading of chronic venous disease in the lower limbs: a consensus statement. In: Gloviczki P, Yao JST (eds) Handbook of Venous Disorders. Chapman and Hall, London, 652–660
14. Linton RR (1953) The post-thrombotic ulceration of the lower extremity: its etiology and surgical treatment. Ann Surg 138:415–432
15. Thomas AMC, Tomlinson PJ, Boggon RP (1986) Incompetent perforating vein ligation in the treatment of venous ulceration. Ann R Coll Surg Eng 68:214–215
16. Field P, Van Boxel P (1971) The role of the Linton flap procedure in the management of stasis, dermatitis and ulceration in the lower limb. Surgery 70:920–926
17. Dodd H (1964) The diagnosis and ligation of incompetent perforating veins. Ann R Coll Surg Engl 34:186–196
18. Labropoulos N, Leon M, Geroulakos G, Volteas N, Chan P, Nicolaides AN (1995) Venous hemodynamic abnormalities in patients with leg ulceration. Am J Surg 169:572–574
19. Mayberry JC, Moneta GL, De Frang RD, Porter JM (1991) The influence of elastic compression stockings on deep venous hemodynamics. J Vasc Surg 13:91–100

Epilogue

"What's past is prologue"

Shakespeare, The Tempest

A superficial glance at this volume would suggest that the final chapter has been written in the story of perforator vein surgery. However, a more thorough study of the contents of the atlas will show that nowhere does Shakespeare's famous line from *The Tempest* better describe the current situation than in perforator vein surgery. Indeed, history is a continuum with no clear beginning and no real end. This is exemplified by profiles in this volume. They go back historically beyond Frederick Trendelenburg to John Gay and also describe surgeons of this century. While Linton Homans, and present-day investigators, including Gerald Hauer and Robert Kistner, are cited, others making important contributions could well have been added.

Evaluation of a new surgical procedure in a reliable scientific manner is a must in today's era of evidence-based medicine. The North American Registry has been an important step forward and more prospective, randomized studies such as the one performed by Cees Wittens and his colleagues in Rotterdam and published in this atlas are beginning to appear. This is salutary, since the problem of chronic venous disease is more complex than this volume describes. Further investigations are needed to establish the contributions of perforator, superficial and deep vein incompetence, alone and in combination, to the pathogenesis of venous ulceration. Only Level I prospective, multicenter studies will provide definite evidence on optimal management of patients with chronic venous disease. Undoubtedly, additional questions on venous pathophysiology will also arise. For example, it is not just outward flow through perforating veins which alters venous pathophysiology, but inward flow from refluxing superficial veins appears to overload the deep venous system and renders it incompetent.

In short, there is much to study in venous pathophysiology in general and in the arena of perforator vein surgery in particular. This volume may serve to open the door to more and presumably well-thought-out investigations. Hopefully, it will challenge new investigators and attract curious scientists to the study of venous disorders.

In some ways, some answer to problems of chronic venous insufficiency are in. For example, endoscopic perforator vein interruption combined with ablation of superficial reflux markedly improves the clinical situation, contributes to rapid ulcer healing and very likey prolongs ulcer-free state. Problems of postoperative cellulitis to rapid ulcer recurrence remain, but these are not nearly as formidable as the postoperative complications of the open Linton procedure, nor as frequent as recurrence of venous ulcer under conservative management. Minimally invasive, endoscopic venous surgery is here so stay and is ready for further, well designed clinical trials.

Perhaps in the future, investigations utilizing venotonic drugs and leukocyte adhesion antagonists will add pharmacologic therapy to the medical procedures of perforator vein interruption. These areas need considerable exploration.

As editors of this volume, we have enjoyed planning the contents, organizing the information, and contacting colleagues who responded generously with time and effort. There is no doubt that the contributors to this atlas join the editors in hoping that this book will stimulate well-planned investigations and provide a background for better care of patients with severe chronic venous insufficiency.

Peter Gloviczki
John J. Bergan

Subject Index